FIRST DO NO SELF-HARM

FIRST DO NO SELF-HARM

Understanding and Promoting Physician Stress Resilience

Edited by

Charles R. Figley

Peter Huggard

Charlotte E. Rees

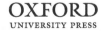

OXFORD
UNIVERSITY PRESS

Oxford University Press is a department of the University of Oxford.
It furthers the University's objective of excellence in research, scholarship,
and education by publishing worldwide.

Oxford   New York
Auckland   Cape Town   Dar es Salaam   Hong Kong   Karachi
Kuala Lumpur   Madrid   Melbourne   Mexico City   Nairobi
New Delhi   Shanghai   Taipei   Toronto

With offices in
Argentina   Austria   Brazil   Chile   Czech Republic   France   Greece
Guatemala   Hungary   Italy   Japan   Poland   Portugal   Singapore
South Korea   Switzerland   Thailand   Turkey   Ukraine   Vietnam

Oxford is a registered trademark of Oxford University Press in the UK and certain other
countries.

Published in the United States of America by
Oxford University Press
198 Madison Avenue, New York, NY 10016

Library of Congress Cataloging-in-Publication Data
First, do no self harm : understanding and promoting physician stress resilience / [edited by] Charles Figley.
    pages cm
Includes bibliographical references.
ISBN 978–0–19–538326–3 (hardcover : alk. paper)   1. Physicians—Job stress.   2. Physicians—Mental health.
3. Resilience (Personality trait)   4. Stress management.   I. Figley, Charles R., 1944– editor of compilation.
RC451.4.P5F56 2013
610.69'5—dc23
2012047889

We dedicate this book to all members of the House of Medicine, including our physician friends and colleagues, who struggle every day to manage the demands of their job. These jobs have very little room for failure: physicians make life and death decisions daily. We hope that this book will provide the clarion call to action: To face head on the deficits of medical education, training, and practice, and to tackle the culture of Medicine, so that the House of Medicine is a safe and healing place for both patients and their physicians.

This book is also dedicated to two people: who were also healers Dr. Dave Cabrera, US Army Medical Corps, co-author, practitioner, researcher, and friend, who would approve of physician's self-care and died in combat October 29, 2011; and Dr. Charlotte Emma Hall, specialist registrar in genitourinary medicine, and friend, who died November 12, 2009 after battling with severe bipolar disorder for a number of years.

CONTENTS

Section 1: STRESS OF BEING A MEDICAL STUDENT: INTRODUCTION
Charlotte E. Rees

Section 2: STRESS OF BEING A PHYSICIAN: INTRODUCTION
Peter Huggard

Section 3: MANAGEMENT OF PHYSICIAN STRESS: INTRODUCTION
Charles R. Figley

Section 4: PERSONAL REFLECTIONS: INTRODUCTION
Charles R. Figley

FOREWORD

JOHN BLIGH AND JULIE BROWNE

> *A distressing feature in the life which you are about to enter, a feature*
> *which will press hardly upon the finer spirits among you and ruffle their*
> *equanimity, is the uncertainty which pertains not alone to our science*
> *and art, but to the very hopes and fears which make us men.*[1]
>
> Sir William Osler

Sir William Osler's words of advice to young doctors, first spoken in 1889, are as pertinent now as they were over a hundred years ago. Stress and distress, now, as then, seem
to be the inevitable and unwelcome bedfellows of learning and practicing medicine.
So it's tempting to ask why it is that even though the existence of distress in medical
students is well known and has been acknowledged for centuries, medical education
research has seemed to advance no further in addressing it than being able to describe
and measure it.

This book, in addition to describing some of the characteristics and consequences
of stress in medical training and practice, provides valuable insights into the reasons for
stress among medical students and doctors. Importantly, it takes major steps forward in
offering new and welcome suggestions for medical education practitioners, especially
those whose work is focused on helping doctors and students in difficulty, on how they
can understand and assist those who are suffering emotional distress to develop a more
resilient approach to learning and practicing medicine.

Osler's words, however, carry with them seeds of both realism and of warning.

First of all is his comment about "finer spirits" suffering the worst distress. Medical
students and doctors tend to be idealists, and perhaps rightly so. They have the privilege of

caring for people at some of the most intense times of their lives. As Iona Heath says, it is the doctor's responsibility to be "always, vehemently on the side of the individual patient, witnessing, and sometimes interpreting, their distress."[2] Doctors bear a burden on behalf of society that they could not carry without a fixed belief that it is worth doing—a belief that, as Osler said, doctors are "here to make the lives of others happier".[1] So if our students care at all about becoming good doctors, they will inevitably suffer along the road to learning, and the more they care, the harder it is likely to be.

Learning medicine is unavoidably stressful as students try, fail, and try again, absorbing new knowledge and pushing their understanding to the limit. And the price of failure is not just personal: it is that ultimately someone may be harmed unnecessarily. Educators, trainers, and curriculum managers do well to remember that there are many fine spirits among their students who need careful handling to ensure that the idealism that underpins their motivation to become doctors is not crushed underfoot as a growing understanding of the realities and limitations of medical practice is acquired.

Second, Osler acknowledges that uncertainty is an inescapable part of medical practice. Medical students and doctors tend to be perfectionists, but this places a tremendous burden on them and the people around them as they constantly seek to avoid error and reduce their own uncertainty. Winston Churchill summed up this attitude of mind in 1925: "To improve is to change, so to be perfect is to change often."[3] Medical students must constantly make and remake themselves as they adopt and assimilate their new identity as a doctor. To slow down the pace just because the rate of change is hard to cope with might make life easier; but it is a solution that, we think, is very hard for most students to accept—let alone the practicing scientists, physicians, and doctors who teach them. The ability to accept uncertainty has become a new requirement for doctors and medical students,[4] but this in itself may become a burden as they strive paradoxically to become the best at accepting uncertainty that they can possibly be.

Third, for Osler, medicine is both a science and an art. Many students come into medicine because they are attracted to the orderliness and purity of science—and why not? Constantly striving to get things right and to improve, seeking after facts and evidence, discovering new knowledge, testing things to breaking point: surely medicine should be like this, or how can we produce enduring improvements and be ready for the next challenge? Yet science is not a matter of black and white; like all human endeavors it is subject to interpretation, debate, and change. Like art, it has its own beauty and complexity. And most doctors understand that science is not the polar opposite, the antidote to art; in clinical practice the two support each other and often merge into one whole. As John Saunders puts it:

The art of caring for patients, then, should flourish not merely in the theoretical or abstract grey zones where scientific evidence is incomplete or conflicting but also in the recognition that what is black and white in the abstract often becomes grey in practice, as clinicians seek to meet their patients' needs.[5]

Science aims at certainty, but the art of medicine, particularly as it is practiced in the presence of human frailty and suffering, forces us to accept that perfection is impossible. These twin tensions are a constant source of stress as students learn to balance the science and art of medical practice, but they are inevitable. The challenge for curriculum planners and teachers is to make them a source of creative, rather than destructive, tension. And it is here that Osler's fourth great insight is revealed when he talks of the "very hopes and fears that make us men."

At the heart of medical practice is the humanity that doctors, students, and patients share. Doctors are, after all is said and done, human. The human in the doctor must speak—and listen—to the human in the patient. As doctors, our students will share joy, relief, grief, and despair with their patients and their families; they will experience the elation that comes from helping people, and the anguish that comes from failing to meet their own and others' expectations. Our challenge as medical teachers is to work with patients, our clinician and scientist colleagues, and our students to produce a curriculum—formal, informal, and, importantly, hidden—that allows students to express and even celebrate their humanity, confront their fears, and prepare them to face and withstand these stresses, not just in medical school and early training, but throughout their careers.

This book is a significant contribution to scholarship on the subject of stress in medical students and doctors. It provides a valuable resource for students, trainees, and practitioners who have faced or are facing difficulties and for all those who work to help colleagues and students who are experiencing hard times. Most of all, it provides a welcome reminder to all medical educators of the need within the medical curriculum to allow students time and space to work meaningfully with patients so that they can acknowledge, understand, and explore the ineffably human side of medical practice.

REFERENCES

1. Osler W. *Aequanimitas, with other addresses to medical students, nurses and practitioners of medicine.* Philadelphia: The Blakiston Company, 1910.
2. Heath I. *The Mystery of General Practice.* London: John Fry Trust, 1995.
3. Churchill WS. *All will be well: good advice from Winston Churchill.* London: Ebury Press, 2011.
4. General Medical Council. *Tomorrow's Doctors.* London: General Medical Council 2009.
5. Saunders J. The practice of clinical medicine as an art and as a science. *Medical Humanities* 2000;26(1):18–22.

ACKNOWLEDGMENTS

The co-editors wish to thank Abby Gross at Oxford University Press for her support throughout the long and fascinating journey to produce this book. We also wish to thank all the contributors to this book and the many reviewers, all of whom are identified by the co-editors individually below.

CHARLES R. FIGLEY

I would like to thank first my support system, starting with Dr. Kathy Regan Figley, my wife, friend, and collaborator, who enabled me to complete this book in good spirits. Dr. Ronald Marks, Dean of the Tulane University School of Social Work, has been an extraordinary supporter in addition to being my boss and friend. In the context of my university, I thank the president of Tulane University, Scott Cowen, and the provost, Michael Bernstein, and Dean of the School of Social Work, Ron Marks for their support scholarship and its applications. Jessica Chynoweth, physician in Albuquerque, New Mexico and my oldest daughter was my inspiration for this book, along with her sister, Laura Figley Lundblom. Jennifer E. MacNeill served as my research assistant in the early stages of the project and was extraordinarily helpful. Vicky Lattone took over where Jenn left off and steered us into the harbor. Reviewers for Section 3 and Section 4 were invaluable. We thank them for their service and recognize in alphabetical order with equal amounts of appreciation for a job well done: Dave Bateman, Dr. Karen DeSalvo, Commissioner of Public Health, City of New Orleans, Frank Rosinia, Stacy Overstreet, Pat Alley, Russell A. Matthews, Jane Parker, Shailesh Kumar, Carol McAllum, Robin Youngson, and Kathy Figley.

PETER HUGGARD

I wish to thank the many international scholars for the generous time they gave to reviewing the six chapters in Section 2. Their peer review comments have been extremely helpful, both to the section editor and to the authors of each chapter. In alphabetical order, my thanks go to Professor Jonathan Cree, Family Medicine Specialist and Director of the Family Medicine Residency Program, Idaho State University, USA; Dr. Wayne Cunningham, General Practitioner and Senior Lecturer, Department of General Practice and Rural Medicine, Dunedin School of Medicine, University of Otago, New Zealand; Dr. J. Eric Gentry, CEO of Compassion Unlimited and Licensed Mental Health Counselor, Sarasota, FL, USA; Dr. John Kennelly, General Practitioner and Senior Lecturer, The Goodfellow Unit, Department of General Practice & Primary Health Care, University of Auckland, New Zealand; Dr. Peter Larmer, Head of Physiotherapy, School of Rehabilitation and Occupation Studies, Faculty of Health and Environmental Sciences, AUT University, Auckland, New Zealand; Dr. Carol McAllum, Palliative Care Specialist and Honorary Lecturer, The Goodfellow Unit, Department of General Practice & Primary Health Care, University of Auckland, New Zealand; Dr. Anne-Thea McGill, Research Clinician, University of Auckland Human Nutrition Unit; and Senior Lecturer, The Goodfellow Unit, Department of General Practice and Primary Care, University of Auckland, New Zealand; Gaeline Phipps, Barrister, Wellington, New Zealand; Professor Geoffrey Riley, Head of the Rural Clinical School, School of Primary, Aboriginal and Rural Health Care, University of Western Australia, Australia; Dr. Geoff Robinson, Addiction Medicine Specialists and Chief Medical Officer at Capital & Coast District Health Board, and Clinical Senior Lecturer, Wellington School of Medicine, University of Otago, New Zealand; Dr. D. Franklin Schultz, Clinical Psychologist, Lakeland, FL, USA; Dr. Josephine Stanton, Psychiatrist, Auckland, New Zealand; Associate Professor Andy Wearn, Director of the Undergraduate Clinical Skills Centre, Faculty of Medical and Health Sciences, The University of Auckland, New Zealand; Dr. Edwin Whiteside, Occupational Medical Advisor and Director of the New Zealand Doctors Health Advisory Group, Wellington, New Zealand; Dr. Peter Woolford, General Practitioner and Honorary Senior Clinical Lecturer, Department of General Practice & Primary Health Care, The University of Auckland, New Zealand. My thanks must also go to two friends and colleagues from whom I have received mentorship and inspiration— Professor Charles Figley and Professor Beth Stamm. I met them both for the first time at the Montreal International Society for Traumatic Stress Studies meeting in 1997. Since then, they have shaped my journey. Also, I thank for their support my colleagues and friends in New Zealand who share the same concerns and teaching and research interests I have, that is, working with health professionals to explore ways of managing the stressors in their professional life. Lastly, to those closest to me—my family Jayne, Katharine, and Samuel, and now our extended family of their partners, Duncan and Fran, and our beautiful grandchildren, Thomas, Anna, and Loren—thank you.

CHARLOTTE E. REES

I would like to thank numerous international scholars for their constructive and timely peer-review of the five chapters in Section 1. In alphabetical order, I would like to thank Dr. Rola Ajjawi, Senior Lecturer in Medical Education, Centre for Medical Education, University of Dundee, UK; Dr. Christine Bennetts, Senior Lecturer in Educational Research Methodology, now retired but previously Graduate School of Education, University of Exeter, UK; Professor D. Jean Clandinin, Professor and Director of the Centre for Research for Teacher Education and Development, The University of Alberta, Canada; Dr. Sayantani DasGupta, Assistant Clinical Professor of Pediatrics, Faculty Member of the Master's Program in Narrative Medicine, Co-Chair, University Seminar in Narrative, Health and Social Justice Columbia University, USA; Dr. Vanessa Druskat, Associate Professor of Organizational Behavior, University of New Hampshire, USA; Dr. Shiphra Ginsburg, Associate Professor, Department of Medicine, Scientist, Wilson Centre for Research in Education, Faculty of Medicine, The University of Toronto, Canada; Dr. Karen Norman, Associate Fellow of the Complexity and Management Centre, Business School, The University of Hertfordshire, UK, and Director of Nursing & Patient Services, Gibraltar Health Authority, Gibraltar; Professor Celia Roberts, Professor of Applied Linguistics, Department of Education & Professional Studies, King's College London, UK; Dr. Nicholas Sarra, Associate Fellow of the Complexity and Management Centre, Business School, The University of Hertfordshire, UK; and finally Professor Jill Thistlethwaite, Professor of Medical Education and Director of the Centre for Medical Education Research & Scholarship, The University of Queensland, Australia. While their peer review comments have been extremely helpful in guiding us as authors in the development of our chapters, any failings of the chapters are completely our own. I would also like to thank my colleagues at the Office of Postgraduate Medical Education, University of Sydney, Australia (2007–2010) and the Centre for Medical Education, University of Dundee, Scotland (2010 onwards) for giving me the time and space to work on this book while I should have been doing other things. I would particularly like to thank Sheila Beckett and Elaine Plenderleith at the Centre for Medical Education for their superb and efficient administrative support. Finally, I would like to thank my support system, my husband Sid and my daughter Kitty. Not only do they help me navigate the stresses and strains of working motherhood but they also help me get a work-life balance. Without you I would be a stressed-out workaholic. I am truly grateful to you both.

CONTRIBUTORS

Alley, Patrick, MBChB, DipProfEthics, FRACS, Clinical Associate Professor of Medicine, Faculty of Medical and Health Sciences, University of Auckland and Rodney Surgical Center's general surgeon, Warkworth, New Zealand

Arroll, Bruce, MHSc, BSc, MBChB, PhD, DipObst, FRNZCPHM, FRNZCGP,Professor,Department of General Practice and Primary Health Care, Faculty of Medical and Health Sciences, University of Auckland, Auckland, New Zealand

Baptiste, Sue, MHSc, OTReg (Ont), FCAOT, Professor, School of Rehabilitation Science, Faculty of Health Sciences, McMaster University, Canada

Baranowsky, Anna, PhD, C. Psych, Traumatology Institute, Toronto, Canada

Bligh, John, Professor and Dean of Medical Education at Cardiff University Medical School, Cardiff, UK

Browne, Julie, External Aff airs Manager at the Wales Postgraduate Deanery based at Cardiff University, Cardiff, UK

Carlin, Nathan, Assistant Professor in the McGovern Center for Humanities and Ethics at Th e University of Texas Health Science Center at Houston, Houston, Texas, USA

Cave, Douglas, Counseling Psychology Consultant and a founding member of the Centre for Practitioner Renewal (CPR) team. He is an Assistant Professor in the Faculty of Medicine at the University of British Columbia, Vancouver, Canada

Chynoweth, Jessica, MD, practicing family medicine physician, board-certified, Isleta Pueblo (American Native American Tribe) Family Clinic outside Albuquerque, NM

Daly, Michele, BSc (Hons), MSc, Research Fellow, Sydney Medical School, University of Sydney, Australia

Dise, Terry L., MD, Associate Professor of Pediatrics, Tulane School of Medicine, Tulane University, New Orleans, Louisiana, USA

Figley, Charles, The Paul Henry Kurzweg, MD Distinguished Chair and Professor in Disaster Mental Health at Tulane University and Graduate School of Social Work Professor and Associate Dean for Research, New Orleans, Louisiana, USA

Frank, Erica, MD, MPH, Professor and Canada Research Chair in Preventive Medicine and Population Health, University of British Columbia, Vancouver, BC, Canada

Hatcher, Simon, BSc, MBBS, MMedSc, MRCPsych, FRA NZCP, MD, Department of Psychiatry, University of Ottawa, Canada

Huggard, Peter, EdD, MPH, MEd(Couns), Senior Lecturer and Director of the Goodfellow Unit, Department of General Practice and Primary Health Care, Faculty of Medical and Health Sciences, University of Auckland, New Zealand

Jovanovic, Alyssa, PhD, Candidate in the Department of Sociology, University of Calgary, Calgary, Alberta, Canada

Kelly, Patrick, BMath (Hons), PhD, Senior Lecturer in Biostatistics, Sydney School of Public Health, University of Sydney, NSW, Australia

Kuhl, David, Founder and Director of the Centre for Practitioner Renewal. He is also an Associate Professor in the Department of Family Practice, Faculty of Medicine at the University of British Columbia, Canada

Kumar, Shailesh, MBBS, MD,FRANZCP, MRCPsych, MPhil, Dip CBT, DPM, Associate Professor, Waikato Clinical School, Faculty of Medical and Health Sciences, University of Auckland, Hamilton, New Zealand

Lamdin, Rain, MBChB, PhD, Clinical Lecturer, Centre for Medical and Health Sciences Education, Faculty of Medical and Health Sciences, University of Auckland; Auckland, New Zealand

Lemaire, Jane, MD, Clinical Professor, Department of Medicine, University of Calgary, Health Sciences, Center, 3330 University Drive NW, Calgary, AB, Canada

Lewis, Natalie J., PhD, Freelance Educationalist and Researcher, Plymouth, UK

Lobelo, Felipe, MD, PhD, Senior Service Fellow, Division of Nutrition, Physical Activity and Obesity Centers for Disease Control and Prevention, Atlanta, Georgia, USA

MacLeod, Rod, MBChB, DRCOG, MMEd, PhD, FRCGP, FAChPM, Senior Staff Specialist in Palliative Care, Hammond Care, Greenwich Hospital, Sydney and Conjoint Professor in Palliative Care, University of Sydney, Australia

McAllum, Carol, MBBS, MGP, MPC, FRNZCGP, FAChPM, FAChSHM, Honorary Senior Lecturer in Palliative Care, Department of General Practice and Primaty Health Care, Faculty of Medical and Health Sciences, University of Auckland, Auckland, and Palliative Medicine Specialist, Hawke's Bay Hospital and Cranford Hospice, Hastings, New Zealand

Monrouxe, Lynn V., BSc (Hons), PGDip, PhD, CPsychol, FAcMEd, Senior Lecturer in Medical Education and Director of Medical Education Research, Institute of Medical Education, School of Medicine, Cardiff University, UK

Moreno-Walton, Lisa, MD, MS, MSCR, FACEP, FAAEM, Associate Professor, Director of Research, Section of Emergency Medicine, Director of Diversity, Section of Emergency Medicine, Louisiana State University Health Sciences Center, New Orleans, USA

Nash, Louise, MBBS (Hons), PhD, FRA NZCP, BA, DipObs, New South Wales Institute of Psychiatry, and University of Sydney, NSW, Australia

Oberg, Erica, ND MPH, Director, Center for Health Policy & Leadership and Assistant Research Professor, Bastyr University, Kenmore, Washington, USA

Pearlman, Laurie Anne, PhD, Clinical Psychologist, Independent Practice, Holyoke, MA, USA

Pearson, Hilary, Counsellor at the Centre for Practitioner Renewal and an Assistant Professor in the Department of Family Practice, Faculty of Medicine at the University of British Columbia, Vancouver, Canada

Rees, Charlott E., BSc(Hons), MEd, PhD, CPsychol, FHEA, FRCP Edin, Professor of Education Research and Director of the Centre for Medical Education, College of Medicine, Dentistry & Nursing, University of Dundee, Dundee, UK

Risdon, Cathy, MD, DMan, CCFP, FCFP, David Braley and Nancy Gordon Chair in Family Medicine, Associate Professor, Family Medicine, McMaster University, Canada

Sallis, Robert, MD, Director, Sports Medicine Fellowship Program, Kaiser Permanente, California, USA

Schmidt, Douglas, PhD, C.Psych, South East Toronto Family Health Team, Toronto Ontario Canada and Toronto District School Board, Toronto, Ontario, Canada

Shakespeare-Finch, Jane, PhD, School of Psychology & Counselling, Institute of Health & Biomedical Innovation, Queensland University of Technology, Brisbane, Australia

Spike, Jeffery, Professor at the McGovern Center for Humanities and Ethics, and Director of the Campus-Wide Ethics Program at The University of Texas Health Science Center at Houston, TX, USA

Stamm, Beth Hudnall, PhD, Institute of Rural Health, Idaho State University, Idaho, USA

Sweeney, Kieran, MA, MPhil, MD, FRCGP, FRSA, Peninsula Medical School, Universities of Exeter & Plymouth, UK

Todd, Fraser C., MBChB, PhD, FRA NZCP, FAChAM, National Addiction Centre, Department of Psychological Medicine, Christchurch School of Medicine and Health Sciences, Otago University, New Zealand

Van Ekert, Elizabeth, BA, DipEd, MMed Hum, Professional Services Advisor, MDA National, Australia

Wallace, Jean E., PhD, Department of Sociology, Faculty of Arts, University of Calgary, Calgary, Alberta, Canada

Whitehead, Paul, Psychologist with the Centre for Practitioner Renewal, and an Assistant Professor in the Department of Family Practice, Faculty of Medicine at the University of British Columbia, Canada

Youngson, Robin, MA, MB ChB, FANZCA, Anesthesiologist, Raglan, New Zealand, Founder of www.HEARTSinHEALTHCARE.com

INTRODUCTION

THE EDITORS

Doctors are human beings and, like the rest of us, must manage work-related stress. Yet doctors are often accused of playing God because they must make life-and-death decisions; often know a patient will die—sometimes long before the patient or the family knows; must live with the memories of split-second decisions often made by instinct; and endure the multitude of patients' pain and suffering every day, day-after-day, ad infinitum. Added to patient-related pressures are colleague-associated demands: a worldwide shortage of physicians places ever-increasing demands on doctors to perform at high levels of productivity and to work longer and harder to care for everyone. These demands, along with the associated day-to-day challenges of physicianship, can take their toll on doctors, thus leading to mental health problems, reduced job satisfaction and productivity, and eventually lowered retention and further compounding workforce shortages. Stress can lead to poor communication between doctors and their colleagues and between doctors and their patients, resulting in poor patient care. In the long run, for doctors to avoid harming patients, they must first do no self-harm. Keeping doctors physically and mentally healthy and personally and professionally productive requires a thorough understanding of the systemic causes and consequences of physician stress. Of equal importance is understanding the role of resilience in terms of the development and sustenance of doctors from the start of their careers as undergraduate medical students to postgraduate training to continuing professional development. No single text has provided this information and guidance—until now.

With this book about physician stress and resilience we aim to send a strong message to the House of Medicine: stress is killing doctors and indirectly their patients, and something has to be done about it. We intend this book to be one such attempt to do something about it. Compiled by a variety of nonclinical and clinical academics, clinicians, and practitioners providing services to doctors-in-need from across the Western world, this book reaches out primarily to medics at all stages of their education continuum so that they can learn to look after themselves and their colleagues. It also addresses practitioners responsible for providing support to medics in their times of need, ranging from academics responsible for the pastoral support of medical students to clinical practitioners involved in recovery programs for physicians. This book focuses on helping this wide range of readers to better understand the sources of stress, methods of coping, and what best promotes resilience across the medical education continuum.

Specifically, the book addresses five interrelated questions via theoretically and empirically driven research and practice-orientated insights from individual, relational, and systems-based perspectives: What stressors do medics experience across the medical education continuum? What are the consequences of stress for multiple stakeholders (e.g. medics, colleagues, patients)? How do medics cope with stressful demands? What strategies can be used to promote resilience among medics? How can we tackle the culture of stoicism and emotional silence in the House of God that encourages doctors' self-harm?

To answer these questions, the book includes twenty-five chapters across four sections, each with its own introductory overview that describes the purpose of the section, gives a brief description of each chapter, and identifies key cross-cutting themes. Section 1, Stress of Being a Medical Student, contains five chapters that attempt to describe the state of medical student stress and resilience across both preclinical and clinical stages of the curriculum, including the transitions between them. These chapters help fill a methodological gap in the literature on medical student stress by drawing on qualitative methodologies underpinned by interpretive approaches. Section 1 chapters, therefore, enable a more thorough understanding of the contextual and socially constructed nuances around medical students' lived experiences of stress and students' various ways of coping, in addition to supportive efforts by faculty and medical schools more generally. Together, the chapters provide numerous recommendations to educational practitioners to help students become resilient in the face of multiple stressors, including the importance of narrative to help students make sense of their stressful experiences, and to make sense of themselves.

Section 2, Stress of Being a Physician, includes six chapters that illustrate the multiple causes of stress for qualified doctors across their continuing education and, especially important, the consequences of stress if left unchecked. These chapters mostly present an individualistic perspective of stress. They speak to academics and practitioners alike to outline the almost infinite range of stressors experienced by doctors, but with a specific focus in two chapters on two particularly distressing experiences that most doctors will face at some point in their career: bearing witness to dying and death and experiencing medico-legal episodes such as complaints. The remaining chapters in Section 2 focus on what can happen if physician stress is unresolved. Introducing important theoretical concepts associated with psychological distress such as burnout, compassion fatigue, and vicarious traumatization, the authors outline the various negative outcomes of stress on physicians' mental health. Together, the chapters illustrate the importance of physicians looking after their own physical and mental health, not only for the good of themselves, but also ultimately for the good of their patients.

Section 3, Management of Physician Stress, includes five chapters that illustrate the range of strategies that physicians employ to cope with stress, as well as formal programs for doctors-in-distress. These chapters mostly speak to practitioners responsible for helping doctors in difficulty. Together, the chapters introduce the concepts of coping and overcoping, outline the range of coping strategies adopted by doctors of different ages and genders, and illustrate a variety of coping strategies, including social support, reflective practice, and humor. Finally, the chapters discuss how resilience can be promoted at both individual and organizational levels through more formal educational and management programs.

Section 4, Personal Reflections, follows the style of essays published in the "A Piece of My Mind" series of the *Journal of the American Medical Association*. In these eight chapters, the authors share their stressful, often "most memorable," experiences related to their own specialties or stage of training. In these narratives, they share what happened during their most stressful experiences, what they did, how they did or did not cope, how the experience made them feel, and what they ultimately learned. The narratives illustrate how these authors tried to make sense of their stressful experiences within the context of their professional roles and how they have been changed through these experiences. By "baring their souls and opening their hearts" (Youngson 2000), these authors help us bear witness to the stressful experiences of doctors. Collectively, these chapters provide a window into the House of Medicine, showing how its occupants find their rhythm in recognizing the costs of stress and the benefits of effective stress management and resilience. The narratives are full of emotional talk, and you may find yourself moved by them.

The book concludes with a chapter in which we revisit the initial five questions posed here and discuss the key themes of the book. We summarize the causes and consequences of stress and the strategies to help doctors cope and become more resilient in the face of stress. We conclude by discussing ways forward: How we can create a new culture in the House of Medicine that fosters doctors doing no self-harm. We hope that this book will stimulate thinking and debate about physician stress and resilience and encourage others to join the worldwide movement to better understand, prevent, and manage the destructive, negative effects of stress that can accompany the delivery of medical services.

FIRST DO NO SELF-HARM

Stress of Being a Medical Student

INTRODUCTION

Charlotte E. Rees

Medical school is a time of significant psychological distress for physicians-in-training

—Liselotte Dyrbye, Matthew Thomas, and Tait Shanafelt (2006)

We know that the processes involved in learning medicine and becoming a doctor are stressful, with stressors typically relating to curricular or personal factors or both. Curricular factors can include academic performance such as work overload and grade competition; sleep deprivation; work-related role problems; interpersonal conflict, including student abuse; patient and clinic responsibilities; challenging patient interactions such as dealing with death and dying; and work-home tensions. Individual factors can include age, gender, ethnicity, professional identity, financial pressures, marital and parental status, personality, and life events such as illness and death in the family (Dyrbye et al. 2006; 2009; Murphy et al. 2009; O'Rourke et al. 2010; Prins et al. 2007). We also know that high levels of stress in students can contribute to a broad range of psychological (e.g. anxiety, depression, substance abuse) and health-related outcomes (e.g. headaches and gastrointestinal disorders) (O'Rourke et al. 2010). Indeed, a recent systematic review of forty articles on medical student distress found that medical students' overall psychological distress was consistently higher than the general population and age-matched peers by later years of training (Dyrbye et al. 2006).

We can see flavors of some of these stressors (and their outcomes) at work in the five chapters in the first section of this edited book. Although the majority of literature on medical student stress employs quantitative methods such as the General Health Questionnaire, Beck Depression Inventory, Maslach Burnout Inventory, and so forth to examine stressors and their impact on psychological outcomes, these measures have been criticized for lacking specificity to ascertain a coherent profile of students' experiences of stress (O'Rourke et al. 2010). Furthermore, few studies exist that explore medical students' stressors via qualitative approaches (Radcliffe & Lester 2003). The empirical contributions within this section (Chapters 1–4) therefore attempt to fill this methodological gap by exploring medical student stress through the use of qualitative methodologies. Rather than being underpinned by a scientific approach bent on establishing statistical relationships between medical student stress and various outcomes, Chapters 1–4 are each underpinned by an interpretive approach aimed at understanding contextual and socially constructed nuances around medical students' lived experiences of stress and coping. While Chapters 1–4 are all underpinned by the same interpretive approach, they draw on different theoretical frameworks and qualitative methods, focus on different levels of training, and examine different stressors experienced by students and different coping strategies.

In Chapter 1, Natalie J. Lewis and I discuss preclinical medical students' distributed emotional intelligence (DEI) within the classroom setting of problem-based learning (PBL) at a new medical school in the United Kingdom. Using video observation and stimulated recall interviews with eight first year medical students and an experienced PBL facilitator, we identify numerous stressors within one PBL group, including students' uncertainties and anxieties about their learning and lack of knowledge and interpersonal conflicts within the group dynamics, such as tension between the students and their facilitator. Critiquing individualist notions of emotional intelligence (EI), we contest the prevailing EI orthodoxy and instead offer an alternative distributed model of EI. We present glimmers of DEI in the chapter, using thick, rich description by way of illustrating how students cope together—often with sophisticated interpersonal dynamics such as humor, laughter, and pauses—within the sometimes fraught setting of PBL.

In Chapter 2, Rain Lamdin discusses stressors arising out of the preclinical to clinical transition for 21 medical students at a traditional New Zealand medical school. Using semistructured interviews with these students—once during their third year (preclinical phase) and again during their fourth year (clinical phase)—Rain identifies numerous stressful experiences around this transition for these medical students. Drawing on Lave and Wenger's sociocultural learning theory (their notions of legitimate peripheral participation and communities of practice), Rain emphasizes the stress caused by being in an unfamiliar environment and having to learn the informal and hidden curriculum of medical work. She also discusses sad and tragic events experienced by students such as the death of patients and tensions between students' personal and professional lives.

This conflict between personal and professional lives is extended to Chapter 3, in which Lynn V. Monrouxe and Kieran Sweeney discuss how students' developing professional identities cause stress for medical students. Using an innovative longitudinal audio-diary method, Lynn and Kieran collected and analyzed personal incident narratives from 17 medical students over a five-year period to explore their professional identity formation. They discuss various stressors arising from tensions between students' personal and professional identities. The three rich and powerful narratives discussed in this chapter include stressful events surrounding illness, dying, and death at the intersection between students' personal and professional worlds, constructed by the authors as *looking onto, living alongside,* and *living with* illness, death, and dying.

In Chapter 4, Lynn Monrouxe and I discuss how medical students employ laughter as a noncontextual coping strategy when narrating stressful professionalism dilemmas they have experienced during medical school. Using 32 group and 22 individual interviews with 200 medical students from each year of three medical schools (England, Wales, and Australia), we identified 833 personal incident narratives of professionalism dilemmas experienced by students, many of which occur in the clinical setting. That professionalism dilemmas were typically recounted with laughter is illustrated by two narratives, both of which surround different stressors concerning intimate examinations (i.e. a student watching a consultant engaging in derogatory humor about an obese patient during an intimate examination and a student conducting an intimate examination without valid patient consent).

What is interesting about these four chapters is that they all indicate the qualitative research method as a therapeutic tool in itself. Indeed, the interviews described in Chapters 1, 2, and 4 and the audio-diary method in Chapter 3 all give students the opportunities to debrief from their stressful experiences with the researcher (and sometimes peers), and they also provided students with a forum for venting their emotions. Moreover, the narrative methods used in Chapters 3 and 4 seemed particularly useful for helping students make sense of their stressful experiences.

At the end of these chapters, authors consistently recommend that medical students should be provided with structured fora as part of their formal curriculum in which to debrief from (and therefore help them cope with) stressful experiences during their medical education.

Such structured forums in which to debrief is an issue taken up in the final chapter of this section. In Chapter 5, Cathy Risdon and Sue Baptiste center on the complexities of the formal, informal, and hidden curriculum and the implications of curricular design on medical student *and* faculty members' stress resilience. Drawing on the principles of complexity theory, the authors describe the development, challenges, and successes of their *Professional Competency (Pro Comp)* curriculum in Canada. They describe the stressors for faculty members and students alike because their weekly tutorials (over a 33-month time frame) require everyone to embrace complexity, uncertainty, and emergent outcomes. Relevant to the other Section 1 chapters, these tutorials are the very enactment of the recommendations made by authors in Chapters 1–4. The weekly "check-ins" at the start of each tutorial provide students with the opportunities to debrief from their stressful experiences in a safe and open forum.

As suggested by Cathy Risdon and Sue Baptise, "stress" and "resilience" are often conceptualized as static concepts to be explored and controlled, and this appears to be the case with much of the current literature on medical student stress within the field of medical education. Instead, we hope that the chapters in this section offer you a glimpse into alternative ways of theorizing and researching medical student stress, resilience, and coping. I think that interpretive approaches and qualitative methodologies are ready for stress research. The question is, are stress researchers ready for them?

REFERENCES

Dyrbye, L.N., Thomas, M.R., Harper, W., Massie, F.S., Power, D.V., Eacker, A., Szydlo, D.W., Novotny, P.J., Sloan, J.A., Shanafelt, T.D. (2009). The learning environment and medical student burnout: a multicentre study. *Medical Education, 43*, 274–282.

Dyrbye, L.N., Thomas, M.R., Shanfelt, T.D. (2006). Systematic review of depression, anxiety, and other indicators of psychological distress among US and Canadian medical students. *Academic Medicine, 81*(4), 354–373.

Murphy, R.J., Gray, S.A., Sterling, G., Reeves, K., DuCette, J. (2009). A comparative study of professional student stress. *Journal of Dental Education, 73*(3), 328–337.

O'Rourke, M.O., Hammond, S., O'Flynn, S., Boylan, G. (2010). The medical student stress profile: a tool for stress audit in medical training. *Medical Education, 44*, 1027–1037.

Prins, J.T., Gazendam-Donofrio, S.M., Tubben, B.J., van der Heijden, F.M.M.A., van de Wiel, H.B.M., Hoekstra-Weebers, J.E.H.M. (2007). Burnout in medical residents: a review. *Medical Education, 41*, 788–800.

Radcliffe, C., Lester, H. (2003). Perceived stress during undergraduate medical training: a qualitative study. *Medical Education, 37*, 32–38.

/// 1 /// DISTRIBUTED EMOTIONAL INTELLIGENCE

A Resource to Help Medical Students Learn in Stressful Settings

NATALIE J. LEWIS AND CHARLOTTE E. REES

INTRODUCTION

Medical students have to learn to cope in the stressful environments in which they are placed during their training. Emotional intelligence (EI) is thought to be useful in terms of helping students and doctors cope, because the ability to manage stress is considered a core part of this construct. However, we think that conventional models of EI are limited in that they frame EI as an internal, static and measurable trait. Such models also assume a simplistic view of stress and fail to consider the importance of context. We have therefore developed an alternative model that reconfigures EI as a distributed, dynamic phenomenon and an emergent property of a complex system. In this chapter, we present some empirical evidence for the emergence of distributed EI in a problem-based learning group (PBL) during a stressful interaction. We also discuss some theoretical implications of distributed EI and offer suggestions on how small group facilitators might begin to work within a collective framework and help students develop the sensitivity required to manage stressful environments.

Salovey and Mayer (1990, cited in Mayer & Salovey, 1997) were the first to define and conceptualize emotional intelligence (EI), as a set of fundamental emotional competencies involving the ability to (1) perceive, appraise, and express emotions accurately, (2) use emotion to facilitate thinking, (3) understand emotion, and (4) regulate emotions to promote emotional and intellectual growth and well-being. Essentially, EI is an emotion recognition and management activity concerned with how we can use our emotions to help us reason, problem-solve, and regulate our behavior. Importantly, the ability to handle stress is considered by all leading EI researchers to be a core part of the construct and characteristic of individuals with "high" levels of EI (Bar-On, 2000; Goleman, 1996; Salovey & Mayer, 1990).

The idea that EI might enable individuals to be more resilient and able to cope with stress is appealing. However, there is a lack of empirical research in this area and, more fundamentally, a lack of clarity surrounding the way in which the construct of EI is conceptualized and measured.

CRITIQUE OF CONVENTIONAL EI

There are several authors, including ourselves, who have provided critical analyses of conventional EI (Conte, 2005; Lewis, Rees, Hudson, & Bleakley, 2005; Matthews, Zeidner, & Roberts, 2002; Zeidner, Matthews, & Roberts, 2009). In brief, currently EI is conceptualized either as intelligence, a narrow set of mental abilities involving the processing of emotional information (Salovey & Mayer, 1990), or as a broad range of personality traits, skills, and personal qualities (Bar-On, 2000; Goleman, 1996; Petrides & Furnham, 2000). Mayer, Salovey, and Caruso (2000) have characterized these different conceptualizations as ability and mixed models, respectively. The different conceptualizations of EI have different associated measurement tools.

Ability EI is measured by use of performance-based tests (i.e., tests designed to assess actual performance of emotional perception, understanding, and management). Mixed models are measured by use of self-report questionnaires that ask individuals to assess their own perceived ability to appraise and manage emotion. Self-report questionnaires, of which there are numerous examples, currently dominate the measurement of EI and suffer from a range of limitations, including response bias and substantial overlap with existing personality constructs. In contrast, there is just one set of "objective" measures of EI (Mayer, Caruso, & Salovey, 2002). Although this test is described as unique and is less confounded by personality, it has a different set of limitations, including problems with the way the test is scored. For example, the use of consensus scoring reduces the test to a measure of conformity in that it merely reflects the particular biases of most people rather than tapping some underlying emotional processing ability (Matthews et al., 2002).

We have seen that EI is assumed to have a positive impact on the ability to manage stress, but it is also thought to be predictive of other important life outcomes with, for example, the potential to enhance academic attainment (Elias et al., 1997) and occupational performance (Caruso, Bienn, & Kornacki, 2006) and improve social relationships (Flury & Ickes, 2006). However, despite almost two decades of rigorous psychometric research, there are inconsistent findings regarding predictive validity. As we discuss in the following section, such inconsistency is evident in the literature on EI and stress.

CONVENTIONAL EI AND STRESS

As mentioned previously, despite stress management being a central component of EI, there is to date a surprising lack of empirical research. The literature available has been comprehensively reviewed (Matthews et al., 2002; Zeidner, Matthews, & Roberts, 2006; Zeidner et al., 2009), revealing a handful of studies offering ambiguous findings. For example, using both self-report and "objective" measures of EI, researchers have found a weak association between EI and coping strategies, with individuals "high" in EI tending to use more adaptive task-focused forms of coping rather than less adaptive avoidance strategies (Matthews et al., 2006; Saklofske, Austin, Galloway, & Davidson, 2007). This association is much stronger or more predictive for self-report measures, suggesting that an individual's confidence in his or her emotional abilities is more important than actual ability in a real-life context (Zeidner et al., 2006). Further, some aspects of self-reported EI may be associated with well-being and low levels of depression and stress (Ciarrochi, Dean, & Anderson, 2002). However, these findings may be explained by the substantial overlap between these self-report measures and personality.

Research using "objective" measures of EI produces much more modest, contradictory, and intriguing findings. For example, EI has been found to be a modest predictor of some stress criteria (Matthews et al., 2006), although it does not predict an individual's ability to cope with laboratory stressors as might be expected. For example, before engaging in a stressful laboratory task, "high" EI was related to lower levels of distress and worry (Matthews et al., 2006). However, while actually performing the task, "high" EI individuals experienced higher levels of distress, suggesting that their coping styles were not more adaptive than those of their lower EI colleagues. EI may also be helpful in reducing stress for certain types of people, specifically those who feel confidence in their ability to deal effectively with difficult situations, but it fails to predict stress for everyone (Gohm, Corser, & Dalsky, 2005). Perhaps the most significant finding from the adaptive EI literature is the mediating influence of social support. Zeidner et al. (2006) suggest that "high" EI individuals may use their EI skills to generate a rich supportive social network around them. This network may in turn act as a protective buffer against stressful situations.

Recognizing the complexity of the coping process, Zeidner et al. (2009) in their review conclude that despite the appeal of the idea that EI is adaptive, "the bulk of the evidence suggests that we cannot identify EI with emotional adaptability" (p. 221). These authors also argue that conventional EI research has failed to address the transactional nature of stress and coping (Lazarus & Folkman, 1984), ignoring the central idea that emotions have to be understood within a specific context. We believe that the lack of predictive validity and inconsistency inherent in the EI and stress research (and in EI research in general) may be due to the research being conducted within a positivist paradigm focused exclusively on psychometric testing and measurement. This methodology, however carefully and rigorously applied, may not be appropriate if, as we have previously argued, that EI is a quality rather than a measurable quantity (Lewis et al., 2005). An alternative interpretative research paradigm recognizes the complexity of a social world composed of human beings who interact, construct meaning, behave intentionally, and exist within a specific social, cultural, and historical context (Crotty, 2004). This methodological framework might offer a better way of understanding EI. The wider educational research community has already recognized the value of alternative paradigms for exploring qualities or complex social phenomena that cannot easily be quantified. We suggest that medical educators would benefit by developing their receptivity to these other ways of knowing with regard to EI research.

We do not think it is possible to separate or isolate EI from context. Indeed, we believe that EI is a product of context. Perhaps the realm of EI can be usefully expanded to take account of this and to include other capabilities that may be of particular relevance in group settings such as the ability to sensitively judge group or team "atmospheres." We think this is part of an important collective and distributed dimension that we have called "distributed EI" (Lewis et al., 2005).

EXPLORING THE LANDSCAPE OF DISTRIBUTED EI

Medical students predominantly learn and work in small-group contexts such as problem-based learning (PBL) and later in clinical teams where the intelligent use of their emotions is paramount. However, the conventional model of EI, conceptualized as an individual, stable, measurable trait, is limited and will have little explanatory or predictive power in group contexts. Indeed, when we started to explore EI, what struck us was the mismatch between the vividness, richness, and complexity of real-life emotional experience within a group context and the narrowness and inadequacy of conventional EI, which failed to capture the intensity, instability, and lightening speed and even the subtlety of emotion. We believe that a reconfigured form of EI, as a distributed, dynamic phenomenon and an emergent property of a complex system (Lewis et al., 2005), offers medical education a rich resource for learning, including helping students learn to cope in the emotionally saturated and stressful environments in which they find themselves.

Within organizational psychology, although Druskat and Wolff (2001) offer a model of group EI, this model is still individualistic in the sense that group EI is conceptualized as an analog of individual EI, a straight transfer from the individual to the group context. Our model (Lewis et al., 2005) is different because we do not think that individual group members simply bring their individual EI to the group. Rather, we think that in shared activity, something qualitatively different emerges, unfolds, and is shaped. In effect, we believe that distributed EI is more than the sum of its parts and that the group context offers unique possibilities for learning. We are not denying the existence or contribution of an individualistic perspective, but we believe that a collectivist perspective can offer particular insights into how groups function. For example, Lingard (2009) discusses the limitations of individualistic notions of competence and highlights how competent individuals can combine to form incompetent teams. Lingard (2009) argues that a collectivist perspective on competence might allow us to better understand why this happens. Similarly, distributed EI offers a better explanatory framework for how groups attempt to work intelligently with their emotions.

As far as it is possible to define distributed EI, we can say that this phenomenon is collaborative and dynamic rather than individual and static and is an emergent property of a complex system operating through time as well as space (Lewis et al., 2005).

In Figure 1.1, the PBL group is an example of a complex system. As the group interacts and engages in shared emotional and cognitive activity, distributed EI emerges out of and is constructed locally through the group dynamic and is managed by the group.

One of the unique possibilities for learning offered by the group context is the central capability of individuals and the group as a whole to sensitively judge or appreciate the "climate" or "atmosphere" in their group or team. Importantly, we believe that the intelligent part of distributed EI is learning how to access, make sense of, and respond appropriately to this distributed and shared affect. For example, an individual clinician who is able to tune in with sensitivity to the "atmosphere" in stressful environments such as in clinical teams may use this information to decide whether to intervene in a procedure. Similarly, an entire group may collectively use such sensitivity to change the way they work and subsequently manage a difficult group meeting more effectively. Here, we see the intersection of individual and collective structures. Group members may tune in individually

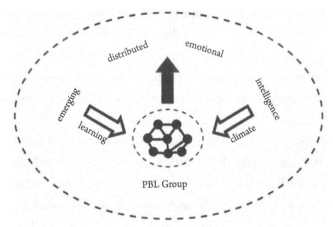

FIGURE 1.1 Distributed Emotional Intelligence Emerging from a PBL Group's Dynamic Activity.

to a group atmosphere, but this atmosphere has to be collectively constructed, and once they have all tuned in, they may collectively respond to and manage it.

We need to make a distinction here between distributed emotion and what we mean by distributed EI, although the two are interconnected. There is a sense in which distributed emotion already exists, forming the background to all our social interactions. We cannot prevent the emergence of shared affect in groups. Indeed, we have common idioms or phrases to describe some of these tangible shared emotional experiences such as tense encounters: "to cut the atmosphere with a knife." Importantly, as discussed earlier, being able to access and then collectively work with or manipulate this shared affect constructively demonstrates the "intelligent" part of collective emotional behavior. Crucially, this "intelligence" lies in the dynamic activity of the group.

As an emergent phenomenon, distributed EI is difficult to manage because it is unstable and unpredictable with atmospheres constantly unfolding, changing, and dissipating according to the group's activity. Importantly, once constructed, distributed EI actually does something. It is formative, creating learning "climates" that, depending on how well the shared affect is managed, may be productive or unproductive.

PBL: THE IMPORTANCE OF CONTEXT FOR DETERMINING STRESS

Regehr (2006) alerts us to a wealth of evidence from the classic social psychology literature that shows the powerful influence of context on human behavior. Yet we cling to what he calls the persistent myth of stability through a reliance on questionnaires designed to measure "stable" characteristics, which then fail to predict how individuals will actually behave in real-life contexts and which cannot hope to capture reality in all its complexity, unpredictability, and messiness. It is often the case that we do not know how we are going to behave in a situation until we are in it. The use of global, generic measures of stress and coping and self-report EI will be of little help in predicting how individuals will react in an actual stressful situation. Similarly, commonly used laboratory stressors such as timed math tasks or public speaking in front of a researcher may not adequately capture or mimic the complexity of real-life stressful situations in which medical students find themselves. Regehr (2006) urges medical educators that it is time to confront the context of our learning and to attend more systematically to that environment. We agree that addressing the context is crucial, and we have examined our distributed model of EI in one dynamic system in medical education: the PBL group. However, as we have discovered, capturing complex "reality" is challenging.

In medical education, PBL is now widely used in medical schools. This is an intensive and structured small-group learning environment that is designed to prepare students for work in the challenging and stressful settings of multiprofessional teams. Studies using questionnaire surveys suggest that compared with traditional medical curricula, PBL is associated with greater well-being in medical and nursing students (Jones & Johnstone, 2006; Kiessling, Schubert, Scheffner, & Burger, 2004). However, it is also a source of stress (Moffat, McConnache, Ross, & Morrison, 2004). As discussed previously, questionnaire surveys will capture only part of the picture, and unfortunately, there is a dearth of research on PBL in context, on what actually goes on inside a PBL group. However, clearly these groups already offer a context for distributed cognition and they are also highly emotional places. In this respect, we believe that they offer the potential for the emergence of a collective and distributed form of EI because it is negotiated and managed in the group and emerges from group process.

In this chapter, we present some empirical findings from the doctoral study of one of the authors (Lewis, 2007) that illustrate how distributed EI emerges in real time during stressful interactions in a PBL group. Because this is ethnographic research situated within the interpretative paradigm (Hammersley & Atkinson, 1995), the excerpt presented is written in the first person and from the point of view of the researcher Natalie Lewis. We revert to dual authorship in the conclusion section. We also discuss some theoretical implications of distributed EI and suggest some possibilities for developing sensitivity to context. However, the alternative framework that we offer presents a challenge to conventional ways of thinking and may also challenge you, particularly if you are comfortable with traditional individualist notions of EI. We live in a culture where it is difficult to escape from an individualist mind-set because the dominant discourse of personal agency is extremely strong and collective and distributed phenomena are by their nature difficult to "see" as they overlay and cut across this. While reading the excerpt in this chapter, we invite you to suspend some of your habitual ways of thinking and to watch the emergence of a "distributed mind" at work. Typically, in individualist research, the actors or individual participants are followed but, as we discuss in the next section, in our study we are following the "object"—in this case, distributed EI—because sometimes the "object" transcends the individual actors.

CAPTURING DISTRIBUTED EI

After obtaining ethical approval, I observed a PBL group for one term as part of a larger ethnography-based doctoral study. Ethnography involves immersing oneself in a particular setting for a period of time and collecting data in a variety of ways (Hammersley & Atkinson, 1995). I used two complementary methods of data collection, with each method providing a partial picture of what occurred: video-recorded observation and audio-recorded interviews. In this chapter, I focus on observational data. Because the camera was fixed and could not capture everything and because, importantly, a camera cannot "feel" the atmosphere, I also sat in the room but outside the group, observing each session and writing supplementary field notes. As I observed sessions, I noted when I felt that a key moment in the group dynamic had occurred, a significant event. This was when I interpreted or felt that something was unfolding or shaping—in effect, evidence of a change in the emotional atmosphere of the group caused by something someone said or did. When these events occurred, I noted the time on the videotape counter and recorded it in my notebook. Immediately after the session, I conducted interviews with the group and later with the facilitator.

In this study, my intention was to become attuned to the psychosocial processes operating in the group; specifically, I wanted to view and then capture a distributed mind at work. In effect, I tried to track an "object" in emergence—that is, distributed EI in a complex activity system (the PBL group). Conventionally, in activity systems (Engeström, 1987), the focus has been on the subjects—the actors in a system. For example, facilitators pay attention to what individuals in the group are thinking or feeling. However, I was trying to follow the object, the distributed mind, and not the subjects, and I tried to capture this through metaphor because my interest was not in measuring or reifying the object. Metaphors are part of our everyday experience (Lakoff & Johnson, 1981). We all use metaphorical language and thinking, including physicians, where metaphor is important in their clinical diagnoses (Bleakley, Farrow, Gould, & Marshall, 2003). In addition, it is through metaphor that we can understand ideas that are difficult to grasp and express. In my study, I have illuminated distributed EI and given a sense of what the "atmosphere" of the group, the shared affect, "felt" like to participants, through their use of metaphor and through my use of textural words. I have also tried to track distributed EI as a dynamic phenomenon moving through time; in an attempt to give you a sense of this, in the scene presented in this chapter, I have used two different columns: one for the raw video transcript (left column) and one for my commentary on it (right column).

In the next section, I present a scene from the PBL group comprising eight first-year medical students (four male and four female students, aged 17 to 19 years, and all white) and one facilitator (white, male, nonclinical, and experienced educator). The scene illustrates distributed EI emerging in a stressful situation.

"The Breakdown of Alcohol" (PBL Session 3)

Time pressure is evident in this session. The group has 15 learning issues to discuss and a workshop to attend immediately afterward. Adding to the pressure, the facilitator also wants to ensure that there is enough time to conduct a group interview afterward. The group members are not very enthusiastic about the workshop but are happy to be interviewed. After a brief discussion about how they identified the learning issues and deciding who will lead the feedback at the end of the session, the facilitator suggests that they work around the group, with each person (given pseudonyms below) taking the lead in turn to "kick start" the discussion on a particular learning issue:

Facilitator: Shall we be very, very concise? Shall we start here?	He points to Ava, who is sitting next to him on his right.
Lily: Oh no!	From this moment, we see the emergence of distributed emotion as the collective anxiety and frustration of the group construct a tense atmosphere.
Facilitator: And just go round in anticlockwise. Just strictly round in order and you, you just kick off, you don't have to do the whole thing; just get the discussion rolling.	He makes a circle shape with his arm indicating the direction. The phrase "strictly round in order" conveys a sense of inflexibility and possible interrogation. Here, the facilitator uses a sporting metaphor—"kick off"—and later in the session he will refer to "throwing googlies." He also refers to getting the discussion "rolling," suggesting movement. This facilitator is a very active individual with a wide range of sporting interests, but his use of metaphor also conveys a sense of trying to motivate and energize the group, to get them engaged and to get things moving.

They begin working through the learning issues, and a rhythm or pattern develops. The facilitator reads out the issue in a loud energetic voice and then looks at the person whose turn it is. All students respond by looking directly back at him, and the interaction and direction of gaze seems locked between student and facilitator. The group has been working steadily through their learning issues but become "stuck" when the facilitator, "throws another googly in" and asks them how alcohol is broken down by the body.

Facilitator: How is it broken down? What does the body do to the alcohol?

Amber: The body uses (unclear) or something like that.

Reading from her notes, she tries to pronounce a word as Ava coughs.

Jack: Breaks it down into water and (unclear)

Last word unclear as Ava coughs again.

Ethan: umm

In agreement.

Facilitator: Straight away?

Silence from the group and a pause before Ethan answers.

Ethan: No

Facilitator: What are the stages then if you take three or four units of alcohol in; how does the body get rid of it?

Ava is still coughing. The facilitator's voice is loud, energetic, and confident. He speaks rapidly.

Leo: You add water to it, don't you? To start with.

In contrast, the group members' voices are much softer and hesitant, as they begin to grapple with this question and search their memories.

Jack: Turns into (unclear) something like that, I don't know.

Leo: It dehydrates you, doesn't it?

Silence from the group. At this point, it seems as if the flow has completely seized up. The atmosphere is tense.

Facilitator: How? Who was at the plenary this morning? This was covered this morning wasn't it, I think?

Jack and Lily put up their hands. The facilitator is frustrated.

Lily: Yeh.

Jack: Oh God! Seriously?

Jack looks round at the group. He was at the plenary but cannot remember this being covered.

Lily: It was.

She laughs.

Facilitator: Believe you me, it was covered this morning.

Said with emphasis and some irritation.

This tense atmosphere now undergoes a fleeting change and distributed EI emerges. The group, having "tuned in" and felt the tension, now responds to and collectively tries to manage this atmosphere through humor as they laugh about their reasons for not attending this morning's plenary. In this way, the tension is dissipated.

Jack: Was that it? Was that the only people? Oh!

Jack looks round the group and shakes his head in mock disapproval that he and Lily were the only ones to go to the plenary and then he looks down. Everyone is smiling sheepishly.

Tom: (unclear)

Tom's voice is quiet but he says why he didn't go and everyone laughs.

Ava: I'm still poorly.

She laughs and the group laughs.

Facilitator: You've got the alcohol in; you've taken on the four hypothetical units. What does the body do to it?

The facilitator then brings them back to the task. Silence follows as they all look directly across at each other.

Tom and Ethan have their hands near their mouths. But something is starting to happen here. The atmosphere is changing again. The group members are now looking at each other. The atmosphere is still tense but it is a different kind of tenseness, a different quality. It suddenly becomes highly charged and this is the moment when distributed EI starts to construct a productive learning climate.

Ethan: (unclear) turning into an aldehyde then, um, hydrating it. So it splits into two sets of CO_2 and water.

He moves his hands apart.

The facilitator has the fat white board marker pen in his hand and is about to give it to Ethan.

Ava: It goes from ethanol to ethanel, doesn't it? And then I can't remember what happens.

Ethan and Jack both talk at once, waving their hands, and Jack is stretching. Ava smiles and bites her bottom lip. Amber starts to open a large textbook.

Ethan: (unclear) hydration. It splits, doesn't it when …

Facilitator: Just put "alcohol" at the top. Bottom? What did it end up as?

Facilitator gives Ava the pen and signals that she should go to the board, which she does. She writes "alcohol" at the top.

Tom has his hand over his mouth and is shaking his head. Lily is looking at the book.

Ethan: (unclear)

Facilitator: Yeah? OK, so we've got the top and the bottom of our grid. What are you going to put in between for that alcohol to be broken down? And a split at the bottom, yeah?

The group now turn in their chairs to face the board where Ava has drawn the grid and two divergent lines to indicate a split at the bottom.

Ava: It's splitting.

She starts writing the pathway in chemical formula, Jack and Ethan helping her by calling out.

Jack: The chemical thing of ethanol is C_2H_2O.

Ava continues to write up the formula as they call it out.

Ethan: (unclear)

Leo: Are we going to, like, do it in two carbons?

He laughs and turns to look at Jack.

The group now grapples with the formula. All of this is fast paced, tense, and energetic.

Jack: Yeah, isn't it like two carbons?

Leo: Yeah, two carbons, so it's—

Jack: C_2H_2O.

Ava: CH_3 to start with, isn't it?

Leo: Yeah.

Ethan: C_2H_5OH.

Ava: And the other one's C_2HOH.

Ethan: Yeah, C_2HOH.

Jack has been trying to work out the formula, writing it on a pad in front of him.

Ava: I think that's right.

Erin: I hate chemistry!

Everyone looks at the board.

Erin throws her pen down on the table in frustration, and there is nervous laughter from the group.

Amber: I had a gap year so I can't remember.

She grins, and Ava continues writing on the board. Everyone is looking.

Ava: Is that right?

Tom: Let's just do it with words.

Ethan laughs.

Tom, who has been quiet up to this point, now offers a way forward.

Facilitator: Yeah. do it with words.

Tom: Words.

He nods his head. Ava asks for the rubber and rubs out the formula, rewriting it in words.

Ava: Ethanol, whoa!

She says and then writes the word "ethanol." Jack sneezes very loudly at this point, causing her to start. He then pretends to wipe the snot from Ethan's sleeve, causing everyone to laugh. The intense atmosphere is temporarily softened with humor.

Ethan: You've just pushed me over the edge.

Jack: Did I?

He grins broadly.

Ethan: Yeah.

Jack: Come on, Ava. You're the one with the pen in your hand!

He grins at Ava, who has been writing away and who now laughs.

Facilitator: No, she's scribing; it's down to us. What do we want her to write next?

The facilitator brings them back to task again.

Ethan: Thing is, I don't know if it does turn into ethanel.

Ethan voices his uncertainty and then receives support from the group.

Lily: I don't think it did.

She is perhaps thinking back to the plenary she attended this morning.

Ethan: No, I don't think it does.

Jack: I don't think it does.

He looks at the facilitator and laughs.

Facilitator: Do we have another emerging learning issue here?

Ava: I'm pretty sure it goes to ethanel.

Ava smiles and everyone is looking at each other.

An individualist perspective would focus on the individual players in this scene and might interpret this extract as depicting an overly controlling, dominant, and time-pressured facilitator, irritated at the lack of preparation and commitment in some of the students.

One extravert student in particular, Jack, attempts to take on the role of informal leader and uses humor to shift attention away from their inadequate preparation for today's session. Because Jack is a popular member of the group, the other students respond to his light-heartedness and laugh at his actions and banter. However, from a collectivist perspective, our focus is different. Our interest is not in individual actors, in this case the facilitator or Jack, but rather with tracking the emergence of distributed EI as an object.

This scene illustrates the emergence of distributed EI as an effect of the group's activity and highlights the dynamic, unstable quality of this phenomenon, which can be tracked through time. The group's activity initially constructs a tense, uncomfortable atmosphere. This is in response to a range of factors, including time pressure, lack of preparation, and associated anxiety and frustration with the facilitator's style of questioning. The first instance of emergence occurs when this atmosphere undergoes a change as the group collectively manages the discomfort through co-constructed humor and laughter, which serve to temporarily release the tension. Although Jack may appear to initiate this, several members of the group make additional utterances, which co-create and prolong the group laughter.

A significant instance of the emergence of distributed EI occurs when the facilitator steps back a little after his initial challenging question and allows the group time and space to grapple with the problem of how alcohol is metabolized in the body. Specifically, a change in the tone and quality of the emotional atmosphere occurs when the group members seem to break out of the constraint of looking at the facilitator and now look at each other instead, engaging in highly charged and collaborative effort.

The atmosphere is still intense and pressurized, but this is a productive pressure and is an example of distributed EI constructing a productive learning climate where the shared affect of the group facilitates their understanding of a difficult concept. The group also exhibits intelligent collective emotional behavior because, rather than withdrawing and allowing themselves to be overwhelmed by the discomfort, they are able to access or tune into the intense atmosphere and respond to and manage it effectively. This is evident in their struggle to work out what they know and do not know about the topic through helping each other with the formula or suggesting ways forward. In addition, the group continues to collectively use humor to manage the atmosphere and to lighten moments of particular intensity and discomfort.

CONCLUSIONS

The scene in this chapter illustrates how EI can be conceptualized as a distributed phenomenon. Specifically, distributed EI is an emergent property of the unique group dynamic, where it is constructed and managed through the group process and not as an individual trait. There is also a higher-order, transcendent quality offered by the group context. This is the ability to appreciate the atmosphere or shared affect of the group, and the "intelligent" part of distributed EI requires cultivating sensitivity to this global phenomenon, which the group itself constructs through activity (Engeström, 1987).

Importantly, distributed EI constructs climates for learning that may be productive or unproductive. It is these climates that offer a rich resource for learning, including learning how to cope in stressful settings. However, we do not want to equate productive learning climates solely with warm comfortable atmospheres. For example, in the excerpt, we see the construction of a highly charged, tense, and stressful atmosphere, which is still educationally productive. Here, the shared affect of the group helps them begin to understand a difficult concept. The group has tuned into this pressurized atmosphere as they collectively try to remember the correct formula and construct the pathway. The group also collectively manages this atmosphere through humor and laughter, which moderate the discomfort. Although it may be something that an individual student or facilitator says or does that acts as an emotional catalyst to trigger the emergence of distributed EI, they are still grounded in a local ecology and co-construct that context.

Because the language of educational research is currently inadequate in terms of being able to discuss emergent and distributed phenomena, we attempted to capture distributed EI through metaphor including the descriptors "atmosphere" and "climate." Interestingly, both of these terms are weather metaphors and the weather is the best known model of a complex system (Lewin, 1999). At the present time, only the language of complexity theory with descriptors such as "turbulence," and "flow" seems appropriate. Complexity theory is beginning to generate some interest in medicine and in medical education (Fraser & Greenhalgh, 2001). Indeed, in Chapter 5, Risdon and Baptiste apply complexity thinking to curriculum development and specifically to the notion of "resilience." Looking at distributed EI through a complexity lens would be an interesting area for further study.

Distributed EI is unpredictable, and it is this unpredictable, unstable, and dynamic quality that means emergence is so difficult to manage. Across the entire study, groups clearly accessed or felt the atmospheres that they had collectively constructed, but they often failed to manage them well. Indeed, some group atmospheres were so highly charged and uncomfortable that the discomfort still resonated with the students, facilitators, and researcher (as observer) long after the sessions. Interestingly, it is precisely the painfulness and discomfort of group atmospheres in a real-life setting that underline the potential of distributed EI as a resource for learning how to cope with stress. However, to capitalize on this resource, medical educators require a fundamental change in their thinking and ways of working. Facilitators might focus on how learning climates emerge initially and then address how they can help students develop sensitivity to context and tune into these difficult atmospheres so that they can subsequently deal with stress more effectively. Facilitators also have to start to question their habitual practice to see how they often contribute to the construction of educationally unproductive learning climates.

Theoretically, re-visioning EI as distributed and emergent, rather than as individual and static, opens up the domain of EI and suggests the possibilities of working within a collective and distributed framework rather than an individualistic one. However, this way of working challenges our individualistic mind-set and requires a completely different focus. The conventional literature on EI reflects the strong influence of organizational psychology and is unsurprisingly steeped in the language of managerial efficiency, with a focus on the selection and improvement of EI (Chernis & Goleman, 2001), on building effectiveness (Druskat & Wolff, 2001), and on measurement (Geher, 2004). The medical education literature has uncritically adopted this view with empirical studies similarly focusing on selection (Carrothers, Gregory, & Gallagher, 2000) and on individual measurement (Stratton, Saunders, & Elam, 2008). This trend seems set to continue with a proliferation of such studies. For example, across the last five years (2009–2013), *Medical Education* and *Academic Medicine*, the leading journals for medical educators and researchers, published eight papers on EI and all have focused exclusively on EI as an individual, stable trait (e.g. Arora et al., 2011; Borges, Stratton, Wagner, & Elam, 2009; Brannick et al., 2009; Carr, 2009). We urge medical educators to familiarize themselves with the critical literature (Conte, 2005; Lewis et al., 2005; Matthews et al., 2002; Zeidner et al., 2009) and to open their minds to other, more complex ways of conceptualizing EI.

We have argued that EI is an unstable, often unpredictable system with an emergent quality, and in this sense we do not think it is possible to measure, fix, or control EI in a conventional way. At a fundamental level, despite much careful and "rigorous" work, the psychometric approach is limited because it fails to capture the complexity of EI in practice. Re-visioning EI as distributed, dynamic, and emergent rather than as individual and static moves us away from the constraints of restricted instrumental thinking and concerns about individual measurement to a wider consideration of how to access and collaboratively manage EI in context. Although the aim of interpretative research such as ethnography is not to generalize to a wider population, we believe that our research findings may be transferable to other settings such as postgraduate groups and clinical teams.

As discussed previously, an individual student's score on a stress management sub-scale on a conventional EI measure will tell us little about how he or she will actually behave in a stressful situation. But how students access and respond to the uncomfortable atmospheres in their groups does have implications for how they will cope with stress in the much more demanding settings of their future careers. Indeed, across this doctoral study, we found that some groups experienced difficulties coping in the relatively benign setting of PBL. They failed to respond to and manage distributed EI effectively and so missed opportunities for learning.

Physicians must have the capacity to work in intense stressful atmospheres such as clinical teams and medical students need to be able to access, make sense of, and respond effectively to what is going on in such settings. Through developing sensitivity to atmosphere and climate, distributed EI may prepare students for work in these real-life contexts. For example, helping students first tune into and notice what is happening in their clinical team may give them the space to respond more sensitively and effectively to a stressful situation, rather than rushing in or floundering and failing to act. As a consequence, such shared "situational awareness" should also increase patient safety (Bleakley, 2006).

A good metaphor for students using a context for learning is research showing how blue fin tuna can increase their speed and maneuverability by exploiting the currents and vortices in the environment that surrounds them (Triantafyllou & Triantafyllou, 1995). The tuna collaboratively use a context, rather than attempt to control and work against, or master that context as individuals. Contrast this approach with a captain steering the ship against a current. Within education theory, there is already a grounding for distributed learning, and distributed EI is consistent with this. In collaborative learning models (Lave & Wenger, 1991), learning activity is distributed across a community of practice and the goal of medical educators is to help students access knowledge that is collaboratively generated and held. Medical educators face a similar challenge in working with distributed EI. Rather than seeking mastery of EI as an individual skill, medical educators should concentrate on developing sensitivity to context in themselves, as well as in students.

Although we cannot offer a set of prescriptive rules regarding how facilitators should work with distributed EI, we can suggest some possibilities. One of the conditions for the potential emergence of distributed EI and the creation of productive learning climates seems to involve the state of tolerance of ambiguity (Furnham & Ribchester, 1995). Facilitators who are better able to tolerate ambiguity are also better prepared to handle emergence, which, as we have seen, is extremely difficult to do. Importantly, facilitators need to feel comfortable with complex and unpredictable situations and be able to hold onto tense and difficult atmospheres and avoid closing down the group flow prematurely. It is in those moments, when everything seems to be falling apart, as the group balances on the edge of chaos, that productive learning can occur. In addition, facilitators need empathy in the sense of being able to monitor and track the changes in the group atmosphere. However, for this to occur, facilitators need to examine and challenge some elements of their habitual practice. PBL groups are complex activity systems where information, knowledge, and expertise are aspects of the total system. However, facilitator education is currently framed by individualistic and static models of emotion and of learning, more consistent with information reproduction than with knowledge production (Bleakley, 2006; Engeström, 1987). Another powerful way of developing sensitivity to context is the use of video recording. We have seen how difficult it is to manage emergent properties, particularly when facilitators are overwhelmed by or deeply engaged with the group dynamic. In this study, video recording became an intervention in itself as facilitators, when viewing the video footage; found confirming evidence for their feelings and, importantly, noticed features of the context, which they were previously unaware of at the time as they struggled with emergence and with managing group atmospheres. This technology, perhaps used as part of a debriefing exercise, would be a valuable tool in helping facilitators learn how to work with emergent and dynamic properties (Forsyth, Carroll, & Reitano, 2009).

In addition, the research method of cooperative inquiry (Heron & Reason, 2001) also has potential in helping facilitators work with distributed EI. This method is particularly suitable for developing professional practice in a landscape of complexity, where it offers the possibility of participants being able to transform their practice over time as they gain new insights from their experiences. It also focuses on the acceptance of emotions and feelings as part of the research process. Importantly, the participative nature of the approach and the sense of ownership it gives to participants also make it uniquely suited to giving EI back to facilitators to explore and work with themselves rather than having a commercially produced conventional EI measurement tool imposed on them.

Medicine is a "cognitive apprenticeship" (Lave & Wenger, 1991), but it is also an affective apprenticeship. Although medicine traditionally values emotional detachment, students will have to work in intense, stressful atmospheres and medical educators must become more familiar with the field of affect. Medical education research also needs to be both more systematic and imaginative, focusing on studies of affect in action in ecologically valid contexts. The work presented in this chapter has begun to map the territory, but further research is needed to capitalize fully on distributed EI as a vital resource for learning how to cope.

REFERENCES

Arora, S., Russ, S., Petrides, K.V., Sirimanna, P., Aggarwal, R., Darzi, A., & Sevdalis, N. (2011). Emotional intelligence in medical students performing surgical tasks. *Academic Medicine, 86*(10), 1311–1317.

Bar-On, R. (2000). Emotional and social intelligence: Insights from the emotional quotient inventory. In R. Bar-On & J. D. A. Parker (Eds.), *The handbook of emotional intelligence* (pp. 363–389). San Francisco, CA: Jossey-Bass.

Bleakley, A., Farrow, R., Gould, D., & Marshall, R. (2003). Making sense of clinical reasoning: Judgement and the evidence of the senses. *Medical Education, 37*(6), 544–553.

Bleakley, A. (2006). Broadening conceptions of learning in medical education: The message from team working. *Medical Education, 40*(2), 150–158.

Borges, N. J., Stratton, T. D., Wagner, P. J., & Elam, C. L. (2009). Emotional intelligence and medical specialty choice: Findings from three empirical studies. *Medical Education, 43*(6), 565–572.

Brannick, M. T., Wahl, M. M., Arce, M., Johnson, H., Nazian, S., & Goldin, S.B. (2009). Comparison of trait and ability measures of emotional intelligence in medical students. *Medical Education, 43*(11), 1062–1068.

Carr, S. E. (2009). Emotional intelligence in medical students: Does it correlate with selection measures? *Medical Education, 43*(11), 1069–1077.

Carrothers, R. M., Gregory, S. W., & Gallagher, T. J. (2000). Measuring emotional intelligence of medical school applicants. *Academic Medicine, 75*(5), 456–463.

Caruso, D. R., Bienn, B., & Kornacki, S. A. (2006). Emotional intelligence in the workplace. In J. Ciarrochi, J. P. Forgas & J. D. Mayer (Eds.), *Emotional intelligence in everyday life* (2nd ed., pp. 187–206). Hove, East Sussex, UK: Psychology Press.

Chernis, C., & Goleman, D. (2001). *The emotionally intelligent workplace: How to select for, measure and improve emotional intelligence in individuals, groups and organisations.* San Francisco, CA: Jossey-Bass.

Ciarrochi, J., Dean, F. P., & Anderson, S. (2002). Emotional intelligence moderates the relationship between stress and mental health. *Personality and Individual Differences, 32,* 197–209.

Conte, J. M. (2005). A review and critique of emotional intelligence measures. *Journal of Organizational Behaviour, 26,* 433–440.

Crotty, M. (2004). *The foundations of social research: Meaning and perspective in the research process.* London, UK: Sage.

Druskat, V. U., & Wolff, S. B. (2001). Building the emotional intelligence of groups. *Harvard Business Review, 79*(3), 80–90.

Elias, M. J., Zins, J. E., Weissberg, R. P., Frey, K. S., Greenberg, M. T., Haynes, N. M., et al. (Eds.). (1997). *Promoting social and emotional learning: Guidelines for educators.* Alexandria, VA: Association for Supervision and Curriculum Development.

Engeström, Y. (1987). *Learning by expanding.* Helsinki, Finland: Orienta Konsultit Oy.

Flury, J., & Ickes, W. (2006). Emotional intelligence and empathic accuracy in friendships and dating relationships. In J. Ciarrochi, J. P. Forgas & J. D. Mayer (Eds.), *Emotional intelligence in everyday life* (2nd ed., pp. 140–166). Hove, East Suzzed, UK: Psychology Press.

Forsyth, R., Carroll, K., & Reitano, P. (Eds.). (2009). Using video in social sciences and health research. *International Journal of Multiple Research Approaches, 3*(3), 214–217.

Fraser, S. W., & Greenhalgh, T. (2001). Coping with complexity: Educating for capability. *British Medical Journal, 323,* 799–802.

Furnham, A., & Ribchester, T. (1995). Tolerance of ambiguity: A review of the concept, its measurement and applications. *Current Psychology, 14*(3), 179–199.

Geher, G. (2004). *Measuring emotional intelligence: Common ground and controversy.* New York, NY: Nova Science.

Gohm, C. L., Corser, G. C., & Dalsky, D. J. (2005). Emotional intelligence under stress: Useful, unnecessary, or irrelevant? *Personality and Individual Differences, 39,* 1017–1028.

Goleman, D. (1996). *Emotional intelligence: Why it can matter more than IQ.* London, UK: Bloomsbury.

Hammersley, M., & Atkinson, P. (1995). *Ethnography: Principles in practice* (2nd ed.). London, UK: Routledge.

Heron, J., & Reason, P. (2001).The practice of co-operative inquiry: Research 'with' rather than 'on' people. In P. Reason & H. Bradbury (Eds.), *Handbook of action research: Participative inquiry and practice* (pp. 179–188). London, UK: Sage.

Jones, M. C., & Johnstone, D. W. (2006). Is the introduction of a student-centred, problem-based curriculum associated with improvement in student nurse well-being and performance? An observational study of effect. *International Journal of Nursing Studies, 43,* 941–952.

Kiessling, C., Schubert, B., Scheffner, D., & Burger, W. (2004). First year medical students' perceptions of stress and support: A comparison between reformed and traditional track curricula. *Medical Education, 38,* 504–509.

Lakoff, G., & Johnson, M. (1981). *Metaphors we live by.* Chicago, IL: University of Chicago Press.

Lave, J., & Wenger, E. (1991). *Situated learning: Legitimate peripheral participation.* Cambridge, UK: Cambridge University Press.

Lazarus, R., & Folkman, S. (1984). *Stress, appraisal and coping.* New York, NY: Springer.

Lewin, R. (1999). *Complexity: Life at the edge of chaos.* London, UK: Phoenix.

Lewis, N. J., Rees, C. E., Hudson, N., & Bleakley, A. (2005). Emotional intelligence in medical education: Measuring the unmeasurable? *Advances in Health Sciences Education, 10,* 339–355.

Lewis, N. J. (2007). *Re-visioning emotional intelligence through a study of small group learning in medical education* (Unpublished doctoral dissertation). University of Exeter, UK.

Lingard, L. (2009). What we see and don't see when we look at "competence": Notes on a god term. *Advances in Health Sciences Education, 14,* 625–628.

Matthews, G., Emo, A. K., Funke, G. J., Zeidner, M., Roberts, R. D., Costa, P. T., Jr., & Schulze, R. (2006). Emotional intelligence, personality and task-induced stress. *Journal of Experimental Psychology Applied, 12,* 97–107.

Matthews, G., Zeidner, M., & Roberts, R. D. (2002). *Emotional intelligence: Science and myth.* Boston, MA: MIT Press.

Mayer, J. D., & Salovey, P. (1997). What is emotional intelligence? In P. Salovey & D. Sluyter (Eds.), *Emotional development and emotional intelligence* (pp. 3–31). New York, NY: Basic Books.

Mayer, J. D., Salovey, P., & Caruso, D. R. (2000) Emotional intelligence as zeitgeist, as personality, and as a mental ability. In R. Bar-On & J. D. A. Parker (Eds.), *The handbook of emotional intelligence* (pp. 92–117). San Francisco, CA: Jossey-Bass.

Mayer, J. D., Caruso, D. R., & Salovey, P. (2002). *The Mayer-Caruso- Salovey Emotional Intelligence Test (MSCEIT),* Version 2. Toronto, Canada: Multi-Health Systems.

Moffat, K. J., McConnache, A., Ross, S., & Morrison, J. M. (2004). First year medical student stress and coping in a problem-based learning medical curriculum. *Medical Education, 38,* 482–491.

Petrides, K. V., & Furnham, A. (2000). On the dimensional structure of emotional intelligence. *Personality and Individual Differences. 29,* 313–320.

Regehr, G. (2006). The persistent myth of stability: On the chronic underestimation of the role of context in behaviour. *Journal of General Internal Medicine, 21*(5), 544–545.

Saklofske, D. H., Austin, E. J., Galloway, J., & Davidson, K. (2007). Individual difference correlates of health-related behaviours: Preliminary evidence for links between emotional intelligence and coping. *Personality and Individual Differences, 42,* 491–502.

Salovey, P., & Mayer, J. D. (1990). Emotional intelligence. *Imagination, Cognition and Personality, 9,* 185–211.

Stratton, T. D., Saunders, J. A., & Elam, C. L. (2008). Changes in medical students' emotional intelligence: An exploratory study. *Teaching and Learning in Medicine, 20*(3), 279–284.

Triantafyllou, M., & Triantafyllou, G. (1995). An efficient swimming machine. *Scientific American, 272*(3), 64–71.

Zeidner, M., Matthews, G., & Roberts, R. D. (2006). Emotional intelligence, coping with stress and adaptation. In J. Ciarrochi, J. P. Forgas, & J. D. Mayer (Eds.), *Emotional intelligence in everyday life* (2nd ed., pp. 100–129). Hove, East Sussex, UK: Psychology Press.

Zeidner, M., Matthews, G., Roberts, R. (2009). *What we know about emotional intelligence: How it affects learning, work, relationships and our mental health.* Cambridge, MA: MIT Press.

/// 2 /// FIRST CLINICAL ATTACHMENTS

Informal Learning and Stressors in the Clinical Environment

RAIN LAMDIN

INTRODUCTION

This chapter provides findings from previously unpublished doctoral research into medical students' professional socialization with respect to the stressors and challenges faced as students enter the clinical environment (Lamdin, 2010). I introduce professional socialization, medical student stress, and contemporary sociocultural learning theory (Lave & Wenger, 1991), the latter of which provides a theoretical background for the research presented. I describe the methods of the study, and the themes developed through the analysis are presented and discussed.

PROFESSIONAL SOCIALIZATION AND SOCIOCULTURAL LEARNING THEORY

The socialization of medical students into the medical profession is more than the acquisition of a body of knowledge, attitudes, and skills, "proved" through the passing of examinations. Medical students learn how to be a doctor, and they learn the "craft" of medicine, which goes beyond the application of medical knowledge (Conrad, 1988). There is no unified theory of medical student socialization into the profession of medicine. Rather, there is a "broad domain of phenomena and theoretical problems" (Levinson, 1967, p. 253). Professional socialization may be considered across three related stages in a professional's career. These stages are anticipatory socialization, socialization during training or education (the period of this study), and post-training or education socialization (Cant & Higgs, 1999).

In this research, I use legitimate peripheral participation (LPP), a sociocultural learning theory of analyzing apprentice-style learning (Lave & Wenger, 1991), because it is relevant in framing clinical experiences within workplace learning (Swanwick, 2005). LPP acknowledges the student as a "legitimate" member of the profession, learning and shifting from the edges or periphery within a social and interactive world, as they move toward full participation. In LPP, medical students on clinical rotations are learning in the workplace—hospitals, clinics, and general practices, or the "community of practice." This community refers to physicians of all levels, other health professionals, peers, patients, and so on, all of whom contribute to medical care and work. No one person or role holds all the knowledge for successful work—in this case, patient care. For work to be undertaken, people of different positions and levels contribute, as they each hold partial and specific information and experience of medical work.

With respect to the apprentice or novice, the emphasis is on what students learn as opposed to what they are taught, and learning will not necessarily be systematically ordered but instead will be varied for each novice depending on the opportunities that arise within the workplace. Becoming a full member means that the novice develops an identity as "apprentice" and their positioning at the peripheries involves relationships of power. Barriers to full engagement can disempower the apprentice. Alternatively, activities and relationships that facilitate participation can empower the learner (Rees, Knight, & Wilkinson, 2007). Newcomers engage with the discourse of the profession, learning the language and culture of the profession. Access is given, or not, to the artifacts of the community of practice (e.g., patient notes), and this will either facilitate or obstruct the learner's participation. While the learner is becoming enculturated into the profession, he or she will work to maintain the culture and at times challenge and alter the culture as he or she brings new knowledge and ways of working. Therefore, there is an interactive constructing relationship between the profession and the novice (Lave & Wenger, 1991).

A medical student's place, on a ward or as a member of a medical team, is not a constant place. The student is a transitory team member, and there is a period of establishing what the student does or does not know and what they can and cannot do. The student must negotiate a place and establish legitimacy each time he or she begins with a new team. (The team itself is a complex and changing place, as people come and go and team membership changes.) As students learn and participate in medical work and in the team, their position changes–shifting to fuller participation. As well as negotiating their place on the team, students need to balance what is required for academic assessment purposes with being a member of the community of clinical care—these two goals may not necessarily be the same and may conflict. This can create considerable effort and stress for the student (Becker, Geer, Hughes, & Strauss, 1961).

Students are enculturated into the medical profession while also challenging it by bringing what is learned in the classroom and their own values and experiences into the clinical environment. When there are differences in what is expected of students in each place, the student will need to manage these differences. Compared with the lay person, medical students have legitimate and privileged access to patients, and this enables students to shift their perception of patients, illness, and disease from lay observer to medical student to physician. LPP provides an approach to considering medical student learning, becoming a member of the medical profession, and understanding the stress experienced by medical students through viewing membership to the profession as a changing process.

Conceptualizing clinical education as an apprenticeship is not without its critics or challenges. The short-term multiple specialty placements that students rotate through during their clinical years are considered to deny the medical student a sense of "belonging to a particular team, continuity of care, support" required for apprenticeship learning (Turner, Collinson, & Fry, 2001, p. 515). Concerns have also been raised with respect to the risks of apprentice-style learning such as the lack of control regarding what students learn from teachers (Howe, Campion, Searle, & Smith, 2004). However, as noted, in medicine and medical practice, knowledge is distributed across many people within the community of practice, so students learn medical work from many different people. LPP is a method of analyzing learning and does not justify or address these challenges but presents them with respect to learning in the workplace or, in this instance, the clinical environment.

FORMAL, INFORMAL, AND HIDDEN CURRICULA

Student learning can be understood through considering three related areas of influence: the formal, informal, and hidden curricula (Hafferty, 1998). The formal curriculum is that which is explicitly taught, for example, in a classroom or at a patient's bedside. However, it has been shown that students learn through informal student–teacher experiences, as well as through the formal curriculum (Arnold, 2002). Values and attitudes, in particular, are learned through informal learning (Stern, 1998). Informal learning is the unanticipated, interpersonal learning that occurs between student and teacher (Hafferty, 1998). It often consists of everyday activities learned through demonstration and imitation (Lave,

1996). The hidden curriculum includes what is commonly understood by the profession (but not usually spoken of). The culture, customs, and rituals implicit to becoming and belonging to the profession are found within the hidden curriculum (Hafferty, 1998; Lemp & Searle, 2004).

Although the divisions of "formal," "informal," and "hidden" are exaggerations of a spectrum of learning processes and curricula (Reber, 1993), they serve to provide a schema for considering student learning and curriculum. In education, the space or separation between the formal and hidden curriculum is problematic. There is a tension for students between the drive to pass exams and what students perceive as knowledge required to be a physician (Becker et al., 1961) and between how they are told to manage their emotions and what is really expected—in the anatomy laboratory, for example (Hafferty, 1991), but also in the clinical environment (Arnold, 2002). Apprenticeship models focus on student learning (rather than teaching), and this can bring students' experiences of stress and tension to the foreground.

MEDICAL STUDENT STRESS AND TRANSITIONS

Becoming a physician is stressful for students (Dyrbye, Thomas, & Shanafelt, 2005; Firth, 1986; Radcliffe & Lester, 2003). The causes of student stress during clinical attachments have been identified as multiple, including talking to patients, presenting cases, dealing with death and suffering, and relationships with seniors (Firth, 1986; Moss & McManus, 1992), as well as a perceived lack of knowledge or application of theoretical knowledge and concerns about fitting into the team (Hayes et al., 2004; Prince, Boshuizen, Van der Vleuten, & Scherpbier, 2005; Radcliffe & Lester, 2003). Intimidation, harassment, and humiliation by consultants and senior staff are also well documented as other sources of stress for clinical students (Baldwin, Daugherty, & Rowley, 1998; Sheehan, Sheehan, White, Leibowitz, & Baldwin, 1990). Increased student workload and responsibility have been identified as stressors in the transition from medical student to junior physician and can be extrapolated as potential stressors for students shifting into the clinical environment (Prince, Van de Wiel, Van der Vleuten, Boshuizen, & Scherpbier, 2004). Stress and anxiety have been associated with potentially detrimental effects on physical and psychological well-being (Mosley et al., 1994; Wolf, 1994) and correlate with negative academic outcomes for students (Linn & Zeppa, 1984) and the increased future risk of mental illness and suicide (Sinclair, 1997).

Entering the clinical environment is a stressful experience for students, even a "culture shock" (Wear, Aultman, Varley, & Zarconi, 2006). Stephenson, Higgs, and Sugarman (2001) suggest that medical students are most vulnerable during the transitional stages of medical education. Pitkala and Mantyranta (2003) suggested that the clinical transition is important for further research, given that this is a time of "intense emotional experiences and rapid development" (p. 155).

There are three major transitions in undergraduate medical training: selection and entry into a medical program; clinical placements or experience; and the graduate's first job on qualification (Bligh, 2002; Cant & Higgs, 1999). When shifting into the clinical environment, students are faced with actual and not the simulated or "well" patients typically common to preclinical education. Students need to adapt to the hospital environment as a place of learning as opposed to the classroom. Teaching styles and expectations differ from the classroom setting, students may feel useless with respect to patient care, and clinical care is unfamiliar (Radcliffe & Lester, 2003). Student learning is often opportunistic depending on the availability of teachers and appropriate patients. Consequently, timetables and learning are flexible compared with the classroom. The clinical environment is a busy social world with heavy staff workloads and unexpected catastrophes and crises to which students must adapt.

Context of the Research

As a physician, I am a member of the medical community that medical students are entering. I trained at the medical school at which the research is based and later worked as a clinical tutor before beginning this research. I am familiar with the medical education culture, both in the hospitals that the students attended and at this medical school specifically. My interest in this area of study developed from observing the different experiences of medical students and how they journeyed through the preclinical to clinical transition. Although my medical education was mostly from the positivist position (Crotty, 2003), I view becoming a physician through an interpretive lens. As with LPP, I see the socialization of medical students as an interactive and constructed process, whereby individuals bring themselves and their experiences, integrating new experiences as they become physicians and are socialized into the profession.

I undertook the research at a New Zealand medical school with a relatively traditionally structured undergraduate curriculum composed of 3 years of classroom, laboratory-based, and small-group learning followed by students completing 3 years of clinical placements in hospitals, clinics, and general practices. I refer to the early years as "preclinical"; however, there are early clinical experiences in those first 3 years. These include the occasional presentation and discussion of patients by physicians, clinical skills teaching, and a clinical methods course encompassing the teaching of patient history and physical examination in small student groups with a medical tutor, in the hospital setting.

The presentation of patients to the class occurred in the lecture theatre and not the clinical environment. Therefore, although the patient was visible to the student, they were sequestered from the clinical context and the community of practice. The physician–teacher took the patient through his or her medical history, and students were given the opportunity to ask the patient questions. This limited student participation with the patient, affirmed the student role as mostly a quiet, and even a passive, learner: very much on the periphery. There were limited opportunities for the teacher to demonstrate the use of equipment and technology (artifacts) to the students. Students could see the application of biomedical sciences to the patient and their illness and the use of medical language.

The clinical skills course was held in a simulated clinical environment but without the full complement of participants of medical work and care. Students had fortnightly sessions working in small groups through tasks of physical examination, reading of radiological material and with the artifacts of medical work (e.g., sphygmomanometer, stethoscope, and so on), under observation and with supervision by tutors. Because of the self-directed nature of learning, students were active participants but removed from the work setting. Students could practice their medical language and skills in a safe environment.

The clinical methods course most closely simulated the students' workplace because it was in the hospital setting. The half-day sessions allowed the students as learners to observe clinical work and the clinical context. With respect to their role or position in the clinical environment, they were legitimately there, but students were not active members of the medical team. They were however surrounded by the language and artifacts of medical work within the community of practice. Students undertook to learn to elicit a case history and learn physical examination skills with patients, but these patients were usually relatively well and practiced in their story telling. Although the clinical methods class most closely simulated their prospective clinical rotations, the sessions were relatively brief and occasional, so students had limited opportunities to observe medical work and no opportunity to contribute to it.

In summary, although early clinical experiences are provided to students, there are significant gaps with respect to sociocultural learning. Students are often sequestered from the community of practice, even outside of the peripheries, and have limited or no opportunities to participate or observe and interact with the community. As Lave and Wenger (1991) have shown, these circumstances limit the apprentice moving to full participation. Therefore, it is in the clinical years that medical students at this New Zealand school undertake their richest learning as legitimate participants engaging with the language, discourse, artifacts, and relationships of clinical work.

Although the medical education literature on student stress is rich, my focus was to build on literature that highlights the importance of transitional periods in medical education (Prince et al., 2005; Radcliffe & Lester, 2003; Stephenson et al., 2001). This study contributes to the literature through applying LPP to students' early clinical experiences, exploring their experiences and demystifying how these experiences can be stressful for students. My research questions asked: What are students' early experiences in the clinical environment? What are their experiences with patients? Where are the stressors for students in this transitional period?

RESEARCH METHODS

Traditionally, professional socialization research in medicine has used participant observation methods (Becker et al., 1961; Fox, 1989; Merton, 1957). However, observational research does not always permit the participants to share their personal experiences and understandings of experiences. Accordingly, I undertook one-on-one, semistructured in-depth interviews with students. After receiving ethical approval from the University Human Subjects Ethics Committee, I invited third-year students, by mail, to participate in the study. Students interested in being interviewed contacted me directly via e-mail or telephone. In the interviews, I asked students to describe their experiences at medical school focusing on their clinical teaching. I asked further questions based on these discussions. About 1 year later, I contacted the same students with a letter asking them to contact me if they were prepared to be interviewed again. In the second interview, I asked students about their experiences on their clinical attachments and with patients and staff. Again, I followed each student's lead as to the direction and progress of the interview. The interviews were audio-taped with each student's consent. The interviews were transcribed by me and a professional transcriber. I proofread all the transcripts as I listened to the audiotapes as the beginnings of the analysis.

DATA ANALYSIS

I used a thematic content analysis to classify students' experiences. Using Borkan's immersion/crystallization method of transcript analysis (Borkan, 1999; Howe, 2008), I read and reread the transcripts to identify and label segments of transcripts to collate developing themes. Incidents applicable to each category were compared and integrated (Lincoln & Guba, 1985). The transcripts were read sequentially as whole transcripts (vertical passes) and as sections common across all the second-interview transcripts (horizontal passes) (Borkan, 1999). These themes were collated together (decontextualized), examined for patterns and relationships within the identified themes, and shaped to present a coherent picture, which was then related back to the field of study (recontextualization). In this chapter, three themes (of 11) that relate to the subject of stress through students' early clinical experiences in the clinical environment are presented. I use participant quotes to give voice and recognition to the participants and their experiences. Pseudonyms are used to maintain student anonymity.

RESEARCH PARTICIPANTS

Of the class of 132 students, 21 students (16%) volunteered to participate. The demographic information and educational experience of participants are presented in Table 2.1.

Results and Discussion

In this section, I discuss the following themes: medical work (which includes aspects of students' informal learning including learning how to work in the clinical environment); sad and tragic patient-related experiences; and bridging professional and personal worlds of the medical students. These three themes were derived from the students' second interviews and reflect aspects of their transition into the clinical environment.

Although students' preclinical teaching was predominantly class and laboratory based with some early clinical experiences, now in their fourth year, medical students were based mainly in the hospital or general practice setting. They spent 4 or 6 weeks attached to various teams (e.g., medical, surgical, psychiatry, emergency medicine, anesthesiology, and general practice). Students attended ward rounds, followed members of

TABLE 2.1 Participant Information

	N
Gender	
Male	7
Female	14
Ethnicity	
Pakeha (Caucasian)	14
Maori	3
Indo-Asian	4
Educational background	
Entered from School	11
Intermediate year	4
Other science degree	2
Health professional experience	4

the team in their work, and clerked or admitted patients arriving in the hospital, clinic, or general practice.

MEDICAL WORK

To undertake medical work to meet formal curriculum assessment requirements (e.g., to complete patient case histories) or to contribute to the work of the medical team, students needed to become familiar with the clinical environment. In this study, being new to this hospital environment was stressful as students needed to familiarize themselves with the hospital, including finding their way around, what they could do, which patients they could talk to, and who the various staff were. Although students were legitimately on the wards, they initially did not feel like they belonged on the ward: "It was quite nerve-wrecking. We still didn't know where we fit in. It was very much tip-toeing around. 'Is it alright if we see this patient?' and we didn't have much confidence" (Andrew). "In the beginning I felt really useless... like a waste of space" (Georgia).

Although medical students are legitimate members of the medical team and are expected to be there to learn, they are novices, in a very peripheral position. There is ambiguity in their status: they are part of the medical community but on the outer edges without the knowledge and experience to participate as a full member. They lack "confidence" and "feel really useless." As the students spent time in the hospital, they reported developing a better understanding of the hospital environment. This assisted them in participating in medical work (shifting from the periphery to a more central position for greater participation) and reduced their perceived stress, as shown in previous research (Pitkala &Mantyranta, 2003). It was important to the students to understand the bigger picture of hospital life, because this gave a context to the practice of medicine: "Osmosis. Just soaking it up on wards and seeing and watching, just keeping all senses open. Seeing what they do, seeing the charts, seeing how the nurses run, who runs what, what does the charge nurse do, what are the nurses expected to do, what are the house officers [junior physicians] supposed to do and stuff like that. Just basic running a hospital" (David).

"Osmosis" is a scientific term that refers to the flow of molecules from more densely occupied areas to less densely occupied areas. David uses this as a metaphor for the flow of information to his less knowledgeable mind through keeping all his "senses open." Although students may feel they are a "waste of space," their presence provides them with a chance to learn about the environment and the work of the various team members. Lave and Wenger (1991) observed this to be important, and when the opportunity to observe was not given to novices, learning was impaired. Despite it not being stated in curriculum documents that it is important for students to know how hospitals function, it is necessary informal learning. To complete their academic work (case histories and logbooks), students need to know when and how to see patients and attend clinics, ward rounds, and so on. Being able to meet their learning objectives and understand the hospital makes it easier and less stressful to be there. Learning how to use the equipment and technology of medical work is part of students' learning and enables their participation: "You have to learn about the computer. I tended to ask the TI [trainee interns—final year students] and house surgeons [junior physicians] (Leah).

This is codified or organizational knowledge that is based within the workplace and is learned informally (Eraut, 2004). Leah asks the junior staff around her who are closest to her in the workplace and apprenticeship hierarchy and with whom she spends time. The trainee interns and house surgeons are experienced novices relative to the students but not yet masters, as are consultants. Computers are part of medical work and provide the novice an opportunity to engage with the technology of medicine. Knowing how to access information on the computer, patient investigation results for example, enables the student to contribute to medical work. The computer is both an object of medical work and a conduit for further learning. This is analogous to the "window" discussed by Lave and Wenger (1991)—it is both visible and invisible, allowing objects to be seen through it, but is also able to be seen itself. Given access to the computer empowers the novice to achieve increased participation. Trish also notes the broad range of knowledge junior physicians had: "They were only first year house surgeons but they seemed to know heaps" (Trish).

Trish's perspective of junior physicians knowing "heaps" acknowledges that, relative to medical students, junior physicians, as full participating members of the community of practice, do know a lot. This is not knowledge of disease and treatment in which neither student nor junior physician is an expert yet, but the knowledge of the work environment. The medical team as a community of practice contributes different aspects to students' learning (Lave & Wenger, 1991) and enables students formal learning so they can complete case histories, examinations and so on, with patients. Becoming a member of the team has been identified as a stressor for students as students struggle to know their role (Prince et al., 2005). As students increased their knowledge and were able to contribute to the community of medical care and work, they were increasingly becoming members of the community, and their anxiety was less evident in the interviews.

In their fourth year, students saw their increased time in the clinical environment as a chance for increased participation in medical work, which they equated with greater opportunities for learning: "It was quite good going down to ED [emergency department] and doing your own histories and examinations and then present the case to the registrar [trainee specialist]. That was really good. You actually felt you were learning something. You can actually do something now" (Marie).

Eliciting and writing the case history and physical examination from a newly presenting patient, compared with writing case histories for academic purposes, is a sign of increased participation. The student is no longer directed to only meet assessment goals but is contributing to the patient's medical record, using medical language and therefore contributing to medical work. Students' place on the wards during the clinical methods course was a passive place with respect to medical work compared with their place in fourth year. Fourth-year medical students are on the periphery compared with physicians but have shifted relative to where they were in third year. The students increased responsibilities represent increased participation and legitimacy with respect to LPP. Mike also noted the difference in seeing patients between third and fourth year: "You do them [clerking or admitting patients] in third year but it's not the same. You didn't have the same pressure to get them right I suppose. Whereas if you are clerking people [now in your fourth year] you need to do them properly" (Mike).

Learning not only takes place as a result of a person's conscious effort but when that knowledge is actively used (Eraut, 1994), as Mike notes. Knowledge is transformed by the learner in the process of using it. For Mike, the context or situational aspect of doing the paperwork like a physician alters his intention as he needs to "do them properly." (It is unclear whether Mike is focused on doing it *properly* for the patient's benefit or if he is being task-oriented. However, getting the task right will improve his communication in the patient's notes and benefit the patient.) Mike is now increasing his contribution to the medical team and undertaking medical work as an apprentice under the supervision of physicians. Permission to contribute to and participate in work indicates acceptance by staff to do so. As students shift from feeling useless to knowing how to use the computer and admit patients, they are shifting to fuller participation. This greater participation reduced students' stress as they found their place on the medical team and were able to contribute to medical work.

SAD AND TRAGIC EVENTS: BEING VERSUS DOING

Medical students enter medical school to help people and "do something meaningful" (Wilhelm, 2002). Although curriculum objectives are often directed at students learning to elicit the case history and examine patients with specific conditions or diseases, students also bear witness to the illness and suffering of patients and their carers. Given that these experiences are part of medical work, they contribute to students' apprenticeship and socialization into the profession. Students' stories of patients reflected profound experiences that distressed students. Students were required to deal with the personal and sad stories of patients that went beyond a current medical problem: "For my last day I had a lady tell me that she didn't want to live anymore and she had had enough and was in pain...I didn't know what to do" (Mike).

Being on the periphery and not having an active role in the clinical environment is a significant medical student stressor (Radcliffe & Lester, 2003). Mike is concerned about what he can "do" and so highlights the tension between "doing" and "being with," particularly in the context of patients' deaths and dying. Students described feeling they were becoming physicians or could see themselves becoming physicians because they could now "do" something like a physician. For students, "doing" includes eliciting patient histories, performing physical examinations, taking blood, and assisting in the operating theater. However, as students listened to patients, they were exposed to patients' stories, which required them to listen and not act or "do": "She was only 60 and she had quite severe Parkinson's disease and was unable to walk. She used to be really active and doing lots of things, playing sports and she's having dementia. Her husband can't cope so you think that's all, but no, I ask her how her children are and they've all died. It's just too terrible and you don't know what to say to things like that.... The other man I met who had been born with congenital adrenal hypoplasia. He was on long-term steroids, so he had long-term problems with infections and things like he had broken every bone in his body just about. Then I asked have you got brothers and sisters? How are they? 'Oh my brother had the same thing as me but he was electrocuted when he was eleven...I've got Crohn's disease and I've got some kind of arthritis". Those two patients I'll never forget. I saw them both in the same day" (Leah).

For Leah, these two patients' stories transcend the medical history she was focusing on. She tried to move to emotionally safer topics (asking about family) to avoid hearing these distressing stories. While the preclinical curriculum includes communication skills training on breaking bad news and death and dying, students are unprepared for such disclosures from patients, perhaps because they are unpredictable in their timing and nature and these conversations involved no clinical supervision. The patient perceives the student as more a legitimate member of the profession than the student sees himself or herself. Also, the earlier small-group classes predated students' experiences with patients, and the combination of unexpectedness and distance from teaching may have contributed to Leah's sense of being unprepared.

Also visible in Leah's quote is her use of medical language. This language is central to medical communication, which is a constituent of medical work and membership to the medical community. As an apprentice, Leah is developing knowledge, understanding practice and socializing into the medical culture. Although Leah and Mike are part of a community of practice, they are in an ambiguous and still peripheral place, legitimately present in the clinical environment but feeling that they do not belong with respect to their role in the patient interaction. They are betwixt and between, as novices are.

The patient who tells a sad life story, who does not want to live anymore, or who has a poor prognosis can be challenging for the medical student. Rather than offering a cure, health professionals offer symptom control, caring, and active listening. To not be able to "do" something for a patient refers to the inability to provide a cure. The students did not identify active listening and caring as "doing." For the student, it may also reflect the tension in not knowing what can or should be done for the patient when there are no further tests to be "done." Students' self-perceptions of becoming a physician have been around their ability to "do" things, and they are now challenged because they are not "doing"; they are listening. Students are in a learning role and do not hold responsibility for patient care but want to be able to "do" something to help, as carers in the community of practice. Rees et al. (2007) have also found students are more comfortable when they are more fully participating as carers in medical communities of practice.

Students are often poorly supported in managing their emotional responses in the clinical environment (Rhodes-Kropf, Carmody, & Seltzer, 2005). Students new to the clinical environment have little or no experience observing others in this position and negotiate their own ways through. Learning how to handle their feelings when confronted with sick and dying patients is important for students, particularly in maintaining empathy with patients (Rosenfield & Jones, 2004). Medical educators have focused on empathy in medical students because of its importance in therapeutic relationships and its association with good physician–patient relationships as well as accuracy in diagnosing illness (Spencer, 2003). Unlike a class on death and dying or communicating bad news, there is no forewarning to what may arise in these patient interactions. There is no control provided by a teacher and no safety in the numbers of a group or class. The boundaries of the interaction are ambiguous compared with the medical history of questions and answers directed toward making a diagnosis of a disease.

Hafferty (1991) observed that students do not discuss their emotional reactions to dying patients or sad experiences with one another in the educational setting, and this parallels the observed detached concern of physicians as other research has found (Fox, 1989; Smith & Kleinman, 1989). The findings in this study do not show medical students feeling emotionally detached. The difference between this study and other research may be due to students in this study not being observed surrounded with their peers and seniors but being interviewed in a private setting without observation by others. In the setting of the current study, there was safety for students to disclose whatever they wished because I had assured them anonymity. Outside of the interviews, students managed their reactions on their own or in their own personal social circles but maintained silence in the medical environment as physicians do (Werner & Kosch, 1976). This silent personal management represents the hidden curriculum of physicians in the clinical environment. For the students, dealing with sad and tragic events had powerful effects on them, and in some instances students questioned their ability to become a physician. They perceived themselves to be inadequate people, rather than inadequately prepared. As novice members of the medical profession, medical students are in an empowered and privileged position to hear these patient disclosures, as are physicians. However, students did not feel prepared for these experiences.

Although illness and dying are common in medicine, medical students are at a relatively early stage in their careers and, like physicians, have to manage their feelings and responses. No student in the current study described seeing any other physician or student managing or dealing with these types of events. In LPP, this is problematic because novices need to see and be around all aspects of work at some time, to learn and move to full participation. The gap for these students probably reflects the short time these students had been in the clinical environment. "Survival skills" have been identified by medical educators as important for enhancing medical student learning in clinical environments (Gordon et al., 2000). However, the list of skills is focused on time management and assertiveness rather than assisting students to manage their emotional responses in these situations. Although this medical school includes ethics, breaking bad news, and death and dying in its professional development course, there appears to be a disconnection for students. What they learn in the classroom is not necessarily applied in the clinical environment during this transitional period. It is also ironic that as members of the health care profession, students were apparently unable to talk with their senior colleagues about their emotional responses to such profound experiences.

BRIDGING PROFESSIONAL AND PERSONAL WORLDS

Even in their early clinical experiences, there were instances when the line between students' professional and personal lives was blurred, as is also discussed in Chapter 3 by Monrouxe and Sweeney. This section addresses students' personal experiences of loss and death of friends and colleagues, where the student had no formal responsibility as a member of the team. The students in this study reported becoming involved or were asked to become involved in clinical situations because they were now medical students. Their place in the medical community permitted legitimate involvement in peoples' lives where otherwise they might not have been involved. One student described grave concerns regarding a friend who was unwell, illness in a family friend who was hospitalized, and, finally, illness in her partner's family. Another student reported two friends dealing with sickness and a life tragedy in the student's personal life. The following describes the unexpected death of a junior physician colleague: "It really affected me actually because the previous three weeks we had been such close good friends and he had helped me out a lot. He was a really good mentor type and then on the last day he took me through all these different IV (intravenous catheters) things and my last tutorial and things like that. Then just to suddenly get a phone call the next day in the next week, that he had died, it was like, how does that happen?" (Marie).

The same student also visited her sick friend in an intensive care unit. For Marie, the junior physician colleague had been a mentor, part of the medical team and community of practice. He had affirmed her legitimate place on the team and assisted her progress from peripheral to a more central member of the community. His death was unexpected and dissonant with his role in Marie's education. The death and dying literature tends to focus on the effect of patients', and not friends' or colleagues' deaths, on students. Although the student stories in this study happened outside of students' formal learning, they were still defined as clinical experiences by the students, illustrating the blurring of professional and personal worlds of students as they become members of the medical profession.

When medical students were involved informally with friends and family who were patients, they took on a different role than when they were being medical students. They had no formal responsibility as a "medical student" part of the medical team involved in the patient's care. However, they used their medical and hospital knowledge with respect to sick friends demonstrating their progression toward full membership of the profession and their changing identity. They traversed two worlds, the medical and the patient or lay world, acting as interpreters and understanding the family's concerns. Paula describes her involvement with family friends where one member had been diagnosed with cancer: "I was struck by the fact that they didn't even know what palliative meant.... No one described any of the medical jargon to them. It was a bit [of] lack of communication really..." (Paula).

Paula was upset in the interview by the apparent lack of communication between the physicians and the family. She was familiar with medical language and so could interpret it for the family and analyze the problems the relatives experienced. This refers to the codified medical information and knowledge about how hospital systems work, what happens to patients, and the meaning of medical language and jargon. This understanding of medical language separates Paula from the lay world now, and by presenting the medical perspective to lay people, Paula demonstrates her membership and participation in the medical community through her insight into the communication and language issues between the medical community and her friends. Being able to have a role with the family was important to her. Friends and family were similarly aware of the student's shift into the medical world and membership in the profession, as shown by their asking for help. However, it can introduce another area of stress for the medical student as they unofficially liaise for family and friends, between the personal and professional worlds or roles. The student's place when being with sick friends and acquaintances in hospital appears to be on a middling ground—between lay person and physician.

CONCLUSIONS

Becoming a physician is a complex process that is often stressful for students. Students are learning a vast body of knowledge, skills, and developing attitudes while becoming physicians. The socialization of a person into the medical profession begins before entering medical school as the applicant considers what it is to be a physician and why he or she wants to be a physician. Transitions are important in medical education because these can be stressful times as the student both legitimately belongs and participates but does not yet know what to do or how to be a physician. The student works within a liminal stage, increasingly shifting to become a full participant, socializing into his or her profession. The extensive formal knowledge that students learn contributes to student stress (Prince et al., 2004) as does the dissonance between the formal and hidden curriculum (Arnold, 2002).

The concept of LPP provides a useful structure for addressing the many and fragmented aspects to student learning in the clinical environment where the learning is both formal and informal and based within a community of practice. Medical work and patient care require cooperation across many health professionals and staff of differing levels of seniority and experience, and these same communities also provide an environment for student learning. Medical students in this study experience and learn this through their transition into the clinical environment.

Participation in medical work gives students the opportunity to "do" like a physician—elicit a case history, write patient notes, monitor investigations, and so on. The apprenticeship model of Lave and Wenger (1991) provides a template for analyzing and understanding student learning in the clinical environment, acknowledging that students learn from many "masters" and learn opportunistically through formal and informal learning. It is seen here that what students informally learn early in the clinical environment is important for them to become a physician. However, it is not without distressing experiences and challenges, as students negotiate their place on the medical team and undertake medical work within the community of practice. Beyond diseases, skills, and pathology, students learn how hospitals function, and students learn their way within and around the hospital. What is learned now will be used and built on through years of clinical practice. As students become familiar with medical care, they master formal and informal knowledge and the hidden ways physicians manage and work, which eases their transitions into new clinical attachments.

As the students in this study work and learn in the clinical environment, they are crossing a threshold from lay person to a member of the medical profession, internalizing the medical culture and being socialized into the medical profession. Their position changes from silent, passive observers and learners on the periphery, to more fully involved participants, understanding and participating in the issues of language between the medical community and lay people, ready to take on responsibility as legitimate members.

On entering the clinical environment, students meet the sad and tragic experiences of medical work. Patients disclose their stories to students as if they are fully participating members of the medical team, when they are still relatively on the periphery, more in the role of student and unable to "help." Conversations with patients could lead students to question their ability to become physicians, as Monrouxe and Sweeney discuss in Chapter 3. In the context of the research interview, students are upset and even distressed at recounting patients' sad stories. The stories and experiences students have with sad or sick patients highlight a known phenomenon of student vulnerability. These are critical incidents, which are defined as any event that overwhelms the usually effective coping skills of a person (Mitchell & Everly, 2000).

Exposure to illness and suffering of patients and their loved ones may lead to the development of maladaptive responses for students. These responses may include not being empathetic with a patient or becoming overinvolved with a patient (Dyrbye et al., 2005). This may have an impact on medical practice and, therefore, the physician–patient relationship. There is an apparent "conspiracy of silence" with regard to physicians' feelings, and so students apparently manage their reactions on their own or in their own personal social circles but in silence within the medical environment as physicians are noted to do (Werner & Kosch, 1976). This is paradoxical because physicians are caring for patients but not seeking support from or giving support to colleagues, with respect to sad and tragic stories and events. The socialization of medical students clearly involves learning and practicing medical work but also the ways physicians manage their feelings and reactions. Students are already receiving and understanding the hidden messages of how to manage their feelings and how to behave, as physicians do—with apparent silence. How students safely manage during these times is important given medical educators' concerns regarding stress and distress within the medical profession (Dyrbye et al., 2005; Dyrbye, Thomas, & Shanafelt, 2006; Radcliffe & Lester, 2003).

Does the stress students experience during their early clinical attachments reflect their peripheral position within the community of practice—that their knowledge and participation are minimal? Or, is the stress due to their shift through their transition into the clinical environment from the very margins as they gain legitimacy and increase toward fuller participation? Certainly being a "waste of space" and not knowing how the hospital works are stressful and challenging. As students can do more, they become part of the team, using the language and participating in the medical work and community. However, as they are increasingly moving to fuller participation, they are seen by others as full participants and what is expected of them increases. Patients disclose their sad and tragic stories because students are members of the community of practice. Students then shoulder patients' sorrows and their own reactions, not knowing "what to do."

Involving medical students in patient care and medical work is important for providing students a context for learning and the opportunity to become legitimate members working toward full participation in the work environment and changing their identities toward becoming physicians. Educating medical students, medical educators, and clinical supervisors as to how and what students learn in the early stages of their clinical experience could benefit student learning. If physicians and health care teams know that participation enhances student learning, greater effort could be made with students, without an added pressure to provide more teaching when people are already busy in their work. Likewise, encouraging students to participate is important particularly in getting through the feeling of uselessness students have when they first begin a clinical attachment. The provision of clinical supervision for students is also required. The relationship between the supervisor and student is most important with respect to assessment and feedback (Kilminster & Jolly, 2000), and this will also be important regarding discussion of emotional matters. Given that this is not a commonly acknowledged aspect of clinical supervision in medicine, care is required. Because students respond to the hidden curriculum or messages, they could be made more vulnerable if asked to behave differently to their seniors. Given that medicine is an exercise in human relationships (Snadden, 2006), supporting students through their experiences would seem a humane approach to benefit student learning and socialization.

REFERENCES

Arnold, L. (2002). Assessing professional behaviour yesterday, today, and tomorrow. *Academic Medicine*, 77(6), 502–525.

Baldwin, D. C., Daugherty, S. R., & Rowley, B. D. (1998). Residents' and medical students' reports of sexual harassment and discrimination. *Academic Medicine*, 71(10), 25–27.

Becker, H., Geer, B., Hughes, E. C., & Strauss, A. (1961). *Boys in white: Student culture in medical school.* London, UK: Transaction Publishers.

Bligh, J. (2002). The first year of doctoring: Still a survival exercise. *Medical Education, 36,* 2–3.

Borkan, J. (1999). Immersion/crystallization. In: B. F. Crabtree & W.L. Miller (Eds.), *Doing qualitative research* (pp. 179–194). Thousand Oaks, CA: Sage.

Cant, R., & Higgs, J. (1999). Professional socialization. In J. Higgs & H. Edwards (Eds.), *Educating beginning practitioners: Challenges for health professional education* (pp. 46–51). Auckland, New Zealand: Butterworth Heinemann.

Conrad, P. (1988). Learning to doctor: Reflections on recent accounts of the medical school years. *Journal of Health & Social Behaviour, 29*(4), 323–332.

Crotty, M. (2003). *The foundations of social research. Meaning and perspective in the research process.* London, UK: Sage.

Dyrbye, L. N., Thomas, M. R., & Shanafelt, T. D. (2005). Medical student distress: Causes, consequences, and proposed solutions. *Mayo Clinic Proceedings, 80*(12), 1613–1622.

Dyrbye, L. N., Thomas, M. R., & Shanafelt, T. D. (2006). Systematic review of depression, anxiety and other indicators of psychological distress among U.S. and Canadian medical students. *Academic Medicine, 81*(4), 354–373.

Eraut, M. (1994). *Developing professional knowledge and competence.* London, UK: The Falmer Press.

Eraut, M. (2004). Informal learning in the workplace. *Studies Continuing Education, 26*(2), 247–273.

Firth, J. (1986). Levels and sources of stress in medical students. *British Medical Journal, 292,* 1177–1180.

Fox, R. (1989). *The sociology of medicine: A participant observer's view.* Upper Saddle River, NJ: Prentice-Hall.

Gordon, J., Hazlett, C., ten Cate, O., Mann, K., Kilminster, S., & Prince, K., et al. (2000). Strategic planning in medical education: Enhancing the learning environment for students in clinical settings. *Medical Education, 34,* 841–850.

Hafferty, F. W. (1991). *Into the valley: Death and the socialization of medical students.* London, UK: Yale University Press.

Hafferty, F. (1998). Beyond curriculum reform: Confronting medicine's hidden curriculum. *Academic Medicine, 73*(4), 403–407.

Hayes, K., Feather, A., Hall, A., Sedgwick, P., Wannan, G., Wessier-Smith, A., et al. (2004). Anxiety in medical students: Is preparation for full-time clinical attachments more dependent in maturity or on educational programmes for undergraduate and graduate entry students? *Medical Education, 38,* 1154–1163.

Howe, K. R. (2008). The third dogma of educational research. In N. K. Denzin & M. D. Giardina (Eds.), *Qualitative inquiry and the politics of evidence* (pp. 97–119). Walnut Creek, CA: Left Coast Press.

Howe, A., Campion, P., Searle, J., & Smith, H. (2004). New perspectives: Approaches to medical education at four new UK medical schools. *British Medical Journal, 329,* 327–332.

Kilminster, S. M., & Jolly, B. C. (2000). Effective supervision in clinical practice settings: A literature review. *Medical Education, 34,* 827–840.

Lamdin, R. (2010). *The professional socialisation of medical students through the preclinical to clinical transition.* Koln, Germany: Lambert Academic.

Lave, J. (1996). Teaching, as learning, in practice. *Mind, Culture and Activity, 3*(3), 149–164.

Lave J., & Wenger, E. (1991). *Situated learning: Legitimate peripheral learning.* Cambridge, UK: Cambridge University Press.

Levinson, D. J. (1967). Medical education and the theory of adult socialization. *Journal of Health and Social Behaviour, 8*(4), 253–265.

Lempp, H., & Searle, C. (2004). The hidden curriculum in undergraduate medical education: A qualitative study of medical students' perceptions of teaching. *British Medical Journal, 329,* 770–773.

Lincoln, Y. S., & Guba, E. G. (1985). *Naturalistic inquiry.* Newbury Park, CA: Sage.

Linn, B. S., & Zeppa, R. (1984). Stress in junior medical students: Relationship to personality and performance. *Journal of Medical Education, 59*(1), 7–12.

Merton, R. K., Reader, G., & Kendall, P.L. (1957). *The student-physician: Introductory studies in the sociology of medical education.* Boston, MA: Harvard University Press.

Mitchell, J. T., & Everly, G. S. (2000). Critical incident stress management and critical stress incident stress debriefings: Evolutions, effects and outcomes. In B. Raphael & J. P. Wilson (Eds.), *Psychological debriefing: Theory, practice and evidence.* (pp. 71–90). New York, NY: Cambridge University Press.

Mosley, T. H., Jr., Perrin, S. G., Neral, S. M., Dubbert, P. M., Grothues, C. A., & Pinto, B. M. (1994). Stress coping and well-being among third-year medical students. *Academic Medicine, 69,* 765–767.

Moss, F., & McManus, I. (1992). The anxieties of new clinical students. *Medical Education, 26,* 17–20.

Pitkala, K., & Mantyranta, T. (2003). Professional socialization revised: Medical students' own conceptions related to adoption of the future physician's role—a qualitative study. *Medical Teacher, 25*(2), 155–160.

Prince, K. J. A. H., Boshuizen, H. P. A., Van der Vleuten, C. P. M., & Scherpbier, A. J. J. A. (2005). Students' opinions about their preparation for clinical practice. *Medical Education. 39,* 704–712.

Prince, K. J. A. H., Van de Wiel, M. W. J., Van der Vleuten, C., Boshuizen, H. P. A., & Scherpbier, A. J. J. A. (2004). Junior doctors' opinions about the transition from medical school to clinical practice: A change of environment. *Education in Health, 17*(3), 323–331.

Radcliffe, C., & Lester, H. (2003). Perceived stress during undergraduate medical training a qualitative study. *Medical Education, 37,* 32–38.

Reber, A. S. (1993). *Implicit learning and tacit knowledge: An essay on the cognitive unconsciousness.* Oxford, UK: Oxford University Press.

Rees, C. E., Knight, L. V., & Wilkinson C. E. (2007). "User involvement is a sine qua non, almost in medical education": Learning with rather than just about health and social service users. *Advances in Health Sciences Education, 12,* 359–390.

Rhodes-Kropf, J., Carmody, S. S., Seltzer, D., Redinbaugh, E., Gadmer, N., Block, S. D., & Arnold, R.M. (2005). "This is just too awful; I can't believe I experienced that…" Memorable students' reaction to their most memorable patient death. *Academic Medicine, 80* (7), 634–640.

Rosenfield, P., & Jones, L. (2004). Striking a balance: Training medical students to provide empathic care. *Medical Education, 38,* 297–933.

Sheehan, H. K., Sheehan, D. V., White, K., Leibowitz, A., & Baldwin, D. C. (1990). A pilot study of medical student abuse: Student perceptions of mistreatment and misconduct in medical school. *Journal of the American Medical Association, 263*(4), 533–537.

Sinclair, S. (1997). *Making doctors: An institutional apprenticeship.* Oxford, UK: Berg.

Smith, A. C., & Kleinman, S. (1989). Managing emotions in medical school: Students' contacts with the living and the dead. *Social Psychology Quarterly, 52*(1), 56–69.

Snadden, D. (2006). Clinical education: Context is everything. *Medical Education, 40,* 97–98.

Spencer, J. (2003). Teaching about professionalism. *Medical Education, 37*(4): 288–289.

Stephenson, A., Higgs, R., & Sugarman, J. (2001). Teaching professional development in medical schools. *Lancet, 357*(9259), 867–871.

Stern, D. (1998). In search of the informal curriculum: When and where professional values are taught. *Academic Medicine, 73*(10), S28–S30.

Swanwick, T. (2005). Informal learning in postgraduate medical education from cognitivism to "culturism." *Medical Education, 39,* 859–865.

Turner, T. H., Collinson, S. R., & Fry, H. S. (2001). Doctor in the house: The medical student as academic, attendant and apprentice? *Medical Teacher, 23*(5), 514–516.

Wear, D., Aultman, J. M., Varley, J. D., & Zarconi, J. (2006). Making fun of patients: Medical students' perceptions and use of derogatory humour in clinical settings. *Academic Medicine, 81*(5), 454–462.

Werner, E. R., & Korsch, B. M. (1976). The vulnerability of the medical student: Posthumous presentation of L. L. Stephens' ideas. *Paediatrics, 57* (3), 321–328.

Wilhelm, K. A. (2002). The student and junior doctor in stress. *Medical Journal of Australia, 177,* S5–S8.

Wolf, T. M. (1994). Stress, coping and health: Enhancing well-being during medical school. *Medical Education, 28*(1), 8–17.

3

BETWEEN TWO WORLDS

Medical Students Narrating Identity Tensions

LYNN V. MONROUXE AND KIERAN SWEENEY

INTRODUCTION

> ...one thing that strikes me like, pretty much once a week is just how much medicine just incorporates so many aspects of your life...and it's just, it's almost like what you're learning socially has almost as much effect on your medical career...it just incorporates so much of yourself and your life...I live with people who do physics and economics and really it's like their academic life is their academic life and their social life is their own but when you're meeting people, and making friends with people who've had a very hard situation or grieving or that kind of thing, and then you're thinking like "right as a doctor this is what I have to deal with" and it's bizarre at times. Kinda wish there could be more of a division but I guess it's a strength in a way.

In this audio diary, Sian reflects on how becoming a doctor "incorporates so much of yourself." Indeed, medical school is not just a site of learning *what*—facts and skills—it is also a site of learning *how*—how to be a doctor. However, people arrive at medical school from a wide range of social, racial, educational, and cultural backgrounds and with a unique set of embodied and primary identities including social and personal identities (Takakuwa, Rubashkin, & Herzig, 2004). Over time, through both taught and "hidden" curricula, students learn attitudes, values, and behaviors expected of them as a physician. As they go through this socialization process, "medical education attempts to 'colonize' the student" (Shapiro, 2009, p. 7), slowly moving them toward fairly homogeneous cultural norms, to their new identities as physicians.

During medical school, students inevitably experience a range of stressful situations. Some are obvious: conducting procedures for the first time, presenting patients to senior colleagues, learning by ritual humiliation, witnessing senior colleagues acting insensitively. Other stressful situations are less obvious. These aspects are often "unheard" by faculty, sometimes even "silenced." Such situations can be classified as a struggle between identities. Perhaps they did not want to be a physician and are at medical school due to external pressures; perhaps they feel that their sexuality has to be hidden for fear of discrimination; or perhaps they encounter personal illness or death and their new status as a future physician causes them difficulties. It is these latter aspects that we focus on-students' narratives of personal encounters with illness and dying.[1] The data we draw on come from our longitudinal solicited audio diary study following 17 students' journeys through a medical school in the United Kingdom. This data collection method provides a unique and intricate insight into how individuals' existing and newly developing identities are negotiated in the face of illness and dying, and how these identities influence each other reciprocally. We begin with a brief overview of identity construction, and the concept of a *narrative identity*, outlining the different ways this has been considered in narrative enquiry. Within this outline we introduce the solicited audio diary as a method for collecting personal incident narratives over time.

IDENTITY CONSTRUCTION

Identity is not something we possess; it is not fixed or static, nor is it singular. Identity construction is a two-way internal-external ongoing process of *becoming*. Through the cognitive and social process of identification with individuals and groups, we make sense of who we are and who we might become in the world (Jenkins, 2008). So through interactions with others in the environment of social institutions (with established ways of doing things), we create complex multidimensional understandings of who we are as individuals and members of groups (Miller, Brewer, & Arbuckle, 2009; Roccas & Brewer, 2002). Sometimes we synergize our identities; sometimes some identities become salient due to contextual demands (Roccas & Brewer, 2002). And some identities are stable, whereas others are malleable (Jenkins, 2008).

---

[1] Although our focus is on encounters with illness and dying, the participants in our study have narrated all of these "identity struggles."

The process of identity construction begins early as we develop primary identities that are prescripted and bestowed on us by others, such as gender (e.g., through the clothes we are given to wear). These identities, culturally circumscribed and conditioned, are embodied through "stylized repetition of acts through time" (Butler, 1988, p. 520). Although gendered identities are not permanent or unchanging, rejection or modification is low. Later identities, such as becoming a physician, are developed through strong internal responses and are more open to negotiation (see Monrouxe, 2010). However, this process of negotiation can cause anxiety and stress.

NARRATIVE IDENTITY

Storytelling is an everyday sense-making activity through which we negotiate and assert our identities. From biographical "big stories" to conversational "small stories," we make meaning of our lives as we recall events, edit and structure those events, and evaluate them (Bamberg, 2006; Georgakopoulou, 2007). Our narratives are produced retrospectively, sometimes drawn from historical and cultural narratives (Monrouxe, 2009a; Schiffrin, 1996), and prospectively for a particular audience: I will tell my story differently to a colleague at work than to a friend over coffee. So the process of becoming incorporates a performative process (e.g., Riessman, 2003). Whether we are conscious of this performance, it is ever present in the pace and the tone of our words, particular ways in which we phrase events (sometimes through the voices or stances of others), in the ways we position ourselves to significant protagonists, and through the metaphors we use.

The notion that narratives play a part in constituting identity is no more apparent than in research investigating people's reactions to chronic illness. In a classic account of narratives of chronic illness experiences, Frank (1995) identifies illness as an interruption to the way things should have been. Frank uses the metaphor of illness as *wrecking* one's life story: the present is not what the past had promised, the future is uncertain. Thus illness is seen as a "call for stories" where "stories have to *repair* the damage that illness has done to the ill person's sense of where she is in life, and where she may be going" (p. 53), restoring a sense of coherence. So, people tell illness stories to reclaim their identities as people (rather than as patients), resisting the colonization of their bodies as the territory of medicine ("clinical material": Frank, 1995, p. 12).

Likewise, we see negative experiences at medical school as a form of *narrative wreckage* for students, also bringing forth a call for stories. Previously held notions of what it is to be a physician (the future they hoped for), along with accompanying values and behaviors, can be shattered in the face of such experiences (Monrouxe, 2009a). Additionally, students' narratives of these experiences are a way to make sense of events that conflict with personal ideology (and so restore a sense of coherence) and a way to resist the "flattening out" and colonization of students themselves, bringing to the fore their own individuality, their own personhood, and their own suffering (Shapiro, 2009; Takakuwa et al., 2004).

The majority of research within narrative enquiry is concerned with the "big" autobiographical narratives of individuals' lives elicited in interviews (such as those elicited by Frank, 1995). Here, researchers encourage the participants to reflect on (often difficult periods of) their lives. Through these life narratives, individuals make sense of themselves, participating in the "doing" of identity. Although the extent to which such narratives reveal the internal states of the person or are shaped by external social events (e.g., the audience) is contested, many researchers consider both aspects through their analyses (Riessman, 2008).

Other researchers consider how people bring off "identity claims in their narrating activities" (Bamberg, 2006, p. 144). These so-called small stories are present in everyday interaction and not direct reflections about who people are. Rather, in and through talk, people establish the content of their story (what happened) along with establishing the social relationships within which their story occurs: "the here and now of the interactive situation" (Bamberg, 2006, p. 144). So, as people relate events to others, they adopt a position that is taken by the interlocutor as a sense of who the speaker is, and ultimately the speaker (with time and practice) adopts this position as a sense of self. Small stories also differ from autobiographical narratives as they often concern recent events. Georgakopoulou (2006) describes these dynamic ongoing narratives as "immediately reworked slices of life that arose out of a need to share with friends what had just happened 'breaking news'" (p. 126). Other small stories include re-tellings, refusals to tell, and deferrals of telling. Research considering identities in this way adopts more ethnographic approaches (e.g., Ochs & Capps, 2001).

APPROACHES TO NARRATIVES AND THE SOLICITED AUDIO DIARY METHOD

Diaries have also been considered as sites of narrative work (Alaszewski, 2006). Participant-recorded diaries provide richly contextualized "documents of lives" to explore unfolding identities (Plummer, 2001). Although most work considers written diaries, we are developing the longitudinal solicited audio diary to investigate the construction of professional identities over time (Monrouxe, 2009a, 2009b; Monrouxe & Sweeney, 2010).

Interestingly, although the solicited audio diary is not a site of talk-in-interaction—participants record their diaries alone—many narratives in our data can be seen as sites of identity work with a performative quality similar to that of small stories (Monrouxe,

2009b). In particular, breaking news is a key feature as diary entries refer to recent, ongoing events in participants' lives. Other features include the narration of hypothetical, future or shared events, re-tellings, and allusions to telling (Georgakopoulou, 2007; Monrouxe, 2009b). Audio diary narratives also contain features reminiscent of autobiographical narratives elicited within interview settings. Although they are recorded without the constraints of direct questioning and observable reactions from the researcher, the researcher is frequently present within participants' narratives as they are recorded in the context of a research project: so, *for* someone else, rather than for themselves (Monrouxe, 2009b). Over time, a relationship between the researcher and participants develops: Participants refer to previous narratives recorded, and a sense of building up shared knowledge between them emerges (Monrouxe, 2009b). However, unlike other forms of narration, due to the physical absence of another, the narrator sometimes forgets the researcher and drifts into a conversation with himself or herself as he or she tries to make sense of events (Monrouxe, 2009b). This unique aspect of the audio diary method suggests that during these moments of self-exploration, of pondering, new *in-the-moment* understandings are being formed by the narrator (Monrouxe, 2009b).

Taken together, the complex dynamics within the narratives recorded during the context of the solicited audio diary call for a multitude of approaches to the understanding of professional identity construction by paying attention to *what* is narrated, *how* narratives are told, and *to whom* and *for what purposes* they are told (Riessman, 2008). So, a number of pertinent questions arise, and in this chapter we focus on the following: What and how do students narrate identity tensions?

INVESTIGATING THE CONSTRUCTIONS OF MEDICAL STUDENTS' PROFESSIONAL IDENTITIES

The setting for this research is a new medical school in England with a 5-year undergraduate curriculum. Early in their first year, students experience clinical placements, which becoming more frequent over time. In year 2, they attend periodic day visits to a general practice surgery. Years 3 to 5 comprise clinically based placements across hospital and community sites. Across the 5 years, students' professional development is fostered via small-group meetings facilitated by clinicians, where students discuss their clinical experiences.

Our study began with the aim of understanding how individuals entering medical education constructed their identities as medical students of today and physicians of tomorrow through the spontaneous stories they conveyed over time. Using the solicited audio diary as our primary means of data collection, we followed the lives of 17 students.

We asked them to record weekly Dictaphone messages, giving them a simple request: "Please tell us a story about something that has happened to you since the last time you left a message and how it has affected the way you think about yourself now and your future role as a doctor."

A "diary entry" was defined as "a recording or group of recordings by any one individual participant in a single day." By the end of 3 years, 353 diary entries were submitted (around 65 hours of recordings). These recordings varied in length, from 10 seconds to 27 minutes 24 seconds (mean 5 minutes 40 seconds). An additional 46 diary entries were submitted in the following eight months from 10 participants continuing with the study.

ANALYTICAL TOOLS

We use a number of interpretive tools for our analysis, including insights from cognitive linguistics, psycholinguistics, and sociolinguistics. The main concepts we draw on come from two perspectives within narrative analysis. The first is inspired by Labov and Waletzky (1967; Labov, 1997), who provide a formal framework for understanding narrative. For the purpose of our analysis, we adopt the definition of a *narrative of personal experience* from Labov (1997, p. 398) as "a report of a sequence of events that have entered into the biography of the speaker by a sequence of clauses that correspond to the order of the original event." Thus, these events will necessarily be evaluated in terms of what they mean to the speaker. This has obvious consequences on how events are reported within the narrative. We also adopt Labov's (1997) definitions of the structural types of clauses within narratives: *abstract*—"an initial clause in a narrative that reports the entire sequence of events of the narrative," *orientation*—"information on the time, place of the events, the identities of the participants and their initial behaviour," *complicating action* "reports a next event in response to a potential question, 'and what happened [then]?'," *coda*—"returns the narrative to the time of speaking," and *evaluation* of the narrative event providing "information on the consequences of the event for human needs and desires" (pp. 402–403). Labov also defined *the most reportable event* which he believed to be central to narrative organizational structure—"the event that is less common than any other in the narrative and has the greatest effect upon the needs and desires of the participants in the narrative [and is evaluated most strongly]" and the *resolution*—"the set of complicating actions that follow the most reportable event" (p. 406).

The second perspective comes from positioning analysis (Bamberg, 2003; Wortham & Gadsten, 2006), which considers how identities are emergent in the small stories of everyday talk-in-interaction through how we position each other in talk. Positioning analysis posits a number of questions, attempting to take the analyst's focus from understanding the specific narrative toward understanding the meaning of that narrative in society. The different levels of positioning analysis address the broad questions—What is the story about? What claims to identity are made? How is this rooted in discourse? So, at one level we consider how characters are established in the narrative and how they are positioned to one another. We then focus on what the narrator is trying to accomplish in their narrative through the strategies they use (e.g., direct reported talk, metaphor, adopted viewpoints). Finally, drawing these together we consider the question, "Who am I vis-a-vis what society says I should be" (Watson, 2007, p. 347).

NARRATING TENSIONS

In previous publications, we have explored the method of data collection and our analysis of narrative storylines in depth (Monrouxe, 2009a, 2009b). In this chapter, we focus on students' struggles between identities that cuts across content themes and narrative storylines as identity struggles appear *in the narration* of a range of events participants reported. During the reporting of events, participants sometimes struggled with making sense of events that called for them to negotiate aspects of their personal identities with their newly developing professional identities. Although participants had difficulties negotiating religious and sexual identities, many identity struggles came to the fore as students narrated personal and professional issues around illness and dying. We focus on three cornerstone narratives here as they emphasize interrelated issues as students grapple with illness and dying, representing different, but common, perspectives. These perspectives reflect the relationship between the narrator and the main protagonist, and so have been classified as *looking onto, living alongside,* and *living with* illness, dying, and death. These cornerstone narratives exemplify stressful events that were commonplace and demonstrate clearly how events impact on medical students' personal and professional identities and how these identities are negotiated during the process of becoming a physician.

Looking onto: Rory's narrative

Rory was a 22-year-old fourth-year student at this time. It was March 8, 2009, when he recorded three messages. He begins by apologizing for his "nasty doom and gloom" messages but stressed that these were the things that "stick in the mind" and were still unresolved. The common focus was illness and dying and the impact that these were having on his future as a physician—indeed, he is now beginning to question his desire to become a physician. We focus on his second message: the first time he witnessed someone dying.[2] Although his narrative concludes with his own concerns about illness, dying, and death (his ultimate evaluation of the event), he begins from the perspective of a medical student *looking onto* these aspects with a patient. As he narrates this powerful event, Rory struggles with his feelings of being overwhelmed as his sense of *self* is changing through his encounters with patients and their lives. Rory begins by describing his first meeting with the patient the day before he died. Using repetition, he emphasizes the time he spent with the patient, his own feelings of knowing the patient, and the patient's relative "wellness." In doing so, he establishes a sense of a developing relationship as he positions himself as an interested and eager medical student talking to a "gentleman" who was dealing with lung cancer. He then quickly moved to the events of the next day:

	COMPLICATING ACTION
1	and the next day during the ward round (.) when we started the
2	ward round somebody mentioned that he was quite ill (.) so he was
3	one of the first patients we actually went and saw and he had
4	*massively* deteriorated overnight
	EVALUATION
5	and it (.) he didn't even *really* seem like the same person there- he was
6	barely moving- struggling and *everything* else that goes along with it
7	(.) not able to eat- able to (.) *barely* move even though his family were
8	there- there was just (.) nobody really- he- nobody could *get* to him
9	and he was *very* (.) isolated >and I think< (2.0) >I can't remember
10	who once said it< but somebody said that we all- we're all born alone
11	and we all die alone (1.0) but it was very (2.0) he *wasn't* the same
12	person that we'd seen the day before and he was quite detached (.)
	MOST REPORTABLE EVENT
13	and erm by the end of the ward round he'd actually passed away (1.0)
14	with us standing (.) more or less around the edge of his bed (1.0)
	EVALUATION
15	and (.) that was (.) quite hard- I mean (2.0)...

So Rory announces that the patient had "massively deteriorated over night" (line 4), and the person he felt that he knew was no longer present (lines 5, 11–12). He then expresses bewilderment and fear that the patient, although surrounded by physicians and family, is alone. In doing so he uses the powerful metaphor of MIND AS A CONTAINER—likening

---

[2] We present brief excerpts, because the narratives are lengthy. We include transcription notes to provide an insight into narration: (.) = micro pause; (1.0) = pause; dash at end of word- = running-on-speech; >at beginning and end< = fast talk; larger and italicised font = emphasis; ((brackets)) = additional comments;...(ellipses) = edited section.

the patient to a physical system that does not interact with its surroundings, where nothing can enter or exit, and is trapped inside its isolating containment (lines 8–9). Drawing on Orson Welles' quote of being born alone and dying alone (lines 10–11), Rory highlights his sense of being unable to help this "isolated" and "alone" patient. This shift in personhood from the "gentleman" dealing with lung cancer, to the person who is "not there" dynamically shifts the positioning between Rory and the patient. Rory is no longer an eager medical student learning about how a patient is living with a disease; he is now a bewildered young man forced to come to terms with a dying patient. The way Rory tells his most reportable event, his witnessing of the death of the patient, is interesting. He avoids directly referring to death, preferring to use the euphemism "passed away." Indeed, although euphemisms are thought to representationally displace topics that evoke negative affect, we can also see how this euphemism resonates with Rory's conceptualization of death as a transition:

EVALUATION

16	I've done a fair few post mortems- I've been along and watched them
17	and (.) discussed all about them and I've seen a fair amount of
18	vivisection there as well (.) and (.) I know what dead bodies look like
19	and they- I don't get the creeped-out thing that- a lot of people get
20	first time- I think I got it to a *smaller* extent but (1.0) I don't have a
21	problem with *bodies* (.) and I don't have a problem with really sick
22	*people* (.) but (.) *that* transition in the middle (.) that was quite hard to
23	then (.) to see this (.) >I don't think I'd ever< *seen* a death before
24	(1.0) an- I'd seen (.) *bodies* and I'd (.) >ev- everything else that goes
25	along with it< I'd never been there at that *moment* (1.0) and (1.0) that
26	*transition* from *person* to *nothing* is quite (.) scary I think- >not very
27	nice< anyway (.)

CODA

28	sorry I've picked two really *big* sort of (.) *moments*- but they are
29	quite (.) *defining* moments

EVALUATION

30	I think 'cause they were both moments when I sort of thought "shhh-"
31	(.) you know (.) "*can* I do this?" (3.0) *but* (3.0) but yeah (3.0) so (.)
32	seeing (.) him (1.0) a-as that *body*- that empty shell was quite…
33	just (.) I didn't *know* what (.) h-h-how I was supposed to *think* or
34	*whether* I was supposed to think or what- what this was supposed to
35	*mean* for me or for *anybody* really- it wasn't (.) I mean I'd only
36	spoken to this person for an hour and a half and even though later
37	some of my (.) peers have said "you know well (.) that hour and a
38	half- may- may have made the difference between his last couple of
39	hours and you know he had somebody to talk to in hospital and you
40	were an ear" and all these things realistically to me it doesn't seem

41   like I had much input to this person's life (.) and yet they had a
42   *massive* impact on mine (.) so (.) it's very hard these (1.0) *people* (.)
43   there's a tendency to think that (.) when you see a doctor you're only
44   seeing them for a few minutes and th- for them it's a day job and you
45   move on- you walk away from it and (.) patients don't affect doctors
46   (3.0) but (.) whereas doctors of course who only spend maybe a few
47   minutes with a patient have a *great* effect on their life- but it's just not
48   true (2.0) because even if you only have a few *moments* with a patient
49   (1.0) their story (.) still feels in some way linked to *you* and *part* of
50   *your story* (2.0) so tha- that's quite (3.0) I mean is- if part of a doctor
51   is going to mean taking on- *being* a doctor means taking on all these
52   different stories *into* me and >*be hanging*< ((laughingly)) around as
53   part of me- that was a big question if I could actually do that (.)

So at the beginning of this excerpt Rory refers to the moment of death being a "transition from person to nothing" (line 26), which he sees as being "scary." Through this expression, and his earlier euphemism of "passing away," Rory draws on the metaphor of LIFE AS A JOURNEY—as he describes how this person has come to the end. Furthermore, Rory's evaluation of his witnessing this man's death focuses on the very aspect that he struggles with the most. So Rory positions himself as someone experienced in the clinical aspects of death: dead bodies, post mortems, and vivisection (lines 16–25), all of which are physical aspects of life and death, safely within the domain of clinical practice in which physicians (and medical students) can intellectualize, pathologize, and act on. However, it is the metaphysical aspect of life and death—dying—that Rory now struggles with. Rory's tone of voice changes. He becomes more pensive: Using frequent pauses, he struggles to find meaning (lines 22–27). His earlier confidence in his own identity as a fearless student undaunted by the sight of dead bodies is challenged as he contemplates the moment of death. Rory briefly steps out of his evaluation of the patient's death, bringing himself and the listener back to the here and now (coda), apologizing again for his distressing stories, and stressing that they are "defining moments" for him (line 29). This unusual shift in frame (the coda typically comes at the end) suggests a need for him to bring his narrative back to the present as he is unable to move forward in his understanding of the past.

Rory then highlights two distinct consequences of these defining moments. The first is expressed through his powerful use of his own directly reported thought "*can* I do this?" preceded by a long sigh, followed by three relatively lengthy pauses, indicating deep reflection (lines 31–32). The second consequence Rory highlights is that seeing someone he felt he knew as an "empty shell" (line 32) caused him to consider his own death (an aspect of his personal identity that he later narrates in depth). Indeed, Rory confesses to feeling lost and confused, searching for a meaning in the events he just witnessed (lines 33–35). He then proceeds to downplay his relationship with the patient, a relationship he had emphasized earlier in his narrative. In addition, it seems that the downplaying of this relationship is due to his frustration that he felt he had done nothing for the patient, yet the patient has had a "massive impact" on his life (line 42).

A common discourse among medical students is that they have chosen medicine to make a difference. Rory clearly feels that he has failed in this aspect: Indeed, it was the patient who had made a difference to *him*. He elaborates on this discourse of making a difference, this time focusing on the physician–patient relationship and challenging the notion that physicians have a great impact on patients' lives but patients do not affect physicians (lines 43–50). As he does so, Rory uses the third person pronoun *you* in a number of ways: to begin with, he uses it impersonally (*you* meaning anyone and everyone): "when *you* see a physician *you're* only seeing *them* for a few minutes" to distance himself from the action of the person seeing a physician (Kamio, 2001), and his use of the pronoun *them* also distances himself from the role of the physician. But Rory tentatively begins to (re)position himself in the role of physician as he continues using the pronoun *them* (referring to physicians) but shifts to using the pronoun *you* (as a physician): "and th- for *them* it's a day job and *you* move on- *you* walk away from it." So this second use of *you* positions Rory in the role of the physician and communicates that the assertion made is a generally admitted truth (Kitigawa & Lehrer, 1990)—that physicians can walk away from patients. Furthermore, as he positions himself in this role, Rory refutes this general *truth* and asserts, "because even if *you* only have a few moments with a patient, their story still feels in some way linked to *you* and part of *your* story." In this excerpt, Rory utters three pronouns—*you, you,* and *your*—meaning *I, me,* and *my,* respectively. This pronoun *use* communicates his own personal *truth* that he wishes the listener to share: this patient had affected him deeply, and so patients affect physicians deeply too. Furthermore, Rory narrates this in an impassioned manner, developing the powerful metaphorical concept of BODY AS A CONTAINER OF THE SELF (Lakoff & Johnson, 1980) by suggesting that his experiences with patients is becoming part of his *self* and that he is embodying the patients' stories. Indeed, the prosodic aspects of his narrative at this point further emphasizes Rory's identity struggle as he emphasizes words, using lengthy pauses and laughter-talk to cope with his recounting of the possibility that this might prevent him from becoming a physician (noncontextual coping, cf. Hay, 2000).

Having evaluated the consequence that witnessing the patient's death has on his developing identity as a physician, Rory begins to consider the consequences it has on himself as a person (not reproduced here for expediency). In doing so, he uses the metaphors DEATH AS AN ENEMY and DEATH AS FAILURE, reflecting Rory's personal and professional identities, which appear to be intertwined. So, death is where medicine fails and death is not only the enemy of medicine, it is also Rory's enemy: "stalking around the corner." At the end of his narrative, Rory shifts from narrating a past event (witnessing a patient's death) to narrating a future event (his own death). Moreover, he positions his own death within his future identity as a physician—a physician who possesses the same vulnerable body as his patient: "figures for cancer and other diseases like that mean that in essence you are going to be infected by some- as a physician you will be affected by something you've treated at some point in your life and that's- that's quite a scary thing to think about." Ultimately, Rory narrates his being filled with patients' stories, those stories linking to his story with their deaths linking to his death. The notion of his witnessing a patient dying, moving from being *infected* to *affected* emphasizing his vulnerability and the "scary thing" of witnessing as an act.

There is something acutely painful and raw about Rory's story. The death of a patient is not necessarily a remarkable event in routine clinical practice (Redinbaugh et al., 2003). But as Rory reminds us, this type of experience causes us to reflect on the frailty of our own humanity. Furthermore, responses like Rory's are not confined to the ranks of the medical student. All physicians will be faced with patients dying, and in primary care these might be patients whom the physician has cared for over several decades (Curtis & McGee, 2000; Ryynanen, 2001). Rory's narrative about the profoundness of witnessing the moment of death is not the only narrative in our data to touch on this subject (see Monrouxe, 2009b). The briefness of students' encounters with patients and their inability to help against the culturally defined backdrop of "wanting to make a difference," to be a "healing doctor," also resonate with other research with medical students (Lamdin, 2010) and ambulance workers (Halpern, Gurevich, Schwartz, & Brazeau, 2009a, 2009b). Furthermore, it is often "the quiet motionless moments that trigger intense distress in ambulance workers" (Halpern et al., 2009b, p. 185), such as the times when action is futile. Further, working within an organizational culture that stigmatizes vulnerability causes additional stress. We see an example of this when we consider Tre's narrative later.

The narrative tension between Rory's personal identity and his developing professional identity comes from an initial perspective of looking *onto* illness, dying, and death. Rory knew the patient by virtue of him being ill and in hospital. Although the patient had a big effect on him, their relationship was purely professional. We now consider Paul's narrative in which he is a good friend with the person who is ill. By virtue of this friendship, we can conceptualize Paul's narrative from the initial perspective of *living alongside* illness.

Living alongside: Paul's narrative

Paul was a 24-year-old fourth-year student when he recorded two narratives one day: both dilemmas concerned friends (for expediency, we only report a brief analysis). In the first dilemma, "Friend A" calls to tell a "funny story" of how he received a needlestick injury while working on a community project. He had not acted on it and had swallowed his blood from the wound. In the second dilemma, "Friend B" e-mailed to say he had been diagnosed with testicular cancer.

When we consider how Paul establishes the characters across his two narratives, there is a stark difference. In the first, Paul constructs his relationship with Friend A with himself as medical expert and his friend as lay member of the public. Paul listens to his friend's jovial story about a needlestick injury. Knowing the dangers involved, he panics, and then panics his friend by explaining the dangers and urging him to go to the emergency department. In his second narrative, Paul does not know the facts about teratomas and testicular cancer. He tells us how Friend B described the situation in detail in his e-mail. However, while Paul conveys to us his initial panic on receiving this news, he admits to not knowing the evidence regarding the treatment of testicular cancer and so positions himself in a supportive (rather than quasi expert) role.

As he evaluates events in his second narrative, Paul uses hypothetical talk, drawing on his medical student identity and to what would have been the case if this was a patient, rather than his friend. In that situation he would take an "active interest" in finding out about the disease, treatment, and prognosis, storing things up in his "memory bank" for his later work as a physician. He emphasizes that he has the means to easily do this right now, in his room, right now. But rather than being actively interested, he is "actively avoiding" the information for fear of discovering a "bleak" outcome. He admits this is partly for himself and partly for his friend, because if the outcome looks bleak, it may inadvertently be conveyed to his friend through his voice. However, in denying himself this knowledge, he is effectively denying his identity as a medical student. Moreover, his active use of texts and e-mails, rather than telephone calls, through which he communicates with his friend suggests that even this state of "not knowing" is troublesome for Paul, possibly fearing that he might be asked for the very information he is avoiding in his role as a *medical student*–friend. As he concludes, we see that this is something that Paul is struggling to reconcile. Through his continual use of rhetorical questions about the benefit of gaining this knowledge, Paul narrates a preference to dwell in ignorance rather than move toward his knowledgeable medical self.

It is important to note that the essence of Paul's narrative of *living alongside* illness, and of what this means to himself, is not the only narrative in our data to touch on this.

For example, during the study, Katie's mother died. She recorded a message telling us that her mother was undergoing an autopsy. Katie was aware of her inner conflict: "Between the idea that as a *doctor* I need to understand, but as a member of the *family* it's all very well to know this stuff in the abstract but to actually think of it as happening to someone who, such a large and important part of your life is- um, I'm not sure that I really wanted to know that much about it."

We have considered narratives where tensions between personal and professional identities have caused students to reappraise who they are, who they will be, and how they negotiate the self in the here and now. Although ultimately they highlight the impact of events on the narrators, they can be seen from the initial perspectives of *looking onto* and *living alongside* illness and dying. We finally turn to a narrative of tensions between identities that comes from the powerful perspective of *living with* illness.

Living with illness: Tre's Narrative

Tre is a 23-year-old fourth-year student at the time of recording. His involvement with the study had been sporadic: months have passed between Tre's diary messages, and he recorded this as a direct result of the researchers contacting him and asking for an update. Tre sent a single message (11 minutes 43 seconds) about his current situation. He has had a difficult year so far; his father had died, and as a result he feels that he is suffering from depression.[3] Furthermore, his identity as a medical student (and physician-to-be) appears to constrain his ability to seek help for this. To provide a deeper insight into the ways in which the audio diary method shapes reflection in these narratives, we bring this aspect to the foreground, as well as commenting on the narrative itself.

Tre begins by addressing the researcher directly and apologizing for not being in touch—a common form of opening for audio diary messages (Monrouxe, 2009b). Following this, he offers an abstract of his narrative: he is going to tell us about ongoing stressful events. Embedded with his initial orientation are some of the difficulties and benefits of the audio diary itself. The difficulties of not knowing "where to begin" or "finding the time" were highlighted. However, he also highlighted a benefit: "I was just lying in bed and I thought 'I'm- instead of having this inner dialogue running through my head, and you know

---

[3] On receipt of this narrative, the first author immediately contacted the participant via e-mail to express her concern regarding his difficulties. She urged the participant to seek help via his pastoral tutor, which the participant did, and a satisfactory resolution to the situation was achieved. The researchers obtained ongoing contact with Tre regarding his consent to use his narrative in this chapter and he has approved our interpretation.

really stressing me out, I should just lay this out for you' I thought 'okay let me make- send a message to Lynn at least that way I'll be able to get it off my chest as well.'" This cathartic aspect of narrating to an absent other has also been noted by other participants.

As Tre begins his narration he reveals how personal time and space have had an impact on his difficulty with depression and his participation in the study. He feels constantly watched, scrutinized, and exposed: "You know you're under scrutiny all day with assessments, then you get home and you don't- I don't- haven't felt that I've had the space." Furthermore, the tensions between anonymity and sharing also appear to have had an impact. Tre says he would like to have recorded a message and shared his story anonymously but is concerned about being overheard by roommates. His subsequent evaluation of this need to conceal his problems is also revealed as he uses the powerful metaphor of MEDICAL EDUCATION AS A GAME, and through the continual assessment process at medical school he feels pressured to win: "You're either satisfactory... or you're excellent... everything was done slickly- your examination was slick and your this was slick and your presentation of findings was slick-... and to do well you just have to, y-you know, you have to be at the top of your game, so you can't let any weakness show." Indeed, his repetition of *slick* to describe every aspect of a "really competent" medical student evocatively captures his feelings of being in a high-pressure environment where anything less is considered a weakness.

In his narration, we see a number of pronoun shifts as Tre moves from using the impersonal *you* and exclusive *we* to the possessive *I* and *me*—sometimes in the same breath—"you don't—I don't." His shift to using *I* and *me* suggests a need to own his dilemma, rather than legitimize it. In doing so, he positions himself as having two separate identities—his personal identity as someone who has suffered the loss of a father and is therefore feeling depressed, which is hidden for fear it will have an impact on his competent, "slick" medical student identity.

Tre continues by moving out of evaluative talk about the pressure of medical education to focus on his experiences of consulting his physician. He says he has frequently consulted with tiredness and lethargy, not wanting to say "I feel depressed" or "medicalize" himself. He contrasts this with his daily interactions with patients where as a medical student he is *required* to "medicalize everything": "so on the one hand you're medicalizing everything and then you come home and you know y-you've got something going wrong with you and you can't help but medicalize yourself and think 'I've got this- this- this- going on' but y-you feel that or what I feel I keep saying you- I feel that I'm not allowed to diagnose myself because I don't have the expertise."

Following his move from talking about patients to talking about himself, Tre displays a meta-cognitive awareness of the way in which he narrates his story: his use of the pronoun *you.* Again, we can see through his shifting pronoun use how Tre narrates his personal (*I*, *me*) identity as someone with depression being in tension with his medical identity (*you*—"you're a medic") as someone who diagnoses. Indeed, his developing identity as "a medic" appears to overshadow facets of his personal identity (Finlay & Fawzy, 2001), namely that of becoming ill and moving into the role of a patient.

Tre positions his personal identity as a patient with respect to his general practitioner: he consults his physician regarding his *symptoms* rather than his depression in the hope that the general practitioner will diagnose him. His evaluation of these events reveals the full extent of his stress, both in the content of his story and in the way in which it is narrated as his narrative reaches an emotional climax: "If I don't pass these [exams] then I'm gonna be asked to leave the bloody course- so that's four years of my life wasted and- and on top of the fact that I'm just s-so emotionally stressed- it was just all getting- erm too much for me but you just don't feel that there's an appropriate outlet (5.0) ((takes a deep breath))." Through his use of the personal pronoun *I*, he explains how it was getting too much for him. He then finally shifts once more to using the impersonal pronoun *you*— possibly meaning "as a medic, *you*" –proclaiming that there is no appropriate outlet for his feelings. Tre's voice is now emotional, and at the end of this excerpt of his narrative Tre pauses for 5 seconds to compose himself.

It is worth noting here that the audio diary method gives space for participants to pause and continue without interruption by others, enabling them to fully direct their own narratives. Following his lengthy pause, Tre suggests that he was about to change the subject slightly and talk about how "meeting ill patients and relatives of ill patients just makes it even more difficult to be ill." He went on to narrate his current situation: a man whose father has passed away but who is trying to undertake an intellectually taxing, time-consuming, and "completely *emotionally* draining" course. He explains how he would like to feel sorry for himself but "then you go outside and you see these beautiful little babies with their smiles on their faces- on the pediatrics ward with these shaved heads and you think '*how* can I feel bad when this kid's got cancer and they- and they are smiling and giggling and l-laughing away.'" He continues his narrative by bringing in further (culturally familiar) stories of optimistic patients and relatives: the man with a terminal brain tumor who is planning to climb a mountain and the courage of relatives of terminally ill patients.

This final excerpt from Tre's narrative powerfully demonstrates the tension between personal and professional identities in the context of personal illness:

RESOLUTION

1	today (.) was the first time I think I've cried in months (1.0)
2	months and months- and I've cried twice in the same day (.)

EVALUATION

3 it was (1.0) it was really cathartic- *yes*- but it was a- a real
4 shock for me because (.) you know I've not been able to express
5 *anything* and it has built up to *such* an extent where I just felt
6 I wanted to *scream* out (.) because no-one's paying any *attention*
7 (.) you know and (.) fortunately I have my faith to stop me doing
8 anything *silly* like- you know- self *harming* (.) *but* (.) I- but I
9 still have this thought in my head that- you know "if I didn't
10 *have* that stopping me (.) then I am >so close to self harming
11 right now< because what else can I do to cry for help?" You know
12 ro- a- how often does a twenty-three year-old guy (.) *go* back- and
13 *go* back- and *go* back- probably I've been I think fifteen times to
14 the GP this year (1.0) ((sniffs)) er- you know wha- what more can
15 a per- a person do rather than actually saying "please help me"
16 >but if you say "please help me"< you know it's >just a sign of
17 weakness< (.) so waiting (.) I think my problem was I was waiting
18 for somebody to say to me (1.0) ">you take some time out< okay
19 yes (.) you know (.) >it's difficult for you< (.) and (.) *I* want
20 *you* to do this" rather than *me* saying it for myself- because if I
21 said it for myself then it's like I'm quitting (.) and (.) *who*
22 (.) which wannabe doctor wants to be seen as a quitter (3.0)

CODA

23 so (2.0) thank you for listening (1.0) >I feel a lot better now<

Tre tells us his crying had been cathartic following months of personal anguish. He mentions self-harming, but we are reassured he will not do this. He continues to emphasize the buildup of his emotions within himself and how he wanted to "scream out" (line 6). As his narrative reaches a crescendo, he proclaims that he has been to his general practitioner about "fifteen times" (line 13). His reluctance to be explicit about his self-diagnosis of depression within these visits appears related to his medical identity. Tre is both "medic" and "patient." Yet his identity as a medic constrains his ability to acknowledge his illness: he feels he cannot feel depressed as there are people worse off and that his illness is situated within a culture that (he believes) will stigmatize it as a "sign of weakness" (lines 16–17). The full extent of the tensions he feels between his identity as a "23-year-old guy" who is suffering depression and his identity as a "wannabe doctor" is narrated in this final evaluation as Tre oscillates between his medical identity and his personal identity, seemingly unable to marry the two.

DISCUSSION

We have presented narratives of medical students' encounters with illness from the initial perspectives of *looking onto, living alongside,* and *living with.* For medical education, these raise a number of issues although we focus on just one here—the indivisibility of students' personal and professional (to be) identities—while developing independently, they interact and influence each other reciprocally—which our participants appear to struggle with at times.

The narratives presented in this chapter illustrate three perspectives of an interior tension within each narrator between two aspects of the self: the student as *clinician-to-be* and the student as *myself*. In each, the narrative tension oscillates between the perceived identities of a physician to which they talk about aspiring—how they see society's prescription of how physicians in general should respond to the narrative plot—and their own preexisting personal identities, with antecedent histories—the *this-is-who-I-am* part of the narrator, struggling to make sense of the unfolding circumstances. The narratives demonstrate how narrators struggle to make sense of a dilemma that begins with a patient, then with a personal friend, and, last, with the narrator himself: although all three are ultimately about their own personal struggle with illness, dying, and death and how this affects their developing professional identities. As we reflect on the importance of these perspectives for medical education, we draw on the works of Polanyi (1958) and Cassell (1991).

At stake here is Polanyi's (1958) central thesis of knowing: no act of comprehension takes place without the active, interior, participation of the knower. Understanding the meaning of witnessing a patient's death for Rory is not an intellectually celibate exercise, but an emotionally and intellectually moving event, which alters his life view and forces him to reflect on his own mortality. Physicians, Rory is showing us, are just frail human beings. They are not immunized by dint of their medical education from the uncertainties of the human predicament. We see the same interplay between an emerging professional identity, and the personal—*this-is-who-I am*—identity for Paul. Paul receives the information about his friend's cancer as a friend and finds himself expressing the natural response in that role (shocked and sad). But he contrasts this with what he perceives to be the professional response of the medical student, and he rehearses what would be his response if this were simply a patient on the ward. Over the course of his narrative, what Paul tells us is that he struggles to get the right balance between these two identities. We can also see that his previous experience with his first friend has affected the way he chooses to act with respect to his predicament with his second friend. Finally, Tre's narrative, sadly, reveals his interior struggle with himself, and his emerging depressive illness. Physicians should not get depressed, pleads his interior *wannabe doctor*, but "I am" responds his *this-is-who-I-am* identity.

These narrators are telling us that, in the process of developing their new professional identities, medical students are not a blank slate on which the novel experiences of medical life are etched. Cassell's (1991) notion of personhood is useful here, helping us to understand this educationally important point. These narrators come to these interactions with a preexisting personhood. They have their own personalities, families, and cultural backgrounds, which are the building blocks of prior understandings of what constitutes wellness, ill health, and dying and of what it means to be a physician. They have their own bodies and, more important, a relationship with their own bodies—a relationship that Tre, for example, struggles to modify in light of his developing identity as a physician. And people do things. They play roles. If, as in Paul's case, one of the crucial life roles— close personal friend—is redefined (am I a *medical student*-friend, or a *person*-friend?), an intense interior struggle ensues.

Thus, professional and personal identities are entwined, interacting and influencing each other while developing independently. The implications of this analysis are clear: Medical educationalists could do well to remember that their students have preexisting personhoods to be understood, taken into account, and recognized as forces that compete with their developing medical identities. Furthermore, students' personal identities interact with their developing professional identities within clinical encounters—influencing students' interactions with patients. As educationalists, we can legitimize and facilitate an understanding of students' developing selves. Although students strive to develop professionally, their personal identities continue to be present: The interplay between identities poses a continuing challenge for students to maintain a healthy balance between the two.

PRACTICAL SUGGESTIONS FOR MEDICAL EDUCATION

We have seen how listening to and analyzing medical students' narratives of personal experiences that hold significance for them can reveal a number of important aspects with respects to their developing professional selves. These aspects go beyond merely listening to *what* is said; they pay attention to *how* their stories are narrated. This provides us with a deeper understanding of how students position themselves with respect to significant others (e.g., physicians, friends, and patients) and how they position their respective personal and professional identities. They also include other aspects of the way in which they tell their stories such as the prosody of talk and the metaphorical concepts that students hold. And, finally, we have considered what this means for medical education by urging educators to engage in a more intimate understanding of the inner word of medical students.

However, students, too, should develop an awareness of their own inner-worlds: bringing together an understanding of how their stories are told and the content of their stories through the development of a narrative competence. Indeed, the development of a narrative competence in medical students can lead to the practice of collegiality, authenticity, and an attunement to patients' best interests (Charon, 2006). We take this idea further and suggest that, by developing a narrative competence in the context of their own narratives, students might also develop reflective practice, including an understanding of what they personally bring to the clinical encounter. Indeed, others have suggested using students' critical incident narratives "as a method for fostering mindfulness and growth" in medical students (Cruess, Cruess, & Steinert, 2009, p. 114), but they work with written accounts (with a focus on *what* is said), which fail to capture the nuances of talk (i.e., *how* it is said).

Following the principle of raising a *reflexive awareness* of the ways in which we talk (Lamerichs, Koelen, & te Molder, 2009), we suggest that medical students would benefit from eliciting and interpreting their own oral narratives of personal experiences, thereby developing their own understanding of the interplay between their developing personal and professional selves. Thus, students could be encouraged to keep a brief personal audio diary of their life as a medical student by recording narratives of events that occur over a short period of time. These could then be analyzed by the students themselves, using the following stepwise approach (reflecting Ricoeur's 1983 articulation of the narrative process). First, the adaptation of an interpretative perspective—rather than seeing narratives as *truths* reflecting a fixed *reality,* students should be encouraged to view them as interpretations and constructions of reality. They should be encouraged to explore aspects of their own *preunderstandings* that inform their narratives—such preunderstandings include a consideration of what human action is, along with categories of thought that encompass semantic meaning: such as our existing commonsense perspective of the world—including social norms.

Second, understanding the process of configuring events into a tellable story: how we configure time within our narrative (temporal scaffolding by identifying the start, middle and end of a story), how *events* are configured into a *story* (emplotment), how the different characters are portrayed in relation to one another (positioning analysis), the ways in which the story is articulated (e.g., metaphor, intonation, pauses, laughter), and how the events are evaluated by the narrator (personal meaning). Understanding these aspects of their personal narratives can help students understand their own roles within their encounters with patients.

Following this, students should be encouraged to consider what their new understanding has for them and their future actions. So, in the context of students' close listening/reading of their personal incident narratives, we might work with them, encouraging them to reflect on new understandings and consider how this might change things for the future.

Finally, we would like to briefly touch on the beneficial effects of students sharing their narratives with significant others. For example, Tre actively sought to narrate his illness story through the medium of the audio diary, albeit to an absent other, as he felt there was nowhere for him to express his intense feelings and to be heard. Indeed, earlier on in the study, Rory himself called the Dictaphone a "cathartic little tool." We believe that these "ad hoc" debriefing opportunities offer methods of coping with stressful and confusing situations by providing a forum for sense-making opportunities along with the feeling of being listened to. Although medical schools sometimes make formal spaces available within which sense-making and the witnessing of students narratives may occur, this is not always sufficient. Students preferred to talk to others who they felt would understand, and with whom they had developed a trusting relationship (e.g., peers, senior colleagues, and us as researchers). Thus, medical educators (and even researchers) need to develop sensitivity to these needs of students in their day-to-day interactions and activities.

CODA

Society currently places physicians under more intense scrutiny than ever before. The audit culture and greater accountability place measurable transactions in clinical care under the spotlight. The stories presented here reveal the interior experience of physician-ship, albeit from novices: capturing experiences and narratives "at the margin." In particular they expose the frailty of the humanity of clinicians-to-be. Although society has the right to demand greater accountability, and to exercise this right through the demands of health care policy, society also has to recognize that clinicians (and clinicians-to-be) are people, too. The practice of medicine has an attritional effect on the practitioner, whose job it is to face illness, dying, and death every day. In recognizing this aspect, legitimizing it, and nurturing the development of medical students within a humanistic framework, we can help tomorrow's physicians develop a healthier relationship with themselves as well as with their patients.

REFERENCES

Alaszewski, A. (2006). *Using diaries for social research.* London: Sage.

Bamberg, M. (2003). Positioning with Davie Hogan—Stories, tellings and identities. In C. Daiute & C. Lightfoot (Eds.), *Narrative analysis. Studying the development of individuals in society* (pp. 135–158). London: Sage.

Bamberg, M. (2006). Stories: Big or small: Why do we care? *Narrative Inquiry, 16,* 139.

Butler, J. (1988). Performative acts and gender constitution: An essay in phenomenology and feminist theory. *Theatre Journal, 40*(4), 519–531.

Cassell, E. (1991). *The nature of suffering and the goal of medicine.* Oxford, UK: Open University Press.

Charon, R. (2006). *Narrative medicine: Honoring the stories of illness.* New York, NY: Oxford University Press.

Cruess, R. L., Cruess, S. R., & Steinert, Y. (Eds.). (2009). *Teaching medical professionalism*. Cambridge, UK: Cambridge University Press.

Curtis, K. K., & McGee, M. G. (2000). An overview of physician attitudes toward death and dying: History, factors, and implications for medical education. *Illness, Crisis, & Loss, 8*(4), 341–349.

Finlay, S. E., & Fawzy, M. (2001). Becoming a doctor. *Medical Humanities, 27*(2), 90–92.

Frank, A. W. (1995). *The wounded storyteller: Body, illness and ethics*. Chicago, IL: University of Chicago Press.

Georgakopoulou, A. (2006). Thinking big with small stories in narrative and identity analysis. *Narrative Inquiry, 16*, 122–130.

Georgakopoulou, A. (2007). *Small stories, interaction and identities*. Amsterdam, Netherlands: John Benjamins.

Halpern, J., Gurevich, M., Schwartz, B., & Brazeau, P. (2009a). Interventions for critical incident stress in emergency medical services: A qualitative study. *Stress and Health, 25*(2), 139–149.

Halpern, J., Gurevich, M., Schwartz, B., & Brazeau, P. (2009b). What makes an incident critical for ambulance workers? Emotional outcomes and implications for intervention. *Work & Stress, 23*(2), 173–189.

Hay, J. (2000). Functions of humor in the conversations of men and women. *Journal of Pragmatics, 32*(6), 709–742.

Jenkins, R. (2008). *Social identity* (3rd ed.). New York, NY: Routledge.

Kamio, A. (2001). English generic we, you, and they: An analysis in terms of territory of information. *Journal of Pragmatics, 33*, 1111–1124.

Kitigawa, C., & Lehrer, A. (1990). Impersonal uses of personal pronouns. *Journal of Pragmatics, 14*, 739–759.

Kuo, S. H. (2003). Involvement vs detachment: Gender differences in the use of personal pronouns in televised sports in Taiwan. *Discourse Studies, 5*(4), 479–494.

Labov, W. (1997). Some further steps in narrative analysis. Retrieved from http://www.ling.upenn.edu/~wlabov/sfs.html

Labov, W., & Waletzky, J. (1967). Narrative analysis. *Journal of Narrative and Life History, 7*, 1–38.

Lakoff, G., & Johnson, M. (1980). *Metaphors we live by*. Chicago, IL: University of Chicago Press.

Lamdin, R. (2010). *The professional socialisation of medical students through the preclinical to clinical transition*. Koln, Germany: Lambert Academic.

Lamerichs, J., Koelen, M., & te Molder, H. (2009). Turning adolescents into analysts of their own discourse: Raising reflexive awareness of everyday talk to develop peer-based health activities. *Qualitative Health Research, 19*(8), 1162–1175.

Miller, K. P., Brewer, M. B., & Arbuckle, N. L. (2009). Social identity complexity: Its correlates and antecedents. *Group Processes Intergroup Relations, 12*(1), 79–94.

Monrouxe, L. V. (2009a). Negotiating professional identities: dominant and contesting narratives in medical students' longitudinal audio diaries. *Current Narratives, 1*, 41–59.

Monrouxe, L. V. (2009b). Solicited audio diaries in longitudinal narrative research: A view from inside. *Qualitative Research, 9*(1), 81–103.

Monrouxe, L. V. (2010). Identity, identification and medical education: Why should we care? *Medical Education, 44*(1), 40–49.

Monrouxe, L. V., & Sweeney, K. (2010). Contesting narratives: Medical professional identity formation amidst changing values. In S. Pattison, B. Hannigan, H. Thomas, & R. Pill (Eds.), *Emerging professional values in health care: How professions and professionals are changing*. London: Jessica Kingsley Publishers.

Ochs, E., & Capps, L. (2001). *Living narrative*. Cambridge, MA: Harvard University Press.

Plummer, K. (2001). *Documents of life 2: An invitation to a critical humanism*. London, UK: Sage.

Polanyi, M. (1958). *Personal knowledge: Towards a post critical philosophy*. Chicago, IL: University of Chicago Press.

Redinbaugh, E. M., Sullivan, A. M., Block, S. D., Gadmer, N. M., Lakoma, M., Mitchell, A. M., et al. (2003). Doctors' emotional reactions to recent death of a patient: Cross sectional study of hospital doctors. *British Medical Journal, 327*(7408), 185.

Ricoeur, P. (1983). Time and narrative, vol. 1. Chicago: University of Chicago Press.

Riessman, C. K. (2003). Performing identities in illness narrative: Masculinity and multiple sclerosis. *Qualitative Research, 3*(1), 5–33.

Riessman, C. K. (2008). *Narrative methods for the human sciences.* Thousand Oaks, CA: Sage.

Roccas, S., & Brewer, M. B. (2002). Social identity complexity. *Personality and Social Psychology Review, 6*(2), 88–106.

Ryynanen, S. K. R. (2001). *Constructing physician's professional identity: Explorations of students' critical experiences in medical education* (Unpublished doctoral dissertation). Oulun Yliopisto (Finland), Finland.

Schiffrin, D. (1996). Narrative as self-portrait: Sociolinguistic constructions of identity. *Language in Society, 25,* 167–203.

Shapiro, J. (2009). *The inner world of medical students: Listening to their voices through poetry.* New York, NY: Radcliffe.

Takakuwa, K. M., Rubashkin, N., & Herzig, K. (Eds.). (2004). *What I learned in medical school: Personal stories of young doctors.* Berkeley, CA: University of California Press.

Watson, C. (2007). Small stories, positioning analysis, and the doing of professional identities in learning to teach. *Narrative Inquiry, 17,* 371–389.

Wortham, S., & Gadsten, V. (2006). Urban fathers positioning themselves through narrative: An approach to narrative self-construction. In A. De Fina, D. Schiffrin & M. Bamberg (Eds.), *Discourse and identity* (pp. 315–341). Cambridge, UK: Cambridge University Press.

4

LAUGHTER FOR COPING

Medical Students Narrating Professionalism Dilemmas

CHARLOTTE E. REES AND LYNN V. MONROUXE

INTRODUCTION

Professionalism dilemmas are common across the medical education continuum. They often challenge medical students' thinking about professionalism and shape their future professionalism attitudes and behaviours. They can also cause medical students significant distress. This chapter discusses what professionalism dilemmas are and their emotional impact on students. It also presents an in-depth analysis of two personal incident narratives around the common dilemma of learning intimate examinations and discusses how students narrate their dilemmas with laughter in order to cope with such difficult and stressful experiences.

Professionalism dilemmas can be described as ethically problematic day-to-day events for learners in which they witness or participate in something that they think is improper, wrong, or unethical (Feudtner, Christakis, & Christakis, 1994). Numerous studies have explored the professionalism dilemmas experienced by students across the medical education continuum, including preclinical and clinical medical students and residents, using various methods such as questionnaires, focus groups, and the analysis of students' ethics essays (Baldwin, Daugherty, & Rowley, 1998; Bissonette, O'Shea, Horwitz, & Routé, 1995; Chiu, Hilliard, Azzie, & Facteau, 2008; Christakis & Feudtner, 1993; Clever, Edwards, Feudtner, & Braddock, 2001; Coldicott, Pope, & Roberts, 2003; Cordingley, Hyde, Peters, Vernon, & Bundy, 2007; Feudtner et al., 1994; Ginsburg, Kachan, & Lingard, 2005; Ginsburg, Regehr, & Lingard, 2003a; Ginsburg, Regehr, & Lingard, 2003b; Ginsburg, Regehr, Stern, & Lingard, 2002; Hicks, Robertson, Robinson, & Woodrow, 2001; Hilliard, Harrison, & Madden, 2007; Kelly & Nisker, 2009; Kushner & Thomasma, 2001; Lingard, Garwood, Szauter, & Stern, 2001; Satterwhite, Satterwhite, & Enarson,1998; Satterwhite, Satterwhite, & Enarson, 2000; St. Onge, 1997). A multiplicity of taxonomies relating to the types of dilemmas experienced by students and residents has arisen from this research, and three are included in Table 4.1. Ultimately, these professionalism dilemmas are common and frequently involve the: "tricky interplay of three often-conflicting aims: to learn medicine, to work as part of the medical team, and to care for patients" (Christakis & Feudtner, 1993, p. 251).

EMOTIONAL IMPACT OF PROFESSIONALISM DILEMMAS

Research has suggested that students who witness or participate in professionalism dilemmas are more likely to behave improperly themselves and to perceive unethical conduct as acceptable (Feudtner et al., 1994; Satterwhite et al., 2000). They also report feeling that their ethical principles have been lost and disappointment with their ethical development (Feudtner et al., 1994). Moreover, professionalism dilemmas can cause students significant dissatisfaction and distress, often expressing emotions such as anger, resentment, and guilt (Baldwin et al., 1998; Christakis & Feudtner, 1993; Feudtner et al., 1994; Monrouxe & Rees, 2012; Rees, Monrouxe, & McDonald, 2013). For example, in a questionnaire survey of 665 third- and fourth-year medical students from six U.S. schools,

TABLE 4.1 Examples of Taxonomies for Types of Professionalism Dilemmas Experienced by Learners

Christakis & Feudtner (1993)	Hicks et al. (2001)	Ginsburg et al. (2003, 2005)
Performing procedures	Conflicts between medical	Communication violations to (or
Being a team-player	education and patient care	about) patients or other healthcare
Challenging medical routines	Responsibilities exceeding	professionals
Knowing the patient as a person	student's capabilities	Individuals resisting expectations of
Witnessing unethical behaviors	Involvement in care perceived	their perceived roles
	to be substandard	Objectification of patients
		Lack of accountability to patients or
		colleagues
		Physical harm to patients or others
		Being caught in the middle of a
		struggle between seniors

67% reported that they felt bad or guilty about something they had done during their clinical learning (Feudtner et al., 1994). Christakis and Feudtner (1993) provided "ward ethics" sessions for students to discuss their professionalism dilemmas. Students reported that the sessions helped to reduce their sense of isolation and anxiety, the authors concluding that the discussions offered support and catharsis, helped the students to regain perspective, recommit to their ideals, and formulate strategies for dealing with future dilemmas. However, students rarely receive such opportunities to discuss their concerns and moral distress in an open and safe forum, meaning that professionalism dilemmas are commonly unresolved (Chiu et al., 2008; Hicks et al., 2001; Hilliard et al., 2007). Indeed, Kelly and Nisker (2009) talk about the increasingly burdensome trend of "moral residue" (i.e., the long-standing psychological effect of failing to perform an ethical action).

PROFESSIONALISM DILEMMAS AND LAUGHTER

The current study aimed to explore personal incident narratives (PINs) of professional dilemmas experienced by medical students from three schools in different countries and their explanations of their own and others' behaviors during these dilemmas. Narratives of actual events are important as they are a key component in the act of sense-making (both for the narrator and for the listener). While some researchers are interested in narratives for this reason, others are interested in narratives as expressions of personal states, as storytelling performances or because they often comprise "manifestations of social or cultural patterns" (Squire, Andrews, & Tamboukou, 2008, p. 6). This chapter focuses on various aspects of how students narrate professionalism dilemmas but mainly centers on the use and function of laughter, adopting an event-centered Labovian approach to our analysis of narratives (e.g., Labov & Waletzky, 1967). Our analysis of laughter is important in the context of narrating professionalism dilemmas for two reasons. First, our analysis of laughter helps to reveal the emotional impact of these situations on our student narrators—insights that would not be wholly apparent from a thematic analysis of what participants say (Wilkinson, Rees, & Knight, 2007). Second, this chapter serves to provide a timely counterbalance to the developing literature in medical education that critiques students' and physicians' humor/laughter in the workplace (e.g. Wear, Aultman, Varley, & Zarconi, 2006; Wear, Aultman, Zarconi, & Varley, 2009). While we do not advocate students' use of derogatory humor, we do hope to emphasize the importance of non-derogatory humor and laughter in this chapter, in terms of facilitating students' coping with common but frequently traumatic professionalism dilemmas.

Laughter has a fundamental communicative role within social interaction. It is not just a behavioral response to humor but instead can be used to construct meaning, identities, and relationships (Billig, 2005; Glenn, 2003; Partington, 2006). Indeed, it can be used strategically in conversation to maintain the face (i.e., positive self-image) of speakers and listeners, particularly during face-threatening acts such as orders, requests, apologies, disapprovals, confessions, and so on (Brown & Levinson, 1987; Goffman, 1967). Hay (2000) developed a taxonomy of humor based on her examination of talk within 18 New Zealand friendship groups. Although she labels this as a taxonomy of the functions of humor, each illustrative example of her three broad classifications (solidarity, power, and psychological functions) includes laughter, so we use her taxonomy here to help explicate some of the potential functions of laughter. In terms of solidarity, we see that laughter and humor can serve to share information about the speaker, to highlight similarities or capitalize on shared experiences, to clarify and maintain boundaries, and to tease. In terms of power, laughter and humor can be used to foster conflict, to control, to challenge and set boundaries, and to tease. In terms of psychological functions, laughter and humor can serve to defend (i.e., identifying weaknesses in self), to cope with a contextual problem (i.e., to cope with a problem arising in the course of conversation), or to cope with a noncontextual problem (i.e., to cope with more general problems). Hay (2000, p. 726) differentiates between the two types of coping, saying, "The first [contextual] copes with problems we need to get through to survive the conversation, and the second [non-contextual] copes with problems we need to get through to survive in life, or a period of our life." Thus, the second can serve to cope with the uncomfortable events that are narrated.

While sociolinguistics studies have examined workplace humor for some time (e.g., Holmes, 2000; Holmes & Marra, 2002a, 2002b) and we have recently examined medical students' laughter to construct identities, power, and gender within learning interactions in the medical workplace (Rees, Ajjawi, & Monrouxe, 2013; Rees & Monrouxe, 2010), to our knowledge, no research has examined students' use and function of laughter when narrating professionalism dilemmas they have experienced. Therefore, this chapter seeks to explore the following questions: What is the function of laughter in medical students' PINs of professionalism dilemmas? Are there any differences in the use and function of laughter across different elements of students' narratives? In particular, we focus on laughter for coping (contextual and noncontextual) to better understand the emotional impact of professionalism dilemmas on medical students.

MAKING SENSE OF PROFESSIONALISM DILEMMAS THROUGH NARRATIVE

We adopt a social constructionist perspective in this chapter, which broadly underpins symbolic interactionism—an approach focusing on how individuals construct and negotiate meaning, social order, and identity through social interaction (Charon, 2007;

Sandstrom, Martin, & Fine, 2006). Within these theoretical perspectives, we conducted 32 focus groups and 22 individual interviews with 200 medical students from each year of three schools in different countries (Australia, n = 38; England, n = 87; and Wales, n = 75). The majority of participants were female (n = 120, 60%), white (n = 166, 83%), and aged between 20 and 24 years (n = 118, 59%). Students from all years of the three schools participated: 41 (20.5%) from year 1, 26 (13%) from year 2, 39 (19.5%) from year 3, 33 (16.5%) from year 4, and 61 (30.5%) from year 5.

All focus groups and interviews began with students discussing their understanding of the term "professionalism" (Monrouxe, Rees, & Hu, 2011), and then narrative interviewing techniques were used to encourage students to recount PINs about professionalism dilemmas. Narratives of personal experience have been described as "a report of a sequence of events that have entered into the biography of the speaker by a sequence of clauses that correspond to the order of the original events" (Labov, 1997, p. 398). All focus groups and interviews were digitally audio recorded and transcribed verbatim. The first-order analysis involved listening to the audio files while reading the transcripts to develop a framework to be used to code all data using Atlas-Ti (Scientific Software Development, GmbH, Berlin, Germany). This framework analysis (Ritchie & Spencer, 1994) includes a consideration of both *what* students say and *how* they say it (Monrouxe & Rees, 2012). Through this first-order analysis, we became aware of participants' laughter and how their laughter seemed to serve multiple functions in the group and individual interviews, most notably coping. Therefore, we decided to go back to our audio files and transcripts to first identify our primary unit of analysis for this study (i.e., the PIN). We chose the PIN as our unit of analysis because we wanted to consider how participants made sense of the professionalism dilemmas through their telling of the whole story, in addition to knowing "what happened" (Monrouxe, 2009; Riessman, 2008). These PINs were identified as reports of *a sequence of events* about a specific dilemma situation that students reported experiencing rather than generalized narratives of a number of conflated events or hypothetical situations. These specific events were therefore assumed to have entered into the speaker's biography and were emotionally and socially evaluated (through the identification of the structure of the narratives) as the raw experience was narrated to an audience (Labov & Waletzky, 1967). Once we had identified our narratives, we coded them using Atlas-Ti as including or excluding laughter. We then coded each episode of laughter within the narratives for the function(s) it appeared to serve.

Of the narratives including laughter, we went back to re-transcribe the two appearing in this chapter (1) in greater detail in terms of laughter and (2) in terms of the different elements of the narrative. In terms of the laughter, we transcribed laughter particles between words such as "ha" and "huh." While we drew on conversational analysis techniques (e.g., Glenn, 2003; Partington, 2006), our analysis is best described as discourse analysis. As with our previous study drawing on insights from interactional sociolinguistics and discourse analysis (Rees & Monrouxe, 2010), we used transcription notes such as ((says laughingly)) instead of transcribing and analyzing laughter particles within words (e.g., "heh huh•hh PLAYN(h)W(h)IZ O(h)R'N ya:h," Jefferson, 1985, p. 29) to give the reader sufficient structure while at the same time preserving the content of the talk (Partington, 2006).

In terms of the structure of the narratives, we identify those elements outlined by Labov and Waletzky (1967), namely the abstract (the summary of the narrative), orientation (details about time, place, participants, etc.), the complicating action (sequence of actions, turning point, problem, etc.), evaluation (the narrator's commentary on the complicating action), and coda (where the narrator returns the audience to the present). We also identify Labov's (1997) "most reportable event" (the least common event in the narrative that has the greatest impact on the narrative participants) and the resolution (the set of complicating actions following the most reportable event; a revision from Labov & Waletzky's original conceptualization as resolution of the plot). This initial structural approach to narrative was important because it enabled us to identify narratives of lived experience rather than generalized narratives, which may or may not have happened. Another advantage of this structural approach is that it enables the identification of different elements within students' narratives (e.g., separating the description of events from the evaluation of events), thus facilitating the comparison of laughter within these elements across narratives (Patterson, 2008). While we draw on Labov's work, not all stories include all elements and the elements sometimes occur in varying sequences (Riessman, 2008).

We prepared a series of questions about laughter on the basis of our reading (e.g., Billig, 2005; Glenn, 2003; Partington, 2006) and asked these questions of our two PINs to enable a comprehensive analysis of laughter: Who laughs? What does the laughter sound like? Is it shared? Where is the laughter situated in terms of narrative elements? What does the laughter accomplish in the social interaction?

STUDENTS NARRATING PROFESSIONALISM DILEMMAS WITH LAUGHTER

We identified and coded 833 narratives relating to professionalism dilemmas. These PINs covered a wide range of professionalism dilemmas experienced by medical students, including ethical dilemmas pertaining to consent and confidentiality, identity dilemmas, and dilemmas about unprofessional behaviors in others such as physicians and peers (Monrouxe & Rees, 2012). Common foci of the narratives recounted by students included dilemmas associated with intimate examinations, death and dying, and the breaking of bad news (Rees & Monrouxe, 2011). Interestingly, laughter was fairly ubiquitous in the recounting of professionalism dilemmas (n = 715, 86%).

It was not unusual for the same episode of laughter within a PIN to serve multiple psychosocial and conversational functions. The different functions of laughter, along with their definitions, were developed by negotiation between both authors. Although based on their immersion in and coding of the data, this process was also influenced by their knowledge of the literature (e.g., Hay, 2000). As with Hay's taxonomy, we found students using laughter to control and assert dominance over others (i.e., power), to share their understanding and support one another (i.e., solidarity), and to cope with the professionalism dilemma itself and its difficult recounting (i.e., noncontextual and contextual coping, respectively). In terms of noncontextual coping, students used laughter to cope with difficult-stressful-embarrassing events they were narrating. In terms of contextual coping, students used laughter to maintain their own and others' "face," coping with various interactional difficulties such as being unable to find the right word for what they were saying, losing their train of thought, being embarrassed because their comment yielded no response from others, smoothing over disagreements and criticisms, asking challenging questions, and so on. In addition to Hay's taxonomy, we found students laughing in response to the narration of incongruent (and therefore comical) situations, and we found them using laughter to end talk and facilitate others' responses to what they were saying. Finally, coupled with identity talk, we found students laughing to construct their personal and professional identities.

Although we identified 715 PINs with laughter, we focus in-depth on two examples only in this chapter. We selected these narratives because they illustrate multiple functions of laughter across a range of different dilemma situations but with the common theme of the intimate examination (Rees & Monrouxe, 2011). The PINs come from two students at different stages of education (year 2 [preclinical] and year 4 [clinical]). They also come from two different schools (A and C). Distinct episodes of laughter are identified within these PINs and they range in size from single laughter particles (e.g., "huh") to shared laughter and laughter-speak between two or more people; thus, they are distinct in that they are bounded by excerpts of talk with no laughter.

" ... THE DOCTOR AND HER ASSISTANT WERE, LIKE, MAKING JOKES"

This narrative was recounted by a second-year student (FS75) in a large (n = 11), all-female focus group at school C. Note that all participants have been anonymized and assigned a label identifying only gender (FS or MS) and participant number in order of recruitment. The PIN was narrated near the start of the discussion and was sandwiched between the narratives of two other students: in the preceding PIN, another student recounted her experience of inadequate consent being taken from a patient in general practice, and in the following PIN, another student recounted her experience of anesthetists making jokes about a morbidly obese patient about to have surgery. This PIN is essentially a conversation between FS75 and the interviewer, with some additional mutterings from other, unidentifiable female students. In this PIN, FS75 recounts the commonly reported dilemma of observing intimate examinations with inadequate consent (Rees & Monrouxe, 2011), with the most reportable event here being FS75 witnessing the gynecologist and her assistant making visual jokes about the hygiene of an overweight patient in the presence of (but out of sight of) the patient. We use the following transcription notes: **bold** = laughter episode; (.) = micro pause; (1.0) = pause in seconds; – = running on talk; ((says laughingly)) = extra detail about how something was said; huh = laughter particle; [] = overlapping talk; _underlined text_ = word said with emphasis; and (…) = unclear speech.

1	INT:	So (.) has anybody else had similar examples?
		EVALUATION
2	FS75:	I felt very uncomfortable when I was doing (.) um- well at the moment- you don't
3		know whether to laugh or just **like ((says laughingly)) hide (.)**
4	FS:	**[huh]**
		ORIENTATION
5	FS75:	[um] they were doing (.) it was cervical smears but if they'd had a positive (.) they
6		came back and (.) were checked (.) and the first one she does it all by the protocol
7		exactly like (.) "this is (.) do you mind if she stays (.) obviously you have to get
8		undressed (.) so (.) you're not going to be hiding much" (.) and then (.)
		COMPLICATING ACTION
9		but after that no one was asked (.)
		EVALUATION
10		**And I was like (.) "okay" ((says laughingly))**
11	FS:	**huh**
12	FS75:	**like (.) "fine" (.) ((says laughingly))**
		ORIENTATION
13		and they were just told to go and get changed and kinda
		COMPLICATING ACTION
14		but like she went **"oh (.) _this_ one's a _really_ healthy one (.) have a look (.)"**
15		**((says in an exuberant tone)) ha ha ha ha ha ha ha ((other students join**
16		**in with this laughter but it is not possible to discriminate between the**
17		**laughter particles of different students))**

EVALUATION

18 ***this poor woman with her legs open ((says laughingly))*** (.)

COMPLICATING ACTION

19 *"yeah (.) look (.) look (.)" ((again said with exuberant tone))*

EVALUATION

20 like like (.) *poor* woman (.) it's bad enough anyway (.) without having a medical

21 student being told (.) *"oh (.) yeah (.) have (.)* do you see this bit right here"

22 *((says in exuberant tone))*

ORIENTATION

23 (.) And (.) a rather large lady came in at one point (.)

EVALUATION

24 and (.) the woman I was *under*neath (.) she was obviously (2.0) like (.) the lady in

25 charge of me was obviously (.) quite a joker (.) she had a good sense of humor (.)

ORIENTATION

26 when the lady came in she obviously (.) *hygiene* wasn't (.) perfect (1.5) and like (.)

27 once they're lying down they can't see you (.)

MOST REPORTABLE EVENT

28 so (.) like (.) the (.) doctor and her assistant were *like* (.) making jokes ((said with

29 trepidation)) (.) ***and (.) like (.) ((says laughingly))*** the patient couldn't *see* (.)

EVALUATION

31 wasn't a problem (.)

ORIENTATION

32 but (.) I could *see* them (.) ((said nervously)) I could see the patient (.)

EVALUATION

33 I just felt uncomfortable that-

34 INT: When you (.) when you said they were making jokes (.) you mean *visually*?

ORIENTATION

35 FS75: Yeah (.) just like (.) ((student holds her nose))

36 FS: pulling faces

37 INT: Holding [their nose]

38 FS75: [holding their nose] ((says quietly)) and just (.) and (.)

MOST REPORTABLE EVENT

39 like (.) when she went they just made a joke (.)

EVALUATION

40 it just (.) it wasn't a problem (.) but (.) I just felt uncomfortable that (.) sh- they

41 shouldn't really have been (.) just telling me to do that (.) as a medical student (.)

42 they should be showing me (.) it (.) it is *fine* (.)

ORIENTATION

43 Friday afternoon (.) their last thing (.)

MOST REPORTABLE EVENT

44 have a joke (.)

EVALUATION

| 44 | | but when I was there *I was just like ((says laughingly))* |
| 45 | INT: | So (.) did you say anything? |

RESOLUTION

46	FS75:	No (.) I was like (.) *"err is that normal?"* ((says laughingly)) huh huh huh
47		huh- *"ah happens (.) some people don't wash as much as others" (.) ((says in*
48		*exuberant tone))*

EVALUATION

49		I was like (.) "oh" huh huh huh- sat back (.) it wasn't (.) like (.) the situation had
50		passed (.) it wasn't (.) anything (.) I would have been undermining them to say (.)
51		"I don't think you should do that" (.)
52	INT:	Mm (.)
53	FS75:	Because it's their job (.) and they do it how they wish (.)

This PIN includes seven episodes of laughter-speak/laughter, the first three episodes being shared between the female narrator and her peers and the remaining being examples of laughter-speak/laughter from the narrator that is not shared by her peers or the interviewer. Note that laughter-speak can be defined as "a form of blended, laughing speech that communicates emotional tone" (Provine, 2000, p. 37, cited in Partington 2006, p. 16). The first episode of laughter-speak comes from the narrator, in which she foregrounds the upcoming complicating actions with her evaluation that she did not know "whether to laugh or just like hide" (see lines 3–4). Her laughter-speak here serves to cope noncontextually with what was a socially embarrassing situation for the student and contextually with her admission to the group that she did not know how to act in this dilemma. Interestingly, her admission to the group that she did not know whether to laugh or hide serves to distance herself from the professionalism lapses she is about to narrate and thereby save her positive face, minimizing the risk that she will be evaluated negatively by her peers and the interviewer. Furthermore, her use of *like* within the phrase "laugh or hide" suggests she was unsure of which word to use. Typically, the phrase is "laugh or cry," which has a high degree of syntactic fixedness (and so the use of *like* in the middle is unusual; Andersen, 2000). The use of *like* and the substitution of *hide* for *cry* therefore suggests that she is reluctant at this point to admit she felt like crying and, along with her use of laughter-speak, further demonstrates that she is troubled within her recounting of these events. Her laughter-speak is shared by an unidentifiable female student, who responds with one brief laughter particle: *"huh"* (see line 4). This brief laughter particle serves to build solidarity with the narrator and tells the narrator that her story will not be judged harshly, thereby encouraging the narrator to continue with her "telling."

The second episode of laughter-speak comes from the narrator during yet more evaluation of the narrative. As she evaluates the situation of the gynecologist not asking patients for their consent for her to be present during their pelvic examinations, she comments: "and I was like 'okay' like 'fine'" (lines 10–12). Her use of *like* (with a referential meaning of "by comparison" or "as if") followed by reported thoughts of herself conveys sufficient ambiguity that the reported thought was actually thought at the time, allowing her to convey her complaint story, which implies a critical stance toward the antagonist—the gynecologist—albeit within the positive words of *okay* and *fine* (Lamerichs & Te Molder, 2009). Furthermore, conveying this through laughter-speak emphasizes her disapproval of the situation and serves to cope both noncontextually with what was a troubling ethical dilemma and contextually with her anxiety that she may be judged negatively by her audience for her apparent passivity within this dilemma. Her laughter-speak is again shared by an unidentifiable female student: "huh" (see line 11), which serves to build solidarity and encourages her to continue with the telling of her story.

The final example of shared laughter in this PIN comes as the student narrates the second complicating action of the narrative: "she went 'oh this one's a really healthy one have a look' ha ha ha ha ha ha ha ha" (lines 14–17). Her exuberant tone, followed by seven open-mouthed laughter particles, serves to cope noncontextually with what was a deeply embarrassing situation for the student. Her laughter also communicates the incongruence of the situation: that the focus of learning centered on what a healthy cervix looked like but did so at the expense of learning about respect for a patient's dignity and feelings. This laughter is shared by numerous peers, probably because of her animated use of direct reported speech, which dramatizes key aspects of the story and mimics the consultant (Niermela, 2005). Indeed, not only does this mimicry lighten the story, but also the enthusiastic tone she uses to mimic the consultant constructs the consultant as an enthusiastic teacher, merely neglectful of the patient's feelings rather than malicious. The shared laughter builds solidarity between the narrator and her peers and encourages her "telling." This laughter is followed by yet more laughter-speak from the narrator: "this poor woman with her legs open" (line 18), which again illustrates the incongruence of the situation and the student's attempts to cope noncontextually with the uncomfortable situation of watching the consultant conduct a pelvic examination while at the same time giving an audible commentary on the look of the patient's cervix in the presence of the patient.

In the next example of laughter-speak, the student narrates the most reportable event in the narrative: "the doctor and her assistant were like making jokes and like the patient couldn't see" (lines 28–29). This laughter-speak serves to cope both noncontextually with what was an uncomfortable ethical dilemma at the time and contextually with her anxiety about revealing such professionalism lapses by senior colleagues during the focus group setting.

The fifth example of laughter-speak from the narrator comes in line 44 at the start of her evaluation: "I was just like." This laughter-speak serves to cope noncontextually with the disturbing event she witnessed. She is then interrupted by a question from the interviewer about whether she did say anything to the consultant and her assistant, to which the student responds with "no I was like" and then some direct reported talk said laughingly: "err is that normal?" and then four soft laughter particles: "huh huh huh huh" (lines 46). This penultimate example of laughter-speak/laughter serves to cope contextually with her awkwardness in recounting her resolution of the story to the interviewer and her peers; indeed, she threatens her own positive face by admitting that she did not say anything to challenge her senior colleagues' professionalism lapses other than to ask a question about whether the patient's poor hygiene was normal.

Her final episode of laughter comes in her evaluation of the story and, in particular, her evaluation of the consultant's comment that some people do not wash as much as others: "I was like 'oh' huh huh huh huh sat back" (line 49). Again, this laughter serves to cope contextually with her awkwardness in recounting her lack of response to the consultant's professionalism lapse to the interviewer and her peers. Her laughter also serves to distance herself from these lapses of her senior colleagues, thereby minimizing the risk to her positive face—that she will be evaluated negatively by her audience. That these final three examples of laughter-speak/laughter are not shared by her peers or the interviewer indicates that they perceive her talk as troubles-talk (i.e., a conversation in which troubles are told, the defining feature of which is the conflict between attending to the trouble and attending to business-as-usual) (Jefferson, 1988).

Within this narrative we have identified seven episodes of laughter and laughter-talk. We can see from the narrator's laughter-speak/laughter in this PIN that she found the experience of observing pelvic examinations and witnessing senior colleagues' derogatory humor around those examinations stressful, and that she also finds the narration of this PIN tricky—these difficulties are emphasized by her micro-pauses and disfluencies such as "um," and "err." Interactionally, laughter was used by the audience as a way of supporting the narrator through her evaluation of the story, thereby demonstrating understanding and solidarity. The narrator's laughter-speak/laughter is situated within four elements of the narrative only: her evaluation of the narrative, and her narration of the complicating action, most reportable event, and resolution. During her evaluation of the events, the narrator used laughter and laughter-speak to cope contextually, enabling her to adopt an opposing stance, thereby distancing herself from the events and maintaining her positive face. Furthermore, she used laughter and laughter-speak to cope noncontextually as she relived her story through her evaluation of these complex events. She used both contextual and noncontextual coping when recounting the complicating action and most reportable event of the narrative, demonstrating her desire to distance herself from the professionalism lapses of her senior colleagues and to cope with the discomfort that this encounter caused her. That her resolution of the event also includes elements of contextual and noncontextual coping indicates that the student may not yet have resolved the unease caused by this encounter.

"HE WAS LYING THERE EXPOSED ON THE TABLE"

This narrative was recounted by a fourth-year female student (FS26) in a mixed-gender (three men and three women) focus group at School A. The PIN was narrated about three-quarters of the way through the focus group and was sandwiched between some generalized talk from two different male students: the first explaining his reluctance to do per rectal examinations (PRs) for the purposes of his learning, and the second bemoaning the difficulties in challenging one's superiors in medicine. This PIN is essentially a conversation between FS26 and the interviewer, with some additional mutterings from other, unidentifiable male students. In this PIN, FS26 recounts her experience of performing a rectal examination on a male patient with inappropriately secured consent:

1	FS26:	On the same note um (.)
2	MS:	Mmm
		ORIENTATION
3	FS26:	I've had to do a few (.) PRs um and it's always been with (.) the doctor (.) err but there
4		was *one* in particular and (.) it was this um (.) *older* (.) man and (.) the doctor did the PR
5		(.) and he sa- uh *he said* "is it okay if the (.) medical student watches" (.) and the guy
6		said "yeah that's fine" (.) and then (.) he did the PR (.) and so he was exposed (.)
		COMPLICATING ACTION
7		and *then* he said "is it okay if the medical student (.) um (.) does it as well" (.)
		EVALUATION
8		but err I just felt a little bit I I (.) you know
		ORIENTATION
9		we did it and he he he did consent
		EVALUATION
10		***but I just thought it was a bit ((says laughingly))*** (.) bad that he didn't ask him (.)
11		before he got exposed
		MOST REPORTABLE EVENT
12		***and it was a bit sort of you know he was lying there ex- exposed on the table***
13		***with his knees up ((says laughingly))*** (.) and then he's asked (.) being asked if a
14		medical student can (.) do a PR as well (.)
		EVALUATION
15		and I just thought it would have been a bit (.) yeah (.) **huh**
16	MS:	[(...)]

17 FS26: [could be a bit more ethically] sound if he'd asked him beforehand rather than

Orientation

18 beforehand he asked "is it okay if she wat- if she observes" (.)

Most Reportable Event

19 and then he didn't actually ask if (.) I could (.) do it as well until (.) he was exposed (.)

20 INT: So

Evaluation

21 FS26: it was a bit
22 INT: So you did do the o-

Orientation

23 FS26: So I but [he]
24 INT: [yeah]

Most Reportable Event

25 FS26: you know he was asking his _back_ basically- **he wasn't asking his face (.) he was**
26 **asking his (.) his back ((says laughingly))** "is it okay if the medical student [has a
27 go as well]"
28 MS: [mmm]

Most Reportable Event

29 FS26: so you can't even see the patient's face whether they're going "uh yeah okay" you can't
30 see that 'cause all you can see is (.) their exposed (.) bottom **huh**

31 INT: **Huh huh** so you don't (.) so you did (.) the examination?

Resolution

32 FS26: Yeah he he consented

Evaluation

33 but it just (.) to me it felt like it could have (.) been asked [beforehand]
34 INT: [Did you] did you say anything to

Orientation

35 FS26: Yeah I I said (.) err (.) th-the doctor asked first and then he said "yes" (.) and then um (.) I
36 you know

Resolution

37 I got the glove on and everything and I came to the patient and I said "um (.) is it okay if
38 (.) I" and so I [asked again]
39 INT: [okay]
40 FS26: and he said "yeah that's fine"

Evaluation

41 INT: Did you mention to the doctor afterwards "perhaps (.) um (.) you might (.) say that (.)
42 **before?" ((says laughingly))**
43 FS26: Um (.) no **mhuh mhuh mhuh mhuh** I probably should have but (.) um no I didn't

44	INT:	Okay but that's quite an interesting one because it kind of cuts into a lot of these it's it's
45		the respectful examination it's the consent issue
46	FS26:	Mmm
47	INT:	um (.) an' it you know its (.) its (.) being asked to (.) do something that (.) you know you
48		fe- feel uncomfortable about really (.) it's kind of (.) cuts across a few of those

This narrative includes seven distinct episodes of laughter-speak/laughter: five from the student, one from the interviewer, and one example of shared laughter between the narrator and interviewer. The first three examples of laughter-speak/laughter come from the student, in which she explains to the interviewer and her peers that the patient was laying on the table with his knees up and bottom exposed, while being asked by the physician whether it was acceptable for the student to conduct a rectal examination. Her laughter-speak in her evaluation, "but I just thought it was a bit" (line 10), serves to cope contextually with her awkwardness about just revealing to the interviewer and her fellow students that she conducted an intimate examination (see line 9, "we did it") with inappropriately secured consent. Her laughter also serves to distance herself from the physician's action, thereby minimizing the risks to her positive face with her audience thinking badly of her. Her second bout of laughter-speak occurs within her recounting of events: "and it was a bit sort of, you know, he was lying there ex- exposed on the table with his knees up" (lines 12 and 13), which serves to illustrate the incongruence of the most reportable event and to cope noncontextually with what was a socially awkward and embarrassing situation for the student. This noncontextual coping is underpinned by her frequent use of semantic qualifiers—*just, a bit,* and *sort of*—which clearly demonstrate a difficulty in retelling the event. Her brief laughter particle at the end of line 15: "huh" serves to cope contextually with her awkwardness in recounting the embarrassing story and encourages a response from her audience. Indeed, an unidentified male student responds to this laughter particle, but his talk is undecipherable because it overlaps with her continuing evaluation of the story.

She later uses laughter-speak again to further emphasize the incongruence of the most reportable event: "he wasn't asking his face he was asking his back" (lines 25–26), and to cope noncontextually with the deeply uncomfortable situation in which she was placed by the physician tutor. This noncontextual coping and reporting of incongruence continues as she completes her narration of the most reportable event with: "huh" (line 30). This also marks the end of her talk and encourages a response from her audience. This laughter particle is shared by the interviewer who responds with two brief laughter particles "huh huh" (line 31), which serves to create solidarity with the student and creates an opening for the interviewer to ask the student a challenging clarification question (i.e., whether she conducted the rectal examination). The interviewer later asks the student another challenging question, this time using laughter-speak at the end of her question: "did you mention to the doctor afterwards 'perhaps you might say that before?'" (lines 41 and 42). This laughter almost serves to preempt any interactional difficulty that may arise from her question; the laughter attempting to neutralize any perception by the student that the question is an attack. However, the question still seems to throw the student, as demonstrated by her response of "um" followed by a micro-pause and then four closed-mouthed laughter particles: "mhuh mhuh mhuh mhuh" (line 43). These laughter particles help the student to cope contextually with her embarrassment at admitting that she did not challenge the inappropriate behavior of the physician tutor. Again, that six of the seven episodes of laughter/laughter speak are not shared suggests that these episodes are perceived as troubles-telling (Jefferson, 1984).

In this PIN we have identified seven episodes of laughter or laughter-speak, one of which was interactional (narrator and interviewer). What is interesting, however, is the laughter and laughter-speak of the narrator in this PIN. Like our previous narrator, this student's laughter-speak/laughter indicates that she found the experience of conducting this rectal examination troubling and that she finds the recounting of this story difficult. These difficulties are further emphasized by her micro-pauses and disfluencies, such as "uh," "um," and "err." Furthermore, in line 18, she quickly repairs the word "watches" with "observes," to make her action of observing a rectal examination sound less voyeuristic. This student's laughter-speak/laughter is only situated within two elements of her narrative: her narration of the most reportable event, and her evaluation of the narrative. Unlike the previous narrator, this student's resolution does not include laughter. Three episodes of laughter/laughter-speak within her evaluation talk function as contextual coping, differing from the functions of evaluation laughter in the previous PIN, whereby evaluation laughter also served a noncontextual coping function. That laughter was not used for noncontextual coping within the evaluation talk by this narrator suggests that her evaluation of events is more straightforward, possibly because she feels less culpable than the previous narrator, who felt included in the "joke," albeit reluctantly. Indeed, the student commented repeatedly that she did secure patient consent for the rectal examination, so this dilemma is possibly less ethically problematic than the previous example. There were three discrete episodes of laughter within the narration of the most reportable event, all of which included laughter for noncontextual coping, demonstrating how the reliving of this event is nevertheless difficult. However, the narrator appears to simultaneously lighten the story through her repeated recounting of incongruence as she narrates events, demonstrating that these events may not have been really traumatic for this student or that she has resolved any discomfort or awkwardness she felt around these events.

CONCLUSIONS

The narratives of medical students at three schools in Australia, England, and Wales covered a broad range of professionalism dilemmas already outlined in the literature (e.g., Christakis & Feudtner, 1993; Ginsburg et al., 2003, 2005; Hicks et al., 2001). The two PINs discussed in depth in this chapter include the experience of one second-year student who witnessed two senior clinicians engaging in derogatory humor about a patient undergoing a pelvic examination and a fourth-year student performing a rectal examination on a patient with inappropriately secured consent; both PINs have the common theme of the intimate examination (Coldicott et al., 2003; Rees & Monrouxe, 2011).

Where our study makes a unique contribution to the literature on professionalism dilemmas is our finding that laughter was fairly ubiquitous in the recounting of students' PINs. The two narratives discussed in this chapter show not only that students use laughter as a response to narrating incongruent (therefore comical) situations but also that their laughter largely serves as a mechanism to cope with stress. Laughter helps them cope with the reliving of the distressing events of the professionalism dilemma (noncontextual coping) and helps them cope with the challenging recounting of the dilemmas, with all the associated interactional difficulties during the interviews (contextual coping).

Although the functions of laughter are consistent with previous research (e.g., Hay, 2000; Wilkinson et al., 2007), this novel context exploring laughter within students' narratives about professionalism dilemmas also brings fresh insights. Interestingly, laughter tended to be situated within four of the narrative elements only—complicating action, most reportable event, evaluation, and resolution, signaling that these elements may be more psychologically problematic for the students than the orientation and coda elements of the narrative (note that none of the orientation and coda elements included laughter in these two PINs). All of the evaluation talk with laughter across the two PINs included laughter for coping (contextual, noncontextual, or both). All of the complicating action and most reportable event talk including laughter served the function of noncontextual coping, suggesting that the reliving of these events is stressful for our students. The resolution talk including laughter served the function of contextual and noncontextual coping, indicating that the first narrator at least may not have resolved her dilemma psychologically. Taken altogether, that laughter is situated within the trickier elements of the PINs emphasizes the emotional impact and emotional burden of professionalism dilemmas on students' well-being as they attempt to make sense of their unpleasant learning experiences. This, coupled with students' emotional talk and their talk *about* emotion during their narratives (Monrouxe & Rees, 2012; Rees, Monrouxe, & McDonald, 2013), suggests that students need better opportunities to discuss their professionalism dilemmas.

As mentioned previously, dilemmas are commonly unresolved in medical students, and this is thought to be due (in part) to inadequate opportunities to debrief (Chiu et al., 2008; Hicks et al., 2001; Hilliard et al., 2007). However, our data indicate that students may lack resolution despite having opportunities to debrief with clinical colleagues immediately after the dilemmas and despite discussing their experiences with friends. Therefore, we urge medical educators to provide students with more structured learning experiences in which to narrate their professionalism dilemmas in an open and safe manner. This could well mirror the narrative methods used in the current study and used in the "ward ethics" sessions described by Christakis and Feudtner (1993), encouraging students to tell their stories and to discuss them with each other and experienced facilitators.

Not only will such sessions help students make sense of (and cope with) stressful professionalism dilemmas, but they will also help them make sense of their developing professional identities: who they are, who they should be, and how they should act. Like other scholars (e.g., Wear et al., 2006, 2009), we do not advocate the use of derogatory humor by medical students and physicians as a coping strategy. However, as Nietzche (1844–1900) stated: "Perhaps I know best why it is man alone who laughs; he alone suffers so deeply that he had to invent laughter." Therefore, we urge medical educators to provide a safe forum for students in which they feel supported in narrating their difficult stories in whatever way they wish. We also urge medical educators not to condemn students if they narrate their dilemmas with laughter as laughter enables students to negotiate the complexities of "telling" their story and helps them navigate the processes of coping with professionalism dilemmas.

REFERENCES

Andersen, G. (2000). *Pragmatic markers and sociolinguistic variation.* Amsterdam, the Netherlands: John Benjamins.

Baldwin, D. C., Daugherty, S. R., & Rowley, B. D. (1998). Unethical and unprofessional conduct observed by residents during their first year of training. *Academic Medicine, 73*(11), 1195–1200.

Billig, M. (2005). *Laughter and ridicule: Towards a social critique of humour.* London, UK: Sage.

Bissonette, R., O'Shea, R. M., Horwitz, M., & Routé, C. F., (1995). A data-generated basis for medical ethics education: Categorizing issues experienced by students during clinical training. *Academic Medicine, 70*(11), 1035–1037.

Brown, P., & Levinson, S. C. (1987). *Politeness: Some universals in language usage.* Cambridge, UK: Cambridge University Press.

Charon, J. M. (2007). *Symbolic interactionism. An introduction, an interpretation, an integration* (9th ed.). Upper Saddle River, NJ: Pearson Prentice Hall.

Chiu, P. P. L., Hilliard, R. I., Azzie, G., & Facteau, A. (2008). Experience of moral distress among pediatric surgery trainees. *Journal of Pediatric Surgery, 43*, 986–993.

Christakis, D. A., & Feudtner, M. A. (1993). Ethics in a short white coat: The ethical dilemmas that medical students confront. *Academic Medicine, 68*(4), 249–254.

Clever, S. L., Edwards, K. A., Feudtner, C., & Braddock, C. H. (2001). Does student's comfort addressing ethical issues vary by specialty team? *Journal of General Internal Medicine, 16*, 560–566.

Coldicott, Y., Pope, C., & Roberts, C. (2003). The ethics of intimate examinations—Teaching tomorrow's doctors. *British Medical Journal, 326*, 97–101.

Cordingley, L., Hyde, C., Peters, S., Vernon, B., & Bundy, C. (2007). Undergraduate medical students' exposure to clinical ethics: A challenge to the development of professional behaviours? *Medical Education, 41*, 1202–1209.

Feudtner, C., Christakis, D. A., & Christakis, N. A. (1994). Do clinical clerks suffer ethical erosion? Students' perceptions of their ethical environment and personal development. *Academic Medicine, 69*(8), 670–679.

Ginsburg, S., Kachan, N., & Lingard, L. (2005). Before the white coat: Perceptions of professional lapses in the pre-clerkship. *Medical Education, 39*, 12–19.

Ginsburg, S., Regehr, G., & Lingard, L. (2003a). To be and not to be: The paradox of the emerging professional stance. *Medical Education, 37*, 350–357.

Ginsburg, S., Regehr, G., & Lingard, L. (2003b). Understanding students' reasoning in professionally challenging situations. *Journal of General Internal Medicine, 18*, 1015–1022.

Ginsburg, S., Regehr, G., Stern, D., & Lingard, L. (2002). The anatomy of the professionalism lapse: Bridging the gap between traditional frameworks and students' perceptions. *Academic Medicine, 77*(6), 516–522.

Glenn, P. (2003). *Laughter in interaction.* Cambridge, UK: Cambridge University Press.

Goffman, E. (1967). *Interaction ritual: Essays on face-to-face behaviour.* New York, NY: Doubleday.

Hay, J. (2000). Functions of humor in the conversations of men and women. *Journal of Pragmatics, 32*, 709–742.

Hicks, L. K., Robertson, D. W., Robinson, D. L., & Woodrow, S. I. (2001). Understanding the clinical dilemmas that shape medical students' ethical development: Questionnaire survey and focus group study. *British Medical Journal, 322*, 709–710.

Hilliard, R. I., Harrison, C., & Madden, S. (2007). Ethical conflicts and moral distress experienced by paediatric residents during their training. *Paediatric & Child Health, 12*(1), 29–35.

Holmes, J. (2000). Politeness, power and provocation: How humour functions in the workplace. *Discourse Studies, 2*, 159–185.

Holmes, J., & Marra, M. (2002a). Having a laugh at work: How humour contributes to workplace culture. *Journal of Pragmatics, 24*, 1683–1710.

Holmes, J., & Marra, M. (2002b). Over the edge? Subversive humour between colleagues and friends. *Humor, 15*, 65–87.

Holt, E., & Clift, R. (2007). *Reporting talk: Reported speech in interaction.* Cambridge, UK: Cambridge University Press.

Kelly, E., & Nisker, J. (2009). Increasing bioethics education in preclinical medical curricula: What ethical dilemmas do clinical clerks experience? *Academic Medicine, 84*(4), 498–504.

Kushner, T. K., & Thomasma, D. C. (Eds.). (2001). *Ward ethics. Dilemmas for medical students and doctors in training.* Cambridge, UK: Cambridge University Press.

Jefferson, G. (1984). On the organization of laughter in talk about troubles. In J. M. Atkinson & J. Heritage (Eds.), *Structures of social action: Studies in conversation analysis* (pp. 346–369). Cambridge: Cambridge University Press.

Jefferson, G. (1985). An exercise in the transcription and analysis of laughter. In T. A. van Dijk (Ed.), *Handbook of discourse analysis; Volume 3: Discourse and dialogue* (pp. 25–34). London, UK: Academic Press.

Jefferson, G. (1988). On the sequential organization of troubles talk in ordinary conversation. *Social Problems, 35*(4), 418–442.

Labov, W. (1997). Some further steps in narrative analysis. *The Journal of Narrative and Life History*. Retrieved from http://www.ling.upenn.edu/~wlabov/sfs.html

Labov, W., & Waletzky, J. (1967). Narrative analysis. Oral versions of personal experience. In: J. Helm (Ed.), *Essays on the verbal and visual arts* (pp. 12–44). Seattle WA: American Ethnological Society/University of Washington Press.

Lamerichs, J., & Te Molder, H. F. M. (2009). "And then I'm really like…": 'Preliminary' self-quotations in adolescent talk. *Discourse Studies, 11*, 401–419.

Lingard, L., Garwood, K., Szauter, K., & Stern, D. (2001). The rhetoric of rationalization: How students grapple with professionalism dilemmas. *Academic Medicine, 76*(10), S45–S47.

Monrouxe, L. V. (2009). Solicited audio diaries in longitudinal narrative research: A view from inside. *Qualitative Research, 9*(1), 81–103.

Monrouxe, L. V., & Rees, C.E. (2012). "It's just a clash of cultures": Emotional talk within medical students' narratives of professionalism dilemmas. *Advances in Health Sciences Education, 17*(5), 671–701.

Monrouxe, L. V., Rees, C. E., & Hu, W. (2011). Differences in medical students' explicit discourses of medical professionalism: Acting, representing, becoming. *Medical Education, 45*, 585–602.

Niermela, M. (2005). Voice directed reported speech in conversational storytelling: Sequential patterns of stance taking. *Journal of Linguistics, 18*, 197–221.

Partington, A. (2006). *The linguistics of laughter. A corpus-assisted study of laughter-talk*. London, UK/ New York, NY: Routledge.

Patterson, W. (2008). Narratives of events: Labovian narrative analysis and its limitations. In M. Andrews, C. Squire, & M. Tamboukou (Eds.), *Doing narrative research* (pp. 22–40). London, UK: Sage.

Provine, R. R. (2000). *Laughter: A scientific investigation*. New York, NY: Viking.

Rees, C.E., Ajjawi, R., Monrouxe, L.V. (2013). The construction of power in family medicine bedside teaching encounters: A video-observation study. *Medical Education, 47*(2), 154–165.

Rees, C. E., Knight, L. V. & Cleland, J. A. (2009). Medical educators' metaphoric talk about their assessment relationship with students: "You don't want to sort of be the one who sticks the knife in them." *Assessment & Evaluation in Higher Education, 34*(4), 455–467.

Rees, C. E., Knight, L. V., & Wilkinson, C. E. (2007). "Doctors being up there and we being down here": A metaphorical analysis of talk about student/doctor-patient relationships. *Social Science & Medicine, 65*(4), 725–737.

Rees, C. E., & Monrouxe, L. V. (2008). "Is it alright if I-um-we unbutton your pyjama top now?" Pronominal use in bedside teaching encounters. *Communication & Medicine, 5*(2), 171–182.

Rees, C. E., & Monrouxe, L. V. (2010). "I should be lucky ha ha ha": The construction of power, identity and gender through laughter within medical workplace learning encounters. *Journal of Pragmatics, 42*, 3384–3399.

Rees, C. E., & Monrouxe, L. V. (2011). Medical students learning intimate examinations without valid consent: A multi-centre study. *Medical Education, 45*, 261–272.

Rees, C.E., Monrouxe, L.V., & McDonald, L.A. (2013). Narrative, emotion, and action: Analysing 'most memorable' professionalism dilemmas. *Medical Education, 47*(1), 80–96.

Riessman, C. K. (2008). *Narrative methods for the human sciences*. Thousand Oaks, CA: Sage.

Ritchie, J., & Spencer, L. (1994). Qualitative data analysis for applied policy research. In A. Bryman & R. G. Burgess (Eds.), *Analysing qualitative data* (pp. 173–194). London, UK: Routledge.

Sandstrom, K. L., Martin, D. D., & Fine, G. A. (2006). *Symbols, selves and social reality. A symbolic interactionist approach to social psychology and sociology*. Los Angeles, CA: Roxbury Publishing.

Satterwhite, W. M., Satterwhite, R. C., & Enarson, C. E. (1998). Medical students' perceptions of unethical conduct at one medical school. *Academic Medicine, 73*(5), 529–531.

Satterwhite, R. C., Satterwhite, W. M., & Enarson, C. (2000). An ethical paradox: The effect of unethical conduct on medical students' values. *Journal of Medical Ethics, 26*, 462–465.

Schiffrin, D. (2006). *In other words. Variation in reference and narrative*. New York, NY: Cambridge University Press.

Squire, C., Andrews, M., & Tamboukou, M. (2008). What is narrative research? In M. Andrews, C. Squire, & M. Tamboukou (Eds.), *Doing narrative research* (pp. 1–21). London, UK: Sage.

St. Onge, J. (1997). Medical education must make room for student-specific ethical dilemmas. *Canadian Medical Association, 156*(8), 1175–1177.

Wear, D., Aultman, J. M., Varley, J. D., & Zarconi, J. (2006). Making fun of patients: Medical students' perceptions and use of derogatory and cynical humor in clinical settings. *Academic Medicine, 81*, 454–462.

Wear, D., Aultman, J. M., Zarconi, J., & Varley, J. D. (2009). Derogatory and cynical humour directed towards patients: Views of residents and attending doctors. *Medical Education, 43*, 34–41.

Wilkinson, C. E., Rees, C. E., Knight, L. V. (2007). "From the heart of my bottom": Negotiating humour in focus group discussions. *Qualitative Health Research, 17*, 411–422.

5

BRINGING COMPLEXITY THINKING TO CURRICULUM DEVELOPMENT

Implications for Faculty and Medical Student Stress and Resilience

CATHY RISDON AND SUE BAPTISTE

INTRODUCTION

Readers of this collection will no doubt be drawn by the diversity of methods, stories, theories and ideas about stress and resilience within the world of physicianship and medical education. This chapter presents a veritable smorgasbord: an account of a curricular "experiment" at McMaster University in Canada which set out to enhance "resilience" for medical students; some theoretical underpinnings drawn from complexity sciences; and some observations which are intended to broaden our concept of what we think we are talking about when we consider issues of stress and resilience in the work of physicians and how this impacts medical education. We start this section by introducing you to the notion of complexity, emergence, as well as implications for ethics, before integrating complexity sciences, curricular processes, and resilience.

Complexity and the Natural Sciences

To begin this exploration, a few working definitions are in order. Perhaps first we can tackle the issue of complexity sciences. The disciplines that are loosely bound under the umbrella of complexity science have long traditions dating back as far as the 1880s to the mathematics of Henri Poincare (Prigogine, 1989). Things started to get interesting as computers began to allow for more powerful computations. Lorenz's famous butterfly effect (i.e. the notion that the flap of a butterfly's wing on one side of the world could influence the initiation of a weather system thousands of miles away) was part of work in the 1960s on weather modeling (Gleick, 1988). Complexity science was integrated into different systems theories and was taken up to help understand and model problems in ecology, computer science, particle physics, and medical biology (to name a few). The term "complex adaptive system" is used to describe a system of agents whose individual actions are not predictable, but whose action has an impact on the context and choice of action for other agents in the system (Gell-Mann, 1994). Key properties for complex adaptive systems include (1) Small disturbances that can lead to large impacts (the so-called butterfly effect): interactions among agents in a system are "co-evolutionary," with an interaction leading to an unknown outcome that, in turn, influences the next interaction, and so on. (2) Requisite variety: systems with more diversity are hardier than those with less diversity or variability. (3) Nonlinearity: the outcomes of interactions among agents produce patterns that cannot be known in advance. These patterns are also thought of as emerging; the result of the self-organizing properties of interaction among agents. (4) Absence of hierarchy or blueprint to determine the overall properties of the system. Instead, each agent within the system is understood to follow a set of simple rules that outline the range of possible behaviors within that system. It is the interactions at the micro level of agents that leads to the emergent properties of the system as a whole.

An example of a complex adaptive system found in nature would be an ant colony (Bonabeau & Meyer, 2001). Within the colony is a group of ants (the agents), each with a specialized function, all performing daily tasks under the influence of their genetic makeup, response to local conditions, and forms of signaling among the ants; the possibilities of their daily tasks provide the simple rules for that type of ant. Without one ant being in control, amazingly intricate structures are formed.

Complex Adaptive Systems in the Social Realm

As complex adaptive systems were explored in more and more branches of the natural sciences, they were soon taken up, unquestioningly, into social and human organizations. Complexity science made sense and, in many ways, felt liberating. Business and health care enterprises were especially quick to adopt complexity science into the thinking of managers and planners (Zimmerman, Lindberg & Plsek, 2001). "Agents" are humans, interacting to form complex adaptive systems. Managing human agents to obtain desired results could be achieved by intervening rationally at the beginning of the change process or teaching effective simple rules that could form the basis of self-organization. Most of the current literature that seeks to link complexity sciences and human enterprise draws upon analogies from complex adaptive systems.

However, the taking up of the natural science analogy of complex adaptive systems to describe people's collective action is problematic in several ways. It is simplistic to imagine human behavior can be governed by simple rules. Even if one could get general agreement to do so, each person comes with a unique history and way of understanding the world. Any rule would be subject to interpretation. From there, significant differences would emerge. Further, rules only have meaning when interpreted within specific local settings and conditions (Taylor, 1993). To interpret a rule is an action, located in the particular; a form of practical reasoning (MacIntyre, 1984) that draws upon a person's response both to what is around them and what they have brought to the situation.

All of our actions are socially embedded—we are interdependent with others in everything we do. Our day-to-day getting along together in shared activity does result in outcomes that cannot be known or planned for in advance; but we would argue it is reductionist and simplistic to think that these actions can be defined or shaped by simple rules. However, when thinking about how humans get along together for such intricate and multifaceted activities as learning to become a physician, the concept of emergence is particularly helpful.

Emergence

Emergence helps us understand how coherence, order, and novelty are possible in the absence of external design, control, or influence (Camazine, 2001). In situations involving people, emergence can be thought of as the patterns of interaction that are made possible by responsiveness, difference, and acts of evaluation or discernment (Stacey, 1996). Human interaction forms ongoing iterations of meaning involving the simultaneous occurrence of action/response that cannot be broken down into cause and effect (Mead, 1934; Bourdieu, 1977). In valuing theories of emergence to explain social behavior, several things happen. One is that the emphasis shifts away from preplanning and design and toward qualities of interaction and participation. Such a shift in causality also opens new ways of thinking about conflict, failure, and blame. Conflict becomes something less to be avoided or managed away—and more an expected dimension of human interaction that invites further curious exploration and inquiry, as illustrated in Chapter 1 of this volume by Lewis and Rees. Failure is not about failures in design or failures to "know better"— but more about unexpected consequences, shifting conditions, or a failure to stay engaged with a process long enough to learn from things that did not go well and perhaps trying something else. With more linear theories of causality, "blame" for an unexpected outcome is usually assigned to the leader or decision maker who failed to plan well enough in advance to assure safe arrival at the desired future state. Fault is located in a person who should have known better. An emergent causality shifts accountability away from a belief in an autonomous controller or designer and locates to the here and now; the critical focus of attention is on the quality of participation and responsiveness.

The Ethic of Engagement

Emergence is often mistaken as chaos—or a laissez-faire attitude that if one just lets go, something will "emerge." However, it is not reasonable to confound a lack of control over outcomes with a belief that nonparticipation will lead to anything desirable. We are more likely to get an outcome we desire by being an active participant in making sense of our actions and participation as we go. It is in our social interactions that we recognize the patterns of themes comprising identity in both ourselves and others (Elias & Schröter, 1991). Patterns might include *teacher, student, leader*; all of these emerge from processes of action that involve intention, choice, and communication. This suggests the need to understand our working together as processes of continued engagement, which involve a paradoxical dance of risk and certainty, knowing and not knowing. We cannot simply act and speak as though we were alone or "right"—if we cannot engage with others, we are cut off from them. However, engagement with others carries the risk of losing ourselves. Challenges arise, differences become highlighted, and the comfort of what is taken for granted becomes unsettled. Furthermore, since we cannot know in advance exactly what is "right," being accountable means sticking around to understand and respond to the results of our actions (Mowles, Stacey & Griffin, 2008). Finding a way into continued engagement with others becomes a form of ethical practice for both the benefit of self and other (Griffin & Stacey, 2005).

In sum, there are many ways of using insights from complexity sciences to understand human behaviors and endeavors. The theories that underpin our thinking in this chapter have been developed by faculty in the University of Hertfordshire's Complexity Management Centre, led by Ralph Stacey, Doug Griffin, and Patricia Shaw (Stacey, Griffin & Shaw, 2000). They call their theory complex responsive processes of relating and emphasize emergence as the key to understanding social patterns, which continue as a result of ongoing action and evaluation and do not arise solely on the basis of design or planning. Instead, actions such as teaching or curriculum planning can be thought of as the enactment of intentions and conversations that, to some extent, organize participants' attention toward some things and away from others—but for all people participating in those activities, how things actually work and feel cannot be known in advance (Stacey & Griffin, 2005; Stacey, 2003).

Emergence, then, can be thought of as a theory of change. In social life, the patterns of both continuity and novelty which arise or emerge from moment-to-moment are formed on the basis of daily, even minute-to-minute, local interaction. In medical school and health care settings, very different people come together in order to achieve things. People of different ages, professions, cultures, and social backgrounds, influenced by their own emotional states, anxieties, and ways of seeing the world, come together to participate in what they each understand "health care," "teaching" or "becoming a doctor" to be. Both rational and irrational things will arise out of these patterns of relating. Some will be expected, some will be surprising, and others will be completely unintended. No one person or group is or can be in control of this patterning. However, all participants have the opportunity to take an interest in everything that happens as a consequence of their participation. All of these observations can serve as "data," which may, in turn, influence subsequent action.

The notion that education results in unintended outcomes is not a new one. John Dewey, one of the earliest education theorists, noted that processes of education may also serve to reinforce or undermine ideals of democracy (Dewey, 1997). Jackson coined the term "hidden curriculum" in 1968 in his exploration of education as a socialization process (Jackson, 1968). Hafferty has explored what this concept means for medical education in his work on the hidden curriculum, also discussed in Chapter 2 by Lamdin. Hafferty has argued that the official or formal curriculum, as defined by centrally produced and sanctioned course materials, outlines, timetables, objectives, and assessment tools, is perhaps less influential than the informal or hidden curriculum, comprising the implicit messages and cultural norms of what actually happens. Simply described, "do as I say" (the formal curriculum) has less of an effect than "do as I do" (the hidden curriculum) (Hafferty & Franks, 1994). This thinking has been foundational in subsequent work examining medical student development (Haidet & Stein, 2006), as well as the teaching and assessment of professionalism (Haidet, 2008). In this chapter's discussion, we revisit the ideas of the hidden curriculum, in contrast to theories of interaction and ideology, as another perspective on how themes of emergence and complexity can be understood in medical curricula.

Complexity Science and Curricular Processes

So where are we? Using complexity science in the way described here, one might understand "curriculum" as a sustained pattern of relating among planners, students, and other members of the medical school community that is under continuous negotiation and enactment. Course outlines, syllabi, and other resources are, in effect, artifacts or idealizations, chosen based on the norms and values of the community choosing and engaging with them. However, it is important to remember that in the movement from an inert page in the syllabus to the lived experience of a medical student or faculty, choices and discernments are made, none of which can be known in advance. Not even a chosen, well-articulated course outline will necessarily guarantee that students will end up learning what is given to them. Also, the official artifacts of medical school—syllabi, timetables, and so forth—only partially describe what is taught and learned during the thousands of hours that comprise medical training. Both official, intended curriculum (e.g. a learning tutorial) and all the learning that occurs that is not official or intended will involve some interactions or discussion that were intended, some that were better than hoped, and probably some that were frustrating, confusing, or even harmful. There is no one person or committee in charge of this. All participants play a role in the emergence of the patterns, but it is only during the moments of live experience that one discovers whether good has resulted. None of it can be known with certainty in advance.

Curricular Processes and Resilience

With this understanding of curriculum, we would also offer a thought about resilience and stress. Stress in itself is neither good nor bad. It can be experienced as an enlivening, creative energy or as a diminishing, demoralizing experience. It can also be difficult to predict: Will my appointment with the difficult patient leave me feeling energized and excited by a therapeutic breakthrough or frustrated by the rut we are in? Either experience can leave me with something to ponder for my next encounter. Since stress is an inevitable experience of human life, notions of stress reduction are problematic. If levels of stress diminished, much of the enlivening stress would be lost, along with the kind that was more distressing. Instead, what might be proposed are methods for gaining distance or perspective on stress as it emerges in daily experience and treating it as a source of potential insight or chance to deepen understanding, not as evidence of failure, poor planning, or incompetence, as illustrated in Chapter 1. This discipline of forming a kind of constructive detachment from harmful stress can be understood as resilience. Instead of seeing resilience as a set of skills to be acquired or a kind of competence that medical schools must ensure appears somewhere in the syllabus, perhaps we can see it as a kind of practice or process that one has the opportunity to experience and learn from during all moments of medical school: a daily engagement with the complicated, messy, uncertain, and exciting moments that come with the experience of medical training and practice. Students are not bystanders in the processes of professionalizing; they are active, full participants in patterns of relating that shape and are being shaped simultaneously by students themselves.[1] We need to engage students in inquiring into their own experiences, including their own processes of coming to terms with their emerging identities as physicians, as discussed in Chapter 3 by Monrouxe and Sweeney.

CASE STUDY: MCMASTER UNIVERSITY'S PROFESSIONAL COMPETENCY CURRICULUM

In this section we describe the basic structure of the McMaster Professional Competency Curriculum, including its historical background, processes of development, and ongoing processes of refinement and implementation.

Background and History

In 2002, the McMaster University M.D. program was approaching middle age. The new dean of the Faculty of Health Sciences commissioned a small group of educators and students to completely reconsider the curriculum in light of current thinking about the education and training of physicians. Several years later, the "Compass Curriculum" was proposed with the first group of students in 2005 (Neville & Norman, 2007).

The portion of the curriculum that addresses the issues raised in this collection was originally coined "the other ologies." The planning committee recognized that there were disciplines of social and methodological science that were difficult to cover within the conventions of the problem-based medical sciences tutorials. Ethics, epidemiology, population health, and communication might need to be taught as mini-courses within the curriculum to ensure that appropriate material was covered.

We were the two curriculum planners appointed to take the recommendations from the "other ologies" report and make something happen. We are a family physician (Cathy) and an occupational therapist (Sue).

Curricular Structure and Content

To begin, we convened several brainstorming and advisory processes, involving patients, students, and full- and part-time faculty. How did people imagine this new curriculum?

---

[1] Of course, the paradoxical pattern of both forming and being formed by patterns of relating is also occurring, at the same time, for all who participate in curricular processes of medical education. The ongoing emergence of coherence/incoherence, intended/unintended is what happens when humans come together for shared action. We all carry on through the interplay of our intentions, communications, and choices.

We felt strongly that students needed to meet weekly for a chunk of time that would allow for meaningful discussion. We proposed three hours a week from the first week of medical school until the start of clerkship. A model predicated on 10 students per group with two facilitators (one M.D. and a person from another clinical discipline such as nursing, social work, or rehabilitation science) was chosen to facilitate the weekly tutorials. These people were designated LFs (longitudinal facilitators) to distinguish them from tutors in other program modules. The course was entitled "Professional Competencies," Pro Comp for short. Tutorials were to last for three hours (the norm for other tutorials) and were to occur at the same time every week, on Tuesday morning. McMaster's M.D. program runs for 33 months in total. The "preclerkship" (from the start of medical school until the start of clerkship) starts in September and finishes the November of the following year, including two months of elective in the summer. Pro Comp tutorials would then run for 15 months (Sept–Nov), with two month's break in the summer. And, unlike their other tutorial groups, which changed each module, the Pro Comp groups would remain intact for the entire preclerkship interval.

To identify the spectrum of content that was to be delivered, we consulted planners responsible for other parts of the curriculum, documents such as CanMEDs (derived from Canadian Medical Education Directions for Specialists, a Canadian outcomes initiative from the Royal College of Physicians and Surgeons of Canada: Frank J, 1996), the Medical School Objectives Project (MSOP: O'Donnell, 1999), plus other literature describing concepts such as relationship-centered care (Tresolini, 1997), interprofessional relationships (Purden, 2005), and client-clinician interaction. We were also influenced by the Indiana University School of Medicine (IUSM) Competency Curriculum (Litzelman & Cottingham, 2007) and borrowed liberally from them to name the domains we had identified as the broad descriptors of what our curriculum would address: ethics and moral reasoning, professionalism, self-awareness and self-care, communication skills, life-long learning, and social determinants of health. For each of these six domains, we appointed a curriculum planner and encouraged each planner to convene a working group to help them develop the goals, objectives, and learning materials for each domain.

Key Curricular Processes: Check-in

With the notion that inquiry into one's own experience is an essential method of evolving medical practice, one of the central features of each week's experience is a check-in. Check-in has been an intentional attempt to hold space for students to bring their own experiences as an object of further study. At the beginning of each session, students are invited to share something that they identify as having some significance to their experience of becoming a physician. It could be taken from their life as a daughter, father, wife, or friend or from an experience within medical training. Check-in occurs as a longitudinal thread of conversation about what it means to become a physician, independent of the specific material intended for any given day's session.

Faculty Development

Teaching the Professional Competencies requires a diverse set of skills. Some familiarity with the content is desired, although each session was planned with background materials to support the LFs. Within each pair, there also needed to be expertise in the teaching of communication skills and the use of standardized patients. Finally, LFs needed to be comfortable managing group processes that are likely to highlight feelings of uncertainty and anxiety. Knowing that each session had a deliberately introduced element of content that was "off the map", LFs needed to be comfortable in helping the group learn from the opportunities afforded by check-in and also find plausible compromises between addressing stated objectives and responding to a compelling situation that may have been brought to check-in. In addition to three days of faculty development offered before the course, LFs were also offered weekly debriefing and supervision sessions to help them address dilemmas, learn from others, and become more aware of how their own anxieties and expectations might be affecting the group experience. The interprofessional pairs were encouraged to meet "offline" to explore their ongoing working together.

Unlike many other teaching experiences, LFs were encouraged and supported to take advantage of learning or teaching moments as they occurred "in vivo" within the group—even if it meant diverging from the pre-identified course material. Often the decisions involved the entire group in an act of discernment about what was most important at any given time. This, of course, provoked a new set of anxieties and frustrations; it was rare that the decisions were unanimously popular. This emphasis on process as content is a riskier form of teaching than sticking unwaveringly to the rulebook and invoked more anxiety for their LFs. Reflecting upon and seeking strategies to enhance their own resilience was an important theme in all the different types of supervision we used. The idea that resilience is a discipline of process and reflection was reinforced for both students and longitudinal facilitators.

FOUR YEARS IN: OBSERVATIONS AND REFLECTIONS

This chapter is based on our experiences, conditioned in a variety of ways as educators, members of the McMaster University faculty, and clinicians. As such, they are simultaneously subjective (related to our own unique histories and expectations) and objective (conditioned by the norms of our professional identities and of the institution within which we work, to name several significant objective influences). Our intention in these observations is to report on findings that we have identified as significant. Our claims for generalizability and validity do not rest on methods involving objectivity. This book makes a contribution to a community of scholars that is taking a thoughtful look at how we understand processes of medical education. Our claims for validity or generalizability will only be realized if, in fact, readers of this chapter are tempted to take up our invitation for further reflection or find our work helpful to a renewed understanding of their own setting.

One of the ways we understand emergence and the interplay of intentions, as described at the beginning of the chapter, is that for everything we set out to do, no matter how clear the thinking and organization might be in advance, things will never turn out as intended or planned. The results of our actions are discovered in the doing of them. There will always be a mix of intended "good," unintended "good," and unintended "bad" outcomes. To report observations from our first four years of involvement with students, we propose organizing our observations according to these headings, sticking to outcomes that we identify as related to the central themes of this collection: stress and resilience. To more roundly illustrate the outcomes, we will preface them, as appropriate, with representative quotes taken from experiences within the curriculum.[2] Experiences of both students and faculty are included here in support of the ideas we explored earlier. The patterns of intention, communication, and discernment comprising identity are continually in motion for all people involved in processes of education.

Intended Good

I. Change in Normative Conversations During Formal Curriculum Time

There has been a significant shift in what constitutes a "normative conversation" within medical training to include self-care, conflicts, uncertainty, and ethical dilemmas.

---

[2] A word about method: It seemed important to allow the reader some insight into the kinds of experiences and conversations that have shaped the observations and arguments outlined in this chapter. Material displayed in italics are not verbatim quotes drawn from any specific source or person. Rather, they may be understood as "subjective generalizations" drawn from many conversations, debriefings, and reflections involving the coauthors, Pro Comp faculty, students, and other faculty members. They are data from our experience only. We are following in a pragmatic tradition, responding to the test Dewey used to assess the validity of scientific inquiry: "Does it end in conclusions which, when they are referred back to ordinary life-experiences and their predicaments, render them more luminous to us, and make our dealings with them more fruitful?". (Dewey, 1929)

When I went home this Christmas, everyone in my family asked about what kind of therapy
my aunt should have for her breast cancer. I am only in first year medicine—I don't know.
But I hate to let them down. What should I say?

On my ER elective last night, I watched my attending tell two parents their son had
been killed. She was so businesslike and cold. Is that what I will become? (first year student
remarks, offered during their check-in)

Students listen to every word my partner, the doctor, says. I am having trouble feeling
like they respect me at all. (LF, during weekly faculty debrief)

The inevitable struggles of both becoming and practicing as a physician are now
on the table, from which to be learned. The challenges of maintaining or modify-
ing one's values and relationships while confronting a series of new demands and
shifts in identity is important enough to be given regular curricular time. As well,
the uncertainties and anxieties of faculty trying to inquire more deeply into their
own experience as educators are normalized as an important topic for regular faculty
meetings.

II. Pressure on Clerkships to Continue Forms of Experiential Learning

It is an irony of Pro Comp (as with many such curricula) that the time over which we
have the most control as central planners is the time where it is actually the least relevant. Another way of putting this is to say we would much rather have students meet
weekly during their clinical clerkship to discuss real clinical experiences and how they
relate to Pro Comp domains. However, clerkships are planned by departments and all
departments are reluctant to give up scarce teaching time to something as intangible
as reflection or inquiry into experience. However, the surgical clerkship has taken an
essence of Pro Comp and offers their students two sessions in which they explore both
an exemplary and a problematic experience they have had during their surgical rotation,
rather like the debrief sessions called for by Rees and Monrouxe in Chapter 4. These
sessions are facilitated by a surgeon and a social worker and have proven enormously
popular with both students and faculty, who have used insights and feedback from student experience to improve the rotation.

The other rotation that students generally experience as emotionally and cognitively intense is internal medicine (IM). A recent cohort of students formed a task
force spontaneously to petition the IM clerkship director for formal time to process
their experiences of internal medicine. This has evoked some anxiety for members of
the department who feel uncertain about accounting for curricular time that is not
described in advance or how to facilitate conversations constructively that might be initiated by strong emotions.

III. We Have Maintained an Explicit Commitment to Both Poles of Knowing/not Knowing, Despite the Anxiety This Creates for Students and Faculty

This is a hard-won success that is difficult to recognize. The pressure from students to provide more structure, certainty, algorithms, and rules is, at times, quite overwhelming. It takes considerable energy to recognize and respect their anxiety and even perhaps to use it for teaching:

I don't understand what we are doing here in this curriculum. Can someone please explain to me what I am supposed to know and then let me know if I have learned it or not? (first year student remark, offered during their check-in)

Their anxiety ("Is this OK? What are we supposed to know? Am I doing the right thing?") is mirrored by ours ("Can we continue to pay so much attention to process? Is this the best way to prepare for professional practice?") There is an ongoing commitment to clarity and quality—but at times it is hard to discern whether learning moments and chances for discovery are lost when we try to explain too much or take all uncertainty out of a decision. The planners and faculty, out of necessity, exist in a chronic state of self-doubt, which is often very stimulating (what is going on here—am I on the right track?) but can also stray into guilt or shame:

I don't know if I am doing the right thing, or not. We had a lot of material to cover today. But when the normally reserved student talked about a deeply impactful moment during check in, I felt it was really important to give him more time. (LF, during weekly faculty debrief)

These experiences can evoke a lot of stress. We have come to understand a mix of complex emotion, including anxiety, as an inevitable outcome of this form of teaching. As previously described, such feelings can be very enlivening and motivating and can also be discouraging and disheartening. However, there are growing numbers of faculty willing to engage in these challenges with students and with one another and to continue to stay engaged in processes of reflection and inquiry. If the curriculum reached a point that the mix of complex emotion was reduced to a state of routine functioning, we would feel something important had been lost. So we consider the fact of being able to tolerate and engage in an ongoing way with experiences of anxiety and not-knowing as a sign of health and resilience for everyone involved in Pro Comp.

Unintended Good

I. Impact on Faculty Development and Promotion and Tenure

Being an LF was the most challenging and rewarding experience of my teaching career. (from an LF, at the end of their first stint)

If I see someone has been an LF, I know they have developed very strong teaching skills.
(from a member of the Faculty Promotion and Tenure Committee)

Being an LF in Pro Comp is now seen as a role in which only very committed and excellent educators participate. Despite the magnitude of commitment, over 50% of the MDs and 80% of the other clinical disciplines return for repeat stints as LFs. (Some degree of turnover is desired to bring new ideas and responses.) Those who do not return to teach Pro Comp have gained nevertheless a strong experience to bring to their other teaching roles.

II. Increasing Student Pride in the Curriculum

Pro Comp is different from everything else we do in medical school—we need to make sure all the incoming students understand how important it is. (from a student member of the Orientation Week committee)

This has taken several years to build. This year, the student advisory group planned a substantial number of orientation week activities to highlight the message that Pro Comp is as important to being a good doctor as their other studies.

The unintended good described above may also be understood as themes of resilience emerging for participants who have direct or indirect experience of Pro Comp as a mechanism that develops teachers, offers meaningful learning, and is something about McMaster that is worthy of pride.

Unintended Bad

I. Dynamics of Exclusion, Potential Marginalization, or Polarization

As we have described, participating in Pro Comp is a huge commitment for both a faculty member and his or her home department. Not all clinical departments have participated. As the traditions and norms of Pro Comp continue to gain credibility, there is a growing chance of creating a kind of "have" and "have not" dynamic that sends a subtle message that Department A is Pro Comp friendly/aware/skilled and Department B is not. Insofar as the processes of inquiry into experience are relevant to all areas of medicine, this kind of schism is potentially problematic.

II. Ongoing Challenge for Its Leaders

This is the shadow side of our commitment to stay in an intentional state of uncertainty and questioning. As already mentioned, providing an ongoing, if rather mild, challenge to prevailing ideologies takes a certain toll. Adequate support and recognition for those who participate in Pro Comp in a leadership position will always be an important component of its long-term sustainability.

DISCUSSION

Clinicians and health science educators are a pragmatic, forward looking group. We are keen to find ways to make things better—and much of the interest in both evidence-based medicine and quality improvement is because we believe in using scientific methods to find generalizable solutions. It can be difficult, therefore, to take seriously any theories or hypotheses that do not claim such generalizability. The case study we have described in this chapter was certainly intended to make an important positive difference. However, the understanding of what we have done, as illuminated by thinking on complexity theories, is tempered by knowing that we were not ever in control[3] of that process and that there continues to be many variables that can impact and influence the net experience of anyone involved in this curriculum. Furthermore, we are as constrained by our relationships, ideals, and beliefs as all the people with whom we work. It makes no sense to think we can step out of our own relationships of interdependence to design something that exists separate from the ongoing interactions that comprise curriculum. If we were to lay claim to anything, it might be to the scientific method proposed by Dewey; a disciplined, ongoing investigation into experience (Dewey, 1910). So in the service of that ongoing investigation, this discussion will continue several key threads of thinking raised earlier in the chapter. Within this case study, how does complexity and emergence relate to the notion of the formal, informal, and hidden curriculum? Does the discipline of ongoing investigation into experience translate into what Fraser and Greenhalgh (2001) term "educating for capability"? Finally, is capability a form of resilience?

Formal, Informal, and Hidden Curriculum

As mentioned earlier, Hafferty's work describing the formal, informal, and hidden curriculum opened a significant body of scholarship in medical education by shedding light on different dimensions of training as a physician. He would probably agree with one of

---

[3] To say we were not in control does not imply that we were without considerable influence. Relations of power between faculty and student tilt in the direction of faculty insofar as our ability to direct attention to certain things and away from others. However, it is not accurate to say we are ever in control. Once our intentions are set in motion, within the social soup of others' intentions and expectations, we can never know, in advance, what might happen.

the central themes of this chapter—simply put, a lot happens in the training of a physician that is neither intended nor planned. For him, the planned, intended, and codified elements of a medical student experience comprise the formal curriculum. The informal curriculum refers to unscripted teaching and learning that occurs outside of preplanned classroom activity. The hidden curriculum refers to the social structures and institutional norms, attitudes, and normative behaviors, all of which have a powerful influence on what gets taken for granted as part of being a doctor. Understanding and even intervening within the hidden curriculum is proposed as a powerful strategy for potentially improving the humanism (Christianson, McBride, Vari, Olson & Wilson, 2007), professionalism (Glicken & Merenstein, 2007), and satisfaction (Arnold, 2007) of medical learners.

To take a specific example that might be thought of as an informal or hidden curriculum issue, we can return to the comments of the student who felt his preceptor had been heartless and cold in breaking bad news. One account would suggest that there was faulty role modeling—that the student was learning that it was okay to break bad news in a perfunctory manner. The hidden curriculum explanation might have to do with the working conditions in the emergency room, the lack of time to spend with patients' families, or perhaps even a failure on the part of medical schools to teach and evaluate communication skills in a manner that translates well into practice through the forming of partnerships between practitioners and patients. In coming to grips with the informal and hidden curriculum, Hafferty and others advocate a redesign of learning environments (Hafferty & Levinson, 2008) in the hope that one can create a learning environment that, in this case, did not transmit a message about how to break bad news. Within this premise is the idea that the learning environment can somehow be isolated and intervened upon as something separate from the learners or teachers who occupy it.

The processual and interdependent view of relating proposed in this chapter takes a slightly different view. As social beings, we continually negotiate/evaluate our interactions with one another—both consciously and unconsciously. All of our actions involve a choice between one thing or another. These evaluative themes framed by norms and values have been described by Griffin and Stacy (2005) as ideology. Ideology is often an unconscious, habitual form of evaluation that expresses the naturalness of an existing way of organizing or interacting. Ideology can be thought of as what is taken for granted. The norms and values that constitute ideology are not located outside of interaction— they arise in that paradoxical relationship of certainty/risk, and continuity/novelty that constitutes human relating.

If we locate causality in local processes of interaction, it makes no sense to formulate a hidden curriculum. Instead, one might understand ideology and power relations as processes that, in the moment-to-moment course of interaction, make it feel natural to pay attention to some things and not to others. In the case just described, one theme of the ideology being expressed is that it is not important for attending physicians (and their medical students) to reflect upon or discuss moments of intense emotion with patients. A related theme might be that acquiring advanced skills in conversations with patients is less important than acquiring advanced skills in resuscitation. In this way of thinking, instead, we might consider curriculum itself as a wide range of processes and practices that emerge from all the interactions comprising medical training. What is often called the formal curriculum (i.e. the syllabi, timetables, computer software, labs, etc.) are actually inert artifacts with no meaning until they are taken up in social interaction.

We would agree with Hafferty and those who have taken up his thinking on the hidden curriculum that there are some themes and processes that comprise medical training and are potentially bullying, dehumanizing, or harmful, as identified in Chapter 4 of this volume. However, we would argue against locating them in generalized abstractions (the hidden curriculum) that can be assumed to be understood or pointed to outside of local processes of interaction. The abstraction "hidden curriculum" is one step removed from the actual experience to which we are trying to pay attention. Taking one's experience seriously (i.e. locating causality in interaction) invites us to pay attention more thoughtfully to here-and-now patterns of relating. In contrast, locating causality in abstract or generalized external forces often leads to a belief that the way to change these patterns is to revisit design: simply rewrite the explicit rules or design new courses or codes that focus on different ways to behave.

Further, we would suggest that the only way to change a pattern of interacting is to inquire directly into that pattern. This is a potentially risky and anxiety ridden business, as it challenges ideologies of what is normal and may prove destabilizing to people who would rather stick to what is taken for granted than venture into unknown territory (similar to the anxiety felt by internal medicine clerkship planners who were reluctant to give students time to discuss their experiences on the ward). Prevailing ideology within the ER setting we described would make it feel very unnatural for a student to approach a preceptor to ask about the shared experience of breaking bad news—or for a preceptor to inquire explicitly into or reflect upon such experience.

Educating for Capability

Fraser and Greenhalgh (2001), as part of a *British Medical Journal* series exploring the relevance of complexity thinking, have written an article in which they suggest that the aim of medical school is not merely to assure competence but also to educate for capability, which they describe as the "extent to which individuals can adapt to change, generate new knowledge, and continue to improve their performance" (p. 799). They suggest that such education should focus on process (i.e. allowing students to define their own learning goals, provide feedback, offer opportunities for reflection) and avoid goals with rigid and prescriptive content. They list a variety of educational strategies that are nonlinear, informal, and unplanned, including storytelling, small group discussion, feedback, experiential learning, role plays, and others.

Much of what they espouse can be found in the Professional Competency Curriculum we describe. We both agree with the educational methods outlined in this article. Where we might differ is in our understanding of the relationship between content and process. Their notion of educating for capability suggests that one can identify a series of processes that will lead to greater capability. Inherent in this suggestion is the optimistic notion that we can use complexity thinking to design in advance a series of educational strategies that will lead to a more capable medical graduate.

Our theory of emergence in this case study of medical education is suggesting more that content and process are inseparable. Other curricular theorists who have explored this possibility include Friere (1970) and Grundy (1987). Curriculum itself is a process or practice in which all participants are simultaneously forming and being formed by their participation. Capability is a kind of idealization which has no meaning until it is taken up and functionalized within specific settings and situations. In the setting of participating in curriculum formation, capability may be understood as one possible outcome of persisting engagement and continuous inquiry, which itself influences the ongoing conversation of how capability is recognized and understood. In other words, capability emerges in social processes as a theme simultaneously shaping and being shaped by curricular practice of all kinds.

TYING IT ALL TOGETHER

So where are we now? If, as proposed, idealizations such as capability, resilience, or even excellence are understood as emergent properties of interaction, which can only be known after the fact (i.e. through reflection upon experience), then the importance of taking our experience seriously becomes paramount. This is a radical challenge to the idea that generalizations precede or govern action. Instead, we are suggesting that enduring generalizations might be found through action and in response to the questions we use to explore our ongoing experience—including the day-to-day interactions of our lives as students and educators. Effecting enduring changes becomes possible, therefore, when we act on our own personal situations, honoring the histories and contexts and perhaps finding ways to recognize and inquire further into the ideologies, norms, and values that make the way we do things feel natural or unquestionable. Even more challenging as an educator is to be open to participating in this practice with our students. This is not a neutral or easy process, as it involves the chance that something that we have used to anchor us—a belief, strongly held value, or defense mechanism—may not stand up to scrutiny or may not be the best course of action in the current situation.

Resilience can be thought of perhaps as another paradox—one named by Elias & Schröter (1987) as "involved detachment". In this setting, it means the ability to be aware of and experience the emotions, values, feelings, experiences, histories in which both ourselves and others find ourselves—and also to be able to hold all of those things up to and for exploration, question, and consideration—again, by both self and other. It is an ability to take a scientific or detached view of both traditional propositional knowledge (i.e. EBM or pathophysiology) but also of our own involved interests, values, and biases. The extent to which a group of people comprising a medical school or involved in medical education can articulate the value of involved detachment and offer opportunities to practice a disciplined inquiry into experience is itself an emergent process, shaped and influenced by local conditions and histories. As we have hoped to demonstrate, the processes that comprise the Professional Competency Curriculum are contested, creative, and contingent, mirroring the practice of medicine itself.

We are not convinced we have it "right"—nor will we ever be. Nor are we arguing that this curriculum be exported or generalized to any other setting. However, using complexity thinking in the way we have demonstrated has begun to help us think of resilience as a verb, rather than a noun. "Resiliencing" might be thought of as the practice of understanding causality as processes of emergence. As medical educators, we have attempted to create and model the ongoing inquiry into experience as daily practice known as the Professional Competency Curriculum. We hope that this chapter has offered a glimpse or two into a way of thinking about your own curricular processes and the other processes that comprise the stresses and joys of professional life.

REFERENCES

Arnold, R. M. (2007). Formal, informal, and hidden curriculum in the clinical years: where is the problem? *Journal of Palliative Medicine, 10*(3), 646–648.

Bonabeau, E., & Meyer, C. (2001). Swarm intelligence: A whole new way to think about business. *Harvard Business Review, 79*(5), 106–114, 165.

Bourdieu, P. (1977). *Outline of a theory of practice.* Cambridge: Cambridge University Press.

Camazine, S. (2001). *Self-organization in biological systems.* Princeton, NJ: Princeton University Press.

Christianson, C. E., McBride, R. B., Vari, R. C., Olson, L., & Wilson, H. D. (2007). From traditional to patient-centered learning: curriculum change as an intervention for changing institutional culture and promoting professionalism in undergraduate medical education. *Academic Medicine, 82*(11), 1079–1088.

Dewey, J. (1910). *How we think.* Boston, MA: D.C. Heath & Co.

Dewey, J. (1929). *The quest for certainty: a study of the relation of knowledge and action*. New York, NY: Minton, Balch.

Dewey, J. (1997). *Democracy and education: an introduction to the philosophy of education*. New York, NY: Free Press.

Elias, N., & Schröter, M. (1987). *Involvement and detachment*. New York, NY: Blackwell.

Elias, N., & Schröter, M. (1991). *The society of individuals*. Oxford: Basil Blackwell.

Frank, J. M. T. P. (1996). Skills for the New Millennium: Report of the Societal Needs Working Group, CanMEDS 2000 Project. *Annals RCPSC 28* 209–216.

Fraser, S. W., & Greenhalgh, T. (2001). Coping with complexity: educating for capability. *British Medical Journal, 323*(7316), 799–803.

Freire, P. (1970). *Pedagogy of the oppressed*. New York, NY: Herder and Herder.

Gell-Mann, M. (1994). *The quark and the jaguar adventures in the simple and the complex*. New York, NY: W.H. Freeman.

Gleick, J. (1988). *Chaos: making a new science*. New York, NY: Penguin.

Glicken, A. D., & Merenstein, G. B. (2007). Addressing the hidden curriculum: understanding educator professionalism. *Medical Teacher, 29*(1), 54–57.

Griffin, D., & Stacey, R. D. (2005). *Complexity and the experience of leading organizations*. New York, NY: Routledge.

Grundy, S. (1987). *Curriculum: product or praxis?* London: Falmer Press.

Hafferty, F. W., & Franks, R. (1994). The hidden curriculum, ethics teaching, and the structure of medical education. *Academic Medicine, 69*(11), 861–871.

Hafferty, F. W., & Levinson, D. (2008). Moving beyond nostalgia and motives: towards a complexity science view of medical professionalism. *Perspectives in Biology and Medicine, 51*(4), 599–615.

Haidet, P. (2008). Where we're headed: a new wave of scholarship on educating medical professionalism. *Journal of General Internal Medicine, 23*(7), 1118–1119.

Haidet, P., & Stein, H. F. (2006). The role of the student-teacher relationship in the formation of physicians. The hidden curriculum as process. *Journal of General Internal Medicine, 21 Suppl* 1 S16–S20.

Jackson, P. W. (1968). *Life in classrooms*. New York, NY: Holt, Rinehart and Winston.

Litzelman, D. K., & Cottingham, A. H. (2007). The new formal competency-based curriculum and informal curriculum at Indiana University School of Medicine: overview and five-year analysis. *Academic Medicine, 82*(4), 410–421.

MacIntyre, A. C. (1984). *After virtue: A study in moral theory*. Notre Dame, IN: University of Notre Dame Press.

Mead, G. (1934). *Mind, self and society*. Chicago, IL: Chicago University Press.

Mowles, C., Stacey, R., & Griffin, D. (2008). What contribution can insights from the complexity sciences make to the theory and practice of development management? *Journal of International Development, 20,* 804–820.

Neville, A. J., & Norman, G. R. (2007). PBL in the undergraduate MD program at McMaster University: three iterations in three decades. *Academic Medicine, 82*(4), 370–374.

O'Donnell, J. F. (1999). The Medical School Objectives Project (MSOP). *Journal of Cancer Education, 14*(1), 2–3.

Prigogine, I. (1989). The philosophy of instability. *Futures, 21*(4), 396–400.

Purden, M. (2005). Cultural considerations in interprofessional education and practice. *Journal of Interprofessional Care, 19 Suppl* 1 224–234.

Stacey, R. D. (1996). *Complexity and creativity in organizations*. San Francisco, CA: Berrett-Koehler Publishers.

Stacey, R. D. (2003). *Strategic management and organisational dynamics: The challenge of complexity*. Harlow, England/New York, NY: Prentice Hall/Financial Times.

Stacey, R. D., & Griffin, D. (2005). *A complexity perspective on researching organizations: Taking experience seriously*. London/New York, NY: Routledge.

Stacey, R. D., Griffin, D., & Shaw, P. (2000). *Complexity and management: Fad or radical challenge to systems thinking?* New York, NY: Routledge.

Taylor, C. (1993). To follow a rule. In C. Calhoun, E. Lipuma, & M. Poston (Eds.), *Pierre Bourdieu: Critical perspectives* (pp. 45–60). Cambridge: Polity Press.

Tresolini, C. P. (1997). Relationship-centered care: its time has come! *Aspen's Advisor for Nurse Executives, 12*(9), 7–8.

Zimmerman, B., Lindberg, C., & Plsek, P. E. (2001). *Edgeware: Insights from complexity science for health care leaders.* Irving, TX: VHA Inc.

Stress of Being a Physician

INTRODUCTION

Peter Huggard

"I think I just had my first look at the enemy. The one I'm training to fight the rest of my life." "Death?" he asked. "Yeah" I replied. "I told Death that I knew it was going to win the war in the end but that I didn't care. I would be dammed if I was going to let it win all the battles."

Daniel J. McCullough (medical student)

Death may be a companion on the journey of physician and healer, and at times it may "win some of the battles." However, is the journey of life a series of battles with death, or is the journey one of living, knowing that death is only the final consequence? Perhaps death does not win the war, rather, it is that final event that takes us all from a state of living into a future state that may be, depending on one's beliefs, one of finality to our existence or the beginning of some new journey.

Not only are there "clinical battles" arising from the complexity of the vast range of ill health experiences possible, but the "battle" or struggle may also be within and arise from prolonged stressors that, unless eliminated or appropriately and effectively managed, can eat away at the healer's very existence, and at times, those closest to him or her. Both the nature of the work of a physician and the character of a physician have been cited as possible causes of distress (Riley, 2004). Potential stressors were reported to include high intensity of work, conflicting time demands, and heavy professional responsibility, as well as frequently working in an environment with reduced physical and social resources, threat of medico-legal action, and limited power to alter work conditions. Riley concluded his article by saying that "the prospect of a lifetime of joyless striving is unacceptable" (p. 353). Many of these stressors and stressful experiences are similar to those discussed in Section 1 of this book and help create the continuum between being a medical student and a physician. Deckard, Meterko and Field (1994), in examining the relationships between physician burnout and personal, professional, and organizational/ work life factors, found that 58% of physicians surveyed reported scores of high emotional exhaustion and that the strongest predictors of emotional exhaustion were workload and the limited degree of influence that physicians had in their work place. A study of general practitioners in the United Kingdom showed that demands of the job and patients' expectations, interference with family life, constant interruptions at work and home, and administrative tasks were the highest predictors of job dissatisfaction (Cooper, Rout, & Faragher, 1989). One of the challenges, therefore, is to reframe the view of clinical practice as being a "battle" to one of being a "privileged companion" to those in need of the healer's special skills and knowledge.

Attention is given to some of the physician stressors (and their possible effects) in the six chapters in this section of this book. These chapters serve to present a summary of both current thinking and the results of recent research into the causes of some of these stressors. The authors are clinicians who have a special interest in identifying what may contribute to physician distress, as well as experience in working with physicians to assist them to manage this distress. In Chapter 6, Rod MacLeod reminds us that caring for people who are dying is an integral part of every doctor's clinical experience and that many doctors experience anxiety and apprehension when faced with the task of providing care for someone who is dying. The chapter examines some of the fears faced by both clinician and patient and describes the nature of hope in a person faced with a major life altering and shortening diagnosis. The work involved is less about the lengthening of life and more about assisting patients to maximize the quality and experience of the time they have remaining. Much of the chapter discusses the concerns and anxieties experienced by physicians; it concludes with discussion of the place of a spiritual dimension in the life of the patient and those caring for them. Some of these experiences for medical students are also described in Chapter 3.

In Chapter 7, Beth Hudnall Stamm, Laurie Anne Pearlman, and I discuss the role that compassion fatigue and vicarious trauma from exposure to distressing experiences can have on physicians. The notion of compassion fatigue and vicarious trauma are relatively recent and are of increasing interest to researchers and those concerned about the emotional and psychological distress that can result from exposure to the trauma of significant others, both patients and colleagues. The messages relayed in this chapter apply not only to physicians but also to all health care workers—both professional and voluntary. However, it is the physicians who are charged with the role of caring for individuals and their families and assisting them to maximize their health and quality of life yet have received little attention regarding their own needs for self-care and well-being. We present recent research that examines the role that resilience, empathy, spirituality, and emotionality may play in helping manage the effects of compassion fatigue. We also discuss the place of compassion satisfaction— the joys and pleasures one receives from one's work—in the work of a physician.

Chapter 8 explores the impact that the medico-legal process has on the health and well-being of the physician, the physician's practice of medicine, and how they relate to their patients. Some practice changes may be for the better, but others may interfere with the exercise of sound clinical judgment. The four authors—Louise Nash, Michele Daly, Elizabeth van Ekert and Patrick Kelly—report the findings of their study of Australian physicians and describe some of the changes to medical practice resulting from involvement in a medico-legal episode, such as a compensation claim, a complaint, an investigation, or a criminal charge. In addition, the study examines the potential for psychiatric morbidity and hazardous alcohol use among physicians. The authors conclude their chapter with important advice for the physician when involved in a medico-legal enquiry regarding their practice.

In Chapter 9, Fraser C. Todd discusses why physician ill-health is of increasing concern. Likely consequences include the potential for risk to patients, as well as physicians' health risks from not attending to their own health needs as promptly as they attend to those of their patients' and therefore presenting late for treatment. A high proportion of physicians who seek help do return successfully to their clinical role. The author examines the prevalence, detection, treatment, and prevention of physician impairment. He concludes with a request that physicians not only take their own health care seriously but also actively engage in changing the culture of their profession by caring for the health of their colleagues.

In Chapter 10, Simon Hatcher continues the theme of physician ill-health by exploring the ways in which physicians become patients and, in particular, why physicians present differently to other professionals. Hatcher describes how to recognize when a physician's health is becoming impaired and what to do when this happens.

Physicians' medical knowledge means that they can knowingly, or unknowingly, distort the presentation of their illness and may engage in self-diagnosis and self-treatment. The author discusses the difficulties in recognizing colleagues' distress and illness, and knowing what to do about it, along with the factors that contribute to the difficulty. He concludes with some practical suggestions of what to do when having a conversation with a physician whose clinical practice appears to be impaired.

In the final chapter of Section 2, Chapter 11, Erica Oberg, Felipe Lobelo, Robert Sallis, and Erica Frank remind us what is, in their view, the most important reason to care about physician health by describing outcomes of their "Healthy Doc = Healthy Patient" program. They present evidence that shows that healthy physicians are more likely to actively engage with their patients around developing and maintaining a healthy lifestyle, and that these patients, as a group, are healthier than the patients of physicians who have a less healthy lifestyle. The preceding chapters in this section all describe evidence of the range and consequence of stressors in the physician's work place. This last chapter clearly informs us that the costs of physician ill health are too high, and that by actively engaging in improving their own health physicians will then improve the health of the populations they care for.

REFERENCES

Cooper, C. L., Rout, U., & Faragher, B. (1989). Mental health, job satisfaction, and job stress among general practitioners. *British Medical Journal, 298*(6670), 366–370.

Deckard, G., Meterko, M., & Field, D. (1994). Physician burnout: an examination of personal, professional, and organizational relationships. *Medical Care, 32*(7), 745–754.

McCullough, D.J. (2000). First Encounter. In R. K. Young (Ed.) *A Piece of My Mind* (pp. 119–121). Hoboken, NJ, USA: John Wiley & Sons.

Riley, G. J. (2004). Understanding the stresses and strains of being a doctor. *Medical Journal of Australia, 18*(7), 350–353.

/// 6 /// MAINTAINING A BALANCE

Doctors Caring for People Who are Dying and their Families

ROD MACLEOD

WHAT DO PEOPLE WHO ARE DYING WORRY ABOUT?

People who are dying worry about further debilitation and dependency and about the loss of dignity that can accompany physical weakness and helplessness; they worry about pain and suffering and about arranging affairs and consequences for dependents. They worry about dying alone and about loss of control, ever changing roles, existential concerns, change in mental functioning, and the possibility or not of an afterlife (MacLeod & Carter, 1999).

Their families, on the other hand, worry about the possibility of not meeting the needs of the person who is dying. They, too, worry about pain and suffering (their own and that of the person they love) and not responding appropriately to the needs of that person. They worry about what death will be like and whether they will be able to carry on without that person in their lives.

All of us who care for people who are dying will have our own particular and personal concerns. Apart from ensuring that we have the appropriate knowledge and skills to deal with whatever events develop, one of the most important things we can do is to ensure that we care or at least have an awareness of the importance of care. This may sound like a fairly obvious statement, but it is worth unpacking for a moment to understand what it entails. In order to care, we should perhaps have the willingness and ability to engender hope in those we are caring for.

THE NATURE OF CARE IN MEDICAL PRACTICE

The concept of care needs to be clarified, as it is clearly a significant part of palliative medicine, yet the concept of care, and what that actually means, remains elusive in medical practice. Care in a medical context has at least two meanings. As a behavior, care is often thought to mean looking after people and attending to their bodily needs. As a motivation it can refer to being fond of someone, feeling sympathy or empathy for him or her, and being concerned for the person's well-being. It could be argued that the best caring professionals show both of these aspects of care in order to maintain a balance in their caring practice (MacLeod, 2001). In the clinical setting, the caring doctor exhibits two primary attributes: receptivity and responsibility (Branch, 2000). It is worth noting, too, that recent work showed that among the nurses who patients perceived as caring are also those who reported being most emotionally affected by the nurse-patient relationship and providing the greatest continuity of care (Perskey et al., 2008). These themes are further expanded, with reference to doctors and how patients perceived their caring, elsewhere in the literature (Janssen & MacLeod, 2010).

THE NATURE OF HOPE

A significant component of the way care is defined is to restore a sense of hope. But what exactly does hope mean in this context? For most people, the concept of hope involves a sense of future. In order to experience hope one must foresee a future for oneself. In his now classic works, Eric Cassell (1976) has written that, for many people who are dying, any notion of time stands still while it continues to move forward for the rest of the world. In discussing the disintegration of the self in his book *The Nature of Suffering and the Goals of Medicine* (1991), he writes of the perceived future that we all have and describes hope as one of the necessary traits of a successful life. He quotes Alasdair MacIntyre's (1979) definition, which is still appropriate today:

> Hope is in place precisely in the face of evil that tempts us to despair, and more especially that evil that belongs to our own age and condition...The presupposition of hope is, therefore, belief in a reality that transcends what is available as evidence.

A reality that transcends what is available as evidence is a tidy phrase to recall when helping to engender hope. It has been suggested that a terminal diagnosis "confronts people with their own mortality and strips them of many of their protective factors," including a "sense of an infinite futuristic hope" (Miyaji, 1993). It could also be argued that the acknowledgment of a "terminal diagnosis" can strip away a number of the protective layers from the doctor caring for that person as well. Most descriptions of hope incorporate some sense of a future, but an excessive emphasis on the future limits the possibilities for exploring the experience of hope in people who are dying who may be viewed by many in the medical profession as having little or no future (Nekolaichuk & Bruera, 1998).

Enhancing or maintaining the quality of life of people who are dying is a main goal of palliative care. It has been acknowledged that one of the most important components in enhancing the quality of life of people who are dying, especially in the Western world, is hope. Of the many attempts at defining hope, another definition that appeals in this context is that of a "multi-dimensional dynamic life force characterized by a confident yet uncertain expectation of achieving good, which is realistically possible and personally significant" (Dufault & Martocchio, 1985). The four central attributes of hope proposed a number of years ago by Farren et al. (1992) based on analyses from a number of disciplines are relevant to this discourse. These attributes are an experiential process, a spiritual process, a rational thought process, and a relational process.

The experiential aspect involves accepting what happens to individuals as part of "being"—what their life is actually like. The spiritual dimension accepts that there is a higher being or a sense of faith or order about something that has yet to be proven; a way of making sense or meaning of the world. The rational thought attribute of hope involves the setting of goals, establishing a sense of one's past, present, and future and maintaining a degree of control. The relational attribute of hope involves a feeling of being connected to others; creating or maintaining a balance between these elements becomes increasingly important at the end of life.

All of us have hope in our lives and the reality that faces many near the end of life is that their hopes have been dashed or will fail to be realized. With that will come a sense for those caring for them of "what would I do in this situation?" This, of course, is the basis of true empathy.

EMPATHY

Janssen, Walker & MacLeod (2008) suggest that empathy is the capacity to enter the subjective world of another. It involves our shared concepts and shared human nature (Gillett, 1993). Empathy should be considered here as having an affective and a cognitive component. It is the capacity to feel as the other person is thought to feel (Darwall's so-called "emotional match-making," 1998). In addition, it involves the abilities to reflect on why the other may feel that way and to show understanding of that feeling (Reynolds & Scott, 2000). Together these two aspects of empathy demonstrate that it is not purely a behavioral response to another person's emotional state, but is also affective and cognitive in nature. They also show that unlike sympathy, empathy has an "understanding" component that introduces a balance between sharing and separation or standing apart from the other (Janssen, Walker & MacLeod, 2008). This is an essential part of a caring patient-doctor relationship—perhaps the art of medicine. It is worthy of note here that showing empathy is not just an essential part of that relationship, it also predicts the reduction of negative patient symptoms and improves patient experiences and satisfaction (Reynolds & Scott, 2000). Knowing that someone cares can and does have a beneficial effect on one's sense of well-being.

PROFESSIONAL ANXIETIES ABOUT CARING FOR PEOPLE WHO ARE DYING

All health care professionals work within a system of health care that may or may not meet the needs of the people it is set up to serve. When someone is dying there may be a sense in which patients and doctors feel that the system "let them down" either due to bureaucratic issues or difficulty in accessing appropriate care. It is sometimes said that hospital teams are not good at "letting go" and families and other health professionals who are not part of that team may feel excluded from the active management of any given situation. In hospitals, it seems that sometimes it is often easier to institute or maintain what could be perceived as futile interventions in the face of impending death than it is to withhold or withdraw treatments at that time.

The fear of overlooking a potentially curable or treatable condition is a particular problem, especially for, but not restricted to, more junior doctors; there is a very real anxiety that accompanies the fear of failing to diagnose potentially manageable (but potentially fatal) situations such as hypercalcemia, vena caval obstruction, or spinal cord compression in people with advanced malignant disease. There is also increasing interest from the media about the apparent increase in iatrogenic disease—doctors are becoming increasingly aware of pharmaceutical side effects and interactions, particularly in this group of people, who often require complex drug regimens. This may be particularly relevant in the development of an evidence base in palliative care, where pharmaceuticals are often prescribed for effects outside their current licensed uses.

Other potentially taxing ethical dilemmas that confront clinicians near the end of life are related to decisions to withhold or withdraw artificial nutrition or hydration, whether or not to undertake cardio-pulmonary resuscitation, and requests for assistance to die and decision making for the "incompetent" patient. For some doctors, apprehension about legal duties and the potential for litigation may influence their own decision making. This apprehension can be alleviated by talking with colleagues who have broader experience and remembering that the balance between the relief of suffering and the maintenance of dignity is perhaps the primary goal of care at the end of life.

Many of these anxieties may be compounded by the doctor's or the patient's and families' belief that "things could have been done better." The patient may have been slow to present with a problem, the doctor may have been slow in diagnosing a problem, or the hospital may have been slow to instigate investigation or treatment at an early stage. Any of these issues can disrupt the therapeutic relationship and therefore the power imbalance between doctor and patient and may increase the anxiety of both parties. Discussion of these issues will be advantageous to all concerned and will create a more likely reduction in anxiety for patient and doctor alike, and so restoring that potential power imbalance between physician and patient.

Much of the focus on well-being and quality of life in the last two decades has been rightly on the patient, but more recently the gaze of interest has been on the medical professionals themselves (Association of Professors of Medicine, 2003). Those authors identify that physicians "now confront the stresses of increasing government regulations, malpractice suits, the business aspects of medicine, increased clinical demands, less time with patients, a rapidly expanding knowledge base, rising student debt, and how to balance their personal and professional lives (p.513)." These stressors equally apply to those who care for the dying. The authors quite rightly point out that the very real concept of physician distress has been identified in the literature for over 20 years but rather than reducing in its effect the changes in modern medical practice seem to have made that burden greater.

TEAMWORK

Working within a multidisciplinary team at the end of life brings challenges and rewards that are quite different from those faced by the sole practitioner working alone because of geographical remoteness or isolation. In palliative care, perhaps one of the most challenging aspects of teamwork is the blurring of roles as an increasing number of health care professionals become involved. In many instances it is not uncommon for a large number of health professionals to be involved in the care of one person and their family. This can lead to a sense of loss of professional control and certainty and the development of situations in which team members are exposed to the emotional reactions of each other, again potentially creating an imbalance. Much of the training and education of doctors is concerned with dealing with certainty, and the biomedical model within which we are taught to work encourages this. It is worth remembering that doctors only took control of the deathbed from the family and the priest in the late 18th century, and it may now be more appropriate to try to ensure that the patient and family engender a greater feeling of control or taking charge—again, redressing the balance.

The role of the doctor in all types of care is one of empowerment of the patient, and this should be no different in people who are close to death. MacLeod & Egan (2007) have reinforced the notion that rather than focusing on medical diagnosis and problems, teams providing specialist palliative care should at least ensure that care is structured around the complexity and disruptiveness of the patients' problems by listening to the voices of those patients (Skilbeck & Payne, 2005)—something of a shift in balance from previous practice, which tended to be more patriarchal. However, as a fallback position "until patients are able to discuss their experiences of illness in shared language, using symptoms and problems remains a starting point for initiating discussions with them" (p.329). There are, however, examples in which the patient voice can be clearly heard; sadly they often tell of inadequacies and problems in the ordering of a caring approach (Armstrong-Coster, 2005). Caring can be learned effectively, though, and nurtured in all of the health care professions.

The ethics of caring assume that connection to others is central to what it means to be human (Branch, 2000)—that "relationships, rather than alienation give meaning to our existence"(p.127). Central to the effective provision of care near the end of life by an interprofessional team is that those people who make up the team create a relationship with each other and assume not only a responsible attitude to their learning and care but also a receptivity to the needs of both their patients and other team members. This may seem like a tall order; however, the creation of an environment where value is placed on each individual irrespective of their profession or their experience is one way of ensuring that a caring and empathetic atmosphere is also created for patients (MacLeod & Egan, 2007).

It is worth acknowledging here that one of the reasons that interprofessional education is potentially different from uniprofessional education is because the values and learning objectives of the participating professions may not be aligned. However, it could be assumed that one aspect that would remain a constant is that there are shared values, particularly with respect to patient (and family) outcomes and that the team would practice with combined or integrated practices so that no one could doubt what the goals of care should be. In other words, teams need to have a shared understanding of what it is they are trying to achieve with each person and their family. In effective palliative care the team is used as a strategy to achieve a goal of improving the quality of life for people whose life expectancy is short. In their writing on the interdisciplinary team Lickiss et al. (2005) have suggested some fundamental prerequisites for effective and efficient teamwork: consensus and clarity regarding goals, objectives, and strategies; recognition of specific personal contributions of each team member; competence of each team member in his or her own discipline and understanding and respect for the competence and role of each team member and procedure; clear definition of tasks and responsibilities-accountability and means of communication within the teams; competent leadership appropriate to the structure and function of the team and the task at hand; procedures for evaluating the effectiveness and quality of team efforts; bereavement care of staff as appropriate; and recognition of the contribution of patients in furthering professional understanding.

The goal of the team then is to maintain a balance of control between the professions and the patient in order to achieve the *patient's* outcomes (desires, wishes, goals, etc.), and in order to achieve this we have to first know what they are. Part of the reality of team-working, though, is that each profession may have different goals of care depending on the various emphases of physical, psychological, social, and spiritual approaches. Consequently these goals must cohere in a shared vision of care derived from the patient narrative, and the team will require a forum in which to articulate this vision. If that team is to be successful, it will need the opportunity to properly reflect on what is being achieved (from the patients' and the practitioners' perspectives). Chris James, a number of years ago, in a review of professional knowledge, suggested that shared reflection with others who understand and can empathize with the professional life of each other is an especially valuable way of optimizing professional practice (James, 1993). This is why mentors, supervisors, preceptors, and critical friends and colleagues of all sorts are particularly valuable. "The non-judgmental conversation between or among collaborative practitioners where experience is reflected upon can be a profound and powerful learning experience for all concerned. Finding ways of encouraging collaborative reflection is an important professional development task." For medicine, with its historical systems of hierarchical relationships, collaborative reflection can be a challenge, one that is being broken down as a better understanding of the importance of collegial support is accepted. Professional supervision, though, has become acceptable and even mandatory in some specialist palliative care teams.

CONCERNS ABOUT MEDICATION

A separate yet distinct area of professional concern for medical practitioners is around the use of medication near the end of life. Despite the widespread use of strong opioid drugs, some doctors still have anxieties about the use of this group of drugs, particularly near the end of life. Principal anxieties about morphine, for example, relate to its sedative properties, its potential respiratory depression, and the potential for addiction, abuse, and euthanasia. In end-of-life care all of these "morphine myths" can be eliminated with meticulous attention to the detail of assessment and symptom management and the appropriate use of other pharmacological agents when necessary. An understanding of the pharmacology and therapeutic benefits of these drugs certainly needs to be gained early on in a doctor's career in order that explanations that are clearly understood about the goal of care and the purpose of the medication can be given to the patient and family. Similar anxieties may arise when considering the use of sedatives, tranquilizers, and hypnotics near the end of life. All of these groups of drugs have a legitimate place in palliative care and should not be withheld because of unjustified fears of shortening life. The doctor has a duty to understand the risks and benefits of each of these classes of drugs and balance them against each other in order to optimize their therapeutic benefit.

CONCERNS ABOUT THE FUTURE

A further source of anxiety is about managing a future that may be uncertain. In medical training, certainty has been the focus of much of what doctors have learned, and certainty is more easily managed than uncertainty. Care planning is easier when a finite time or goal is involved, and it is also easier for some clinicians to maintain hope when a greater degree of certainty is apparent. Roberts (2005) points out that for a number of reasons physicians seem "to have grown averse to predicting the future for patients and families even when asked directly. (p.261)" She points out that "when we know what is ahead of us we are freer to live more fully today (p.262)"—this could be as true for the patient and family as it is for the doctor. One of the challenges for clinicians is not to make unreal offers such as "there's no need to suffer" or "we'll make this better." Statements such as how we expect people to die need to be guarded, and once again the anxious doctor can inadvertently create anxiety for others while trying to alleviate it. For example, the use of the metaphor of dying as "going to sleep" can create huge disquiet for people as they get weaker and less able to stay awake. Attempts by the doctor to alleviate his or her anxiety by trying to explain all the possibilities of what might happen can also increase the patient's anxiety. Rather, as Roberts points out, we should expect physicians to listen, to ask previously unasked questions ("what do *you* think is going on?"), and to be honest, not to offer unrealistic hope but to face reality and offer a commitment to accompany people until the end of their life.

PERSONAL ANXIETIES

The anxieties of the doctor can also be felt on a much more personal level. For those people dealing with death and dying on a regular basis, the experience of repeated loss can be wearying. It can also seem burdensome for those who deal with death and dying infrequently. Working within a multidisciplinary team and with people who are dying can also mean doctors and others are subjected to strong emotions on a regular basis.

For many the challenge to medical idealism increases anxiety. The fact that the care of people who are dying, in some ways, forces us to face our own mortality and our own limitations, both personally and professionally, can produce a feeling of frailty. This can be exaggerated by a personal identification with the person who is dying.

For some, the intimacy that develops between patient and doctor near the end of life can be a threat. Generations of doctors have been told to "keep your distance," yet people near the end of life are vulnerable and often have feelings of helplessness. Intimacy is something that they often need, and this intimacy can take professional carers by surprise. Feelings of hopelessness and vulnerability may also be shared by the doctor. Although intimacy often does take us by surprise and may hold great promise for feeling connected to others, it is often accompanied by the fear that we may be overwhelmed by another's suffering (Barnard, 1995). "The fear of our own undoing in confrontation with chaos and disintegration is at the core of the fear of intimacy in palliative care" (p.22), and it is not until we can express and share these feelings that they can be addressed. Our ability to care and get close to people we are caring for may be influenced by attachment theory; how a person relates to others can be predicted by their experiences of attachment to others from infancy and all the way through their development. John Bowlby (1969/1982) suggested that there are four components of attachment: the desire to be near the people we are attached to; returning to the attachment figure for comfort and safety in the face of a fear or a threat; the attachment figure acts as a base of security from which to explore; and separation from that figure will induce anxiety.

Differing forms of attachment style can influence how we relate to others (Janssen et al. 2008). In institutional settings such as hospitals or hospices, patients (and families) can be vulnerable and apprehensive, thus increasing their need to feel attached to someone who is caring for them. Thompson and Ciechanowski (2003) have shown that an understanding of a patient's attachment style can make effective primary care more likely, and it is likely to be no different in end-of-life care in any setting. We need to ensure also that we have a good understanding of our own attachment style—a secure clinician is unlikely to become overwhelmed or to feel insecure when faced with a seemingly clingy or overanxious person they are caring for.[1]

---

[1] Attachment style questionnaires are available on the internet often based on the work of Mary Ainsworth.

Essentially, the four central tasks of clinical medicine are discovering what the matter is, finding the cause, determining a management plan, and predicting the future—all functions that can create a sense of imbalance if not attended to effectively. However, uncertainty is intrinsic to the nature of diagnosis and therapy, and in order to help reduce uncertainty we must know more about the processes that surround the life of people who are dying. This emphasizes the need for more undergraduate and postgraduate training for people in end-of-life care. At an undergraduate level the experience can be variable to say the least (Lloyd-Williams & MacLeod, 2004). But there is little doubt that the key to effective learning about the care of people who are dying is to learn *from* those people who are dying themselves (Janssen & MacLeod, 2010). Janssen and MacLeod's study sought to hear what patients approaching death had to say about their interactions with doctors and the care they felt they had been given so that doctors of the future could learn how to demonstrate that care more effectively. Using semistructured interviews they encouraged people dying of cancer to share their experiences and perspectives on care within the patient-doctor relationship. They demonstrated that participants' recollections of times with doctors showed that *authentic* demonstrations of care begin with those doctors looking for common ground with the patient as a fellow human being and individual above all else. The psychological and physical suffering that resulted from allowing stereotypical assumptions and behaviors to shape doctor-patient interaction was clear from the voices of those interviewed. Those authors call for a greater emphasis on transformative educational experiences (for examples see MacLeod & Egan, 2009) and on narrative medicine (for examples see Charon, 2001a, 2001b, 2004). They suggest that both approaches require students to acknowledge and act on the events that are the patients' experiences. Transformative learning happens when learners become critically aware of their own tacit assumptions and expectations, often in a "disorienting" manner, reflect on those and those of their patients, assess the way they interpret or understand those assumptions, and in this case perform a clinical action (care) in a different manner (Janssen & MacLeod, 2010). This increased awareness endorses the approach of the reflective practitioner—reflection being a key to achieving and maintaining a balance.

Ultimately, the anxiety of coping with the failure of medical treatment can, for some, challenge their beliefs in what it is they are trying to do. Many curricula have been developed to try to help clinicians acquire the skills and knowledge to provide effective care (for some examples see Hylton Rushton et al., 2009, Cairns et al., 2005),[2] but despite this,

---

[2] One effective example is to be found at the Australian Palliative Care Curriculum for Undergraduates (PCC4U) Project website www.pcc4u.org which gives up-to-date information on the PCC4U project including the aims, objectives and what the expected outcomes can be.

health professionals generally report deficiencies in their perception of being able to care for people near the end of life, with psychosocial and spiritual care being particularly singled out as being problematic. One of many novel approaches has been the "Being with Dying" professional training program (Halifax et al., 2006). This builds on contemplative practices that regulate attention and emotion, promote calm and resilience, reduce stress, and cultivate emotional balance. Some have used Tibetan Buddhist traditions to "demonstrate practical ways in which the wisdom and compassion of the Buddhist teachings can be of benefit to those facing illness or death and also to their families and caregivers" (Wasner et al., 2005, p100). Other examples include the use of poetry (for example see MacLeod, 2002, Coulehan & Clary, 2005), literature (for example Killick, 2009), or daily spiritual experiences and training (Holland & Neimeyer, 2005). There seems little doubt that the ability to see ways to consolidate and understand experiences around death and dying do help to equip practitioners to cope with it all more effectively.

SPIRITUALITY

There is also no doubt that there is an increasing interest and acknowledgement of the importance of our spiritual dimension both for the patient and for the carer (and that includes the professional carer, Sinclair et al., 2006). There has been confusion about the term "spirituality" in much of the literature; the word itself is derived from the Latin *spiritus* meaning something that is within the body, therefore providing the life force. It could be regarded as central to the domain of human existence that lies beyond the material— the aspect of life that gives a sense of meaning, connection, integrity, and hope (Wasner et al., 2005). Evidence of the lack of a universally agreed understanding of spirituality is seen in a recent Canadian analysis of spirituality definitions in palliative care, finding 71 articles and subsequent definitions (Vachon et al., 2009). These were helpfully categorized into 11 dimensions that make sense of what could be a complex notion: meaning and purpose in life, self-transcendence, transcendence with a higher being, feelings of communion and mutuality, beliefs and faith, hope, attitude toward death, appreciation of life, reflection upon fundamental values, the developmental nature of spirituality, and its conscious aspect.

So it is easy perhaps to see that this is a significant element of our life and work in end-of-life care. Despite this there is little in the medical education literature or practice about spirituality and its significance in health. Medical schools in the United States are perhaps furthest ahead in this area, thanks mainly to the pioneering work of Christina Puchalski (for examples see Puchalski 2006a, 2006b, 2007, 2009). As Puchalski and others have demonstrated, there is now good evidence that spiritual care training for palliative care professionals can produce significant and sustained improvements in compassion toward the dying, compassion toward oneself, attitude to one's family, satisfaction with work, reduction in work-related stress, and in attitudes toward colleagues (see also for example Wasner et al., 2005).

CONCLUSION

Caring for one's self physically, psychologically, and spiritually will help in the practice of palliative care, bringing with it a sense of psychological and spiritual balance and a reduction in the number of anxieties and stressors that can accompany such work. Appropriate education and training in every aspect of palliative care is essential as a basis for this aspect of medical work. The development of a personal spiritual or religious philosophy, combined with a positive sense of self-regard and self-awareness, will all contribute to a sense of emotional well-being and a more balanced approach to care.

Working with people who are dying is at the same time a rewarding and a challenging aspect of any doctor's professional (and personal) life, and it is not something that any doctor should do on his or her own. Supportive teamwork and the development of realistic expectations of what that team can provide will help in the overall reduction of many of the anxieties identified in this chapter and therefore help practitioners maintain a balance in their professional practice. Care for people who are dying is also an area where many clinicians find that professional supervision and mentoring can be beneficial. The challenge for all carers is to be able to identify both personal and professional anxieties and limitations and deal with them. Facing one's own mortality, sharing control, facing challenges to one's own beliefs, and learning to *be* with patients, not just doing things for them, will enable doctors to maintain a balance and face those challenges more effectively, therefore encouraging a more humane and rewarding approach to the care of people who are dying.

REFERENCES

Armstrong-Coster, A. (2005). *Living and dying with cancer*. Cambridge University Press: Cambridge.

Association of Professors of Medicine (2003). The well-being of physicians. *American Journal of Medicine* 114, 513–519.

Barnard, D. (1995) The promise of intimacy and the fear of our own undoing. *Journal of Palliative Care* 11(4), 22–26.

Bowlby, J. (1969/1982) *Attachment and Loss Vol 1: Attachment*. New York: Basic Books.

Branch, W.T. (2000) The ethics of caring and medical education. *Academic Medicine*, 75, 127–132.

Cairns, W., Adler, J., Agar, M., Auret, K., Brogan, R., Brooksbank, M. et al.(2005). *Curriculum for the training and professional development of specialists in palliative medicine*. Sydney, Australia: Australasian Chapter of Palliative Medicine and Royal Australasian College of Physicians.

Cassell, E. (1976). *The Healer's Art*. Cambridge, Massachusetts: MIT Press.

Cassell, E. (1991). *The Nature of Suffering and the Goals of Medicine*. Oxford: Oxford University Press.

Charon, R. (2001a). Narrative medicine: Form, function and ethics. *Annals of Internal Medicine, 134,* 83–87.

Charon R. (2001b). Narrative medicine: A model for empathy, reflection, profession and trust. *JAMA, 286,* 1897–1902.

Charon, R. (2004). Narrative and medicine. *New England Journal of Medicine, 350,* 862–864.

Coulehan, J. & Clary, P. (2005). Healing the healer: Poetry in palliative care. *Journal of Palliative Medicine* 8(2); 382–389.

Cushing, H. (1926). *The life of Sir William Osler*. New York: Oxford University Press.

Darwall, S. (1998). Empathy, sympathy, care. *Philosophical Studies, 89,* 261–282.

Dufault, K. & Martoccio, B. (1985). Hope: Its spheres and dimensions. *Nursing Clinics of North America. 20,* 379–391.

Farren, C.J., Wilken, C.S. & Popovich, J.M. (1992). Clinical assessment of hope. *Issues in Mental Health. 13,* 129–138.

Gillett, G. (1993). "Ought and well-being." *Inquiry, 36,* 287–306.

Halifax, J., Dossey, B. & Rushton, C. (2006). *Compassionate care of the dying: An integral approach*. Santa Fe, NM: Prajna Mountain Publishers.

Holland, J.M. & Neimeyer, R.A. (2005). Reducing the risk of burnout in end-of-life care settings: The role of daily spiritual experiences and training. *Palliative and Supportive Care, 3,* 173–181.

Hylton Rushton, C., Sellers, D.E., Heller, K.S. et al (2009). Impact of a contemplative end-of-life training program: Being with dying. *Palliative and Supportive Care, 7,* 405–414.

James, C.R. (1993). *Professional knowledge: what do we know?* Paper presented to English National Board Professional Conference, London, September 1993. Proceedings of the ENB. ENB, London.

Janssen, A.L. & MacLeod, R.D. (2010). What can people approaching death teach us about how to care? *Patient Education and Counseling 81*(2), 251–256.

Janssen, A., Walker, S. & MacLeod, R.D. (2008). Recognition, Reflection, and Role models: Critical elements in the education of care. *Palliative and Supportive Care 6*(4), 389–395.

Killick, A. (2009). Illuminating the path: What literature can teach doctors about death and dying. *Palliative and Supportive Care, 7,* 521–526.

Lickiss, J. N., Turner, K.S. & Pollock, M. L. (2005). The interdisciplinary team. In D. Doyle, G. Hanks, N. Cherny & K. Calman (Eds). *Oxford textbook of palliative medicine* (pp. 42–46). Oxford: Oxford University Press.

Lloyd-Williams, M. & MacLeod, R.D. (2004). A systematic review of teaching and learning in palliative care within the medical undergraduate curriculum. *Medical Teacher, 26*(8), 683–690.

MacIntyre, A. (1979). Seven traits for designing our descendants. *The Hastings Centre Report, 9,* 5–7.

MacLeod, R.D. & Carter, H. (1999). Health professionals' perception of hope: Understanding its significance in the care of people who are dying. *Mortality, 4*(3), 309–317.

MacLeod, R.D. (2001). On reflection: Doctors' learning to care for people who are dying. *Social Science & Medicine, 52,* 1719–1727.

MacLeod, R.D. (ed). (2002). *Snapshots on the journey—an anthology of poems through death and remembrance*. Wellington: Steele Roberts.

MacLeod, R. & Egan, A. (2007). Interprofessional education. In B. Wee, & N. Hughes (Eds). *Education in palliative care—building a culture of learning* (pp. 235–251).Oxford: Oxford University Press.

MacLeod, R.D. & Egan, A.G. (2009). Transformation in palliative care. In J. Mezirow & E. Taylor (Eds). *Transformative learning in action: Insights from community, workplace and higher education* (p. 111–121). San Fransisco: Jossey-Bass.

Miyaji, N.T. (1993). The power of compassion: Truth telling among American doctors in the care of dying patients. *Social Science & Medicine, 36*(3), 249–264.

Nekolaichuk, C.L. & Bruera, E. (1998). On the nature of hope in palliative care. *Journal of Palliative Care, 14*(1), 36–42.

Perskey, G. J., Nelson J. W., Watson, J. & Bent, K. (2008). Creating a profile of a nurse effective in caring. *Nursing Administration Quarterly, 32*, 15–20.

Puchalski, C. M. (2006a). *A time for listening and caring: Spirituality and the care of the chronically ill and dying.* Oxford: Oxford University Press.

Puchalski, C. M. (2006b). Spirituality and medicine: Curricula in medical education. *Journal of Cancer Education, 21*(1), 14–18.

Puchalski, C. M. (2007). Spirituality and the care of patients at the end-of-life: An essential component of care. *Omega, 56*(1), 33–46.

Puchalski, C.M. (2009). Physicians and patients' spirituality. Ethical concerns and boundaries in spirituality and health. *Virtual Mentor, 11*(10), 804–815.

Redinbaugh, E.M., Sullivan,.A.M., Block, S.D. et al (2003). Doctors' emotional reactions to recent death of a patient: cross sectional study of hospital doctors. *British Medical Journal, 327*, 185–190.

Reynolds, W. J. & Scott, B. (2000). Do nurses and other professional helpers normally display much empathy? *Journal of Advanced Nursing, 31*, 226–234.

Roberts, J. (2005). Describing the road to death. *British Medical Journal, 5*, 261–262.

Sinclair, S., Pereira, J., & Raffin, S. (2006). A thematic review of the spirituality literature within palliative care. *Journal of Palliative Medicine, 9*(2), 464–479.

Skilbeck, J.K. & Payne, S. (2005). End of life care: a discursive analysis of specialist palliative care nursing. *Journal of Advanced Nursing, 52*(4), 325–334.

Thompson, D. & Ciechanowski, P.S. (2003). Attaching a new understanding to the patient-physician relationship in family practice. *Journal of the American Board of Family Practice, 16*, 219–226.

Wasner, M., Longaker, C., Fegg, M.J. & Borasio, G.D. (2005). Effects of spiritual care training for palliative care professionals. *Palliative Medicine, 19*, 99–104.

Vachon, M., Fillion, L., & Achille, M. (2009) A conceptual analysis of spirituality at the end of life. *Journal of Palliative Medicine, 12*(1), 53–59.

PHYSICIAN STRESS

Compassion Satisfaction, Compassion Fatigue and Vicarious Traumatization

PETER HUGGARD, BETH HUDNALL STAMM, AND LAURIE ANNE PEARLMAN

INTRODUCTION

A considerable number of physicians are struggling with professional distress due to their working conditions and professional experiences (Balch, Freischlag & Tait, 2009). Stress and burnout have been linked to the quality of patient care. A study of 115 medical residents found that 76% met criteria for burnout and that these physicians were significantly more likely to report suboptimal patient care at least monthly (Shanafelt, Bradley, Wipf, & Back, 2002). The work, and the environment in which a physician practices their art and science, have been cited as possible causes of distress (Riley, 2004). Riley reported the emotional climate of the "professional life" of a doctor as high intensity of work, conflicting time demands, heavy professional responsibility, frequent work in an environment with reduced physical and social resources, threat of medico-legal action, and limited power to alter the work conditions. He summarized this as working in an environment with a "lack of control or lack or reward in the face of unrelenting effort" (p. 350). He concluded his article by saying that "the prospect of a lifetime of joyless striving is unacceptable" (p. 353).

There may be punitive or stigmatizing consequences for resisting or "pushing back" against a life of "joyless striving." Center and colleagues (2003), in their American

Foundation for Suicide Prevention consensus statement published in the Journal of the American Medical Association, concluded that there were punitive outcomes for physicians acknowledging and seeking treatment for mental health problems. These punitive problems include stigma as well as censure by licensing boards and removal of patient care practice privileges. A core recommendation of the consensus statement is that there should be an organizational and peer culture change to reduce the stigma and increase mental health help-seeking among physicians. One of these changes is recognizing the problem of the effect of providing care to the physicians themselves.

The Effect of Work-related Stress on Physicians

Research examining the effects of work on physicians emerged as a coherent body of literature in the late 1980s and early 1990s. Emotional exhaustion was identified as a significant consequence of the work of a physician. Deckard and colleagues (Deckard, Meterko & Field, 1994) found that, 58% of doctors reported scores of high emotional exhaustion, and that high workload and a low degree of influence were the strongest predictors of emotional exhaustion. Environmental factors leading to physician stress have been reported to include the demands of the job and patients' expectations, interference with family life, constant interruptions at work and home, and administration tasks, which were the highest predictors of job dissatisfaction (Cooper, Rout, & Faragher, 1989; Sutherland & Cooper, 1993).

Physician-in-training experience may expose young physicians to individual and program training demands, such as the tendency to work excessive hours, and may promote an overdeveloped sense of responsibility as well as a trait of compulsive perfectionism. All of these factors are also thought to contribute to physician stress. A common response to this stress is to work harder, which can lead to emotional isolation, and an inability to seek collegial support and guidance (Kam, 1998). Other authors have suggested the inclusion of specific aspects in physicians' training such as sessions which allow trainees to examine their beliefs and attitudes towards being a physician. These beliefs and attitudes include the way in which physicians emotionally respond to their patients and to challenging clinical situations and aim to promote the acknowledgement of their own needs and the development of strategies to effectively care for themselves (Novack et al., 1997).

Healthcare Self-Neglect as a Result of Physician Stress

Physicians often neglect to arrange for their own medical care, particularly by not having their own general practitioner (Kay, Mitchell, & Del Mar, 2004; Pullen, Lonie, Lyle,

Cam & Doherty, 1995; Richards, 1999; Rogers, 1998). Richards's (1999) study showed that many New Zealand doctors claimed to be working under substantial stress, and, although many reported having a family doctor, relatively few had regular checkups. This later finding was also reported by Rogers (1998) who described physicians' behavior model towards their own medical care as one that included delusion, denial and delay, self-investigation, self-diagnosis, self-treatment, and self-referral. He believed that this may explain the behaviors of doctors not seeking help and their difficulty in entering into a patient role. Rogers ascribed this pattern to a medical culture which appeared to foster and construct inappropriate health-seeking behaviors in doctors, and postulated that the application of a behavioral change model could facilitate the doctor-as-patient role.

These findings appear to shed light on the difficulties found in the duality of the role of doctor and patient and may explain, at least in part, the difficulty experienced by doctors in acknowledging their own needs and taking action that will provide them with the same level of medical care enjoyed by their patients. A study that attempted to identify data on doctors' health and their health maintenance behavior described the lack of such data as "surprising, if not disgraceful" (Kay et al., 2004, p. 369). An anonymous questionnaire asking about past emotional distress that was sent to doctors in a large London teaching hospital found that professional help was rarely sought and that the doctors did not appear to access available professional help even when it was available. Nonprofessional help was reported as coming from family and friends and doctors had difficulty disclosing psychological problems (King, Cockcroft, & Cooch, 1992).

A number of these studies have highlighted the consequence of failing to address the interpersonal interaction between doctor and patient as a contributor to stress and burnout, with some researchers reporting as many as 25% of doctors experiencing some psychiatric morbidity and burnout (Dowell, Hamilton, & McLeod, 2000; Dowell, Westcott, McLeod, & Hamilton, 2001; Ramirez et al., 1995; Ramirez, Graham, Richards, Cull, & Gregory, 1996; Snibbe, Radcliffe, Weisberger, Richards, & Kelly, 1989). Garelick et al. (2007) showed that depression, anxiety, interpersonal relationships, self-esteem, and work-related issues were the most common reasons that doctors present with mental health problems at specialist services for doctors. In this study of 121 doctors, 9% of the participants were identified as severely psychiatrically distressed.

Increased Suicide Risk for Physicians under Stress

In addition to the emotional distress noted above, Garelick et al. (2007) found 42% of the 121 physician survey respondents reported being at some risk of suicide. An international meta-analysis revealed that male physicians had an increased risk of suicide of 1.41 and females at 2.27 when compared with the general population (Schernhammer & Colditz, 2004). In an epidemiological study using U.S. death and census data from 1984 to 1992 Petersen and Burnett (2008) concluded that white female and older white physicians and dentists had increased suicide rates compared to the general population. Center and colleagues (2003), in their consensus statement, attributed the increased suicide risks among physicians to emotional and psychological problems typically caused or exacerbated by their work as physicians.

Together these studies paint a compelling picture of the difficulty that doctors face in their work and in managing their own health needs. In particular, there is an individual and work culture reluctance to identify and utilize appropriate resources for emotional and psychological support. This is perhaps due, as Center et al. (2003) concluded, to stigma and punitive outcomes. For a doctor to continue to work in an emotionally-charged environment, he or she will need well-developed coping mechanisms. These include the development of positive psychological states, the establishment and utilization of appropriate social support networks, a process in which they can talk about the suffering of their patients, and a degree of hardiness and resiliency. An absence of resiliency and emotional competence, in the face of difficult work, would appear to contribute to a physician's stressful existence.

THE POSITIVE AND NEGATIVE ASPECTS OF PROVIDING CARE

Workers who feel committed to or responsible for helping people who are suffering can have both positive and negative experiences and even changes in their ways of interacting with the world as a result of their work as helpers. Ongoing efforts to help others who have been hurt can lead to changes in a person's day-to-day relationship with their work, their ability to conduct their work, and their overall psychological, physical, and spiritual well-being reaching far beyond the work setting. Some negative and positive aspects are related to providing care in general and some are related to providing care to trauma survivors in particular.

Three people defined the landscape of the negative, as well as the positive aspects of caring, each offering language to describe the terrain. Figley (1995) introduced the concept of compassion fatigue (CF), Pearlman the concept of vicarious trauma (VT; McCann & Pearlman, 1990), and Stamm (1995/1999) focused on secondary traumatic stress (STS). Both Stamm (Stamm, 2002) and Pearlman (McCann & Pearlman, 1990; Pearlman & Caringi, 2009; Pearlman & Saakvitne, 1995) later recognized the positive, and transformative, aspects of caring. Stamm focused on compassion satisfaction and the positive aspects relating to providing care, and Pearlman on the rewards of doing the work (Saakvitne & Pearlman, 1996) and the vicarious transformation that can occur in physicians (Pearlman & Caringi, 2009). Other authors have conceptualized certain positive changes resulting from trauma work as vicarious posttraumatic growth (Arnold, Calhoun, Tedeschi, & Cann, 2005) or vicarious resilience (Hernández, Gansei, & Engstrom, 2007).

Some authors correctly noted inconsistencies in the conceptualization and measurement of CF and VT and made attempts to separate the definitions (cf. Baird & Kracen, 2006; Wilson & Thomas, 2004). While there are differences, the constructs are not competitive but each contributes to the overall understanding and articulation of the positive and negative aspects of caring. Vicarious traumatization and transformation speak to the traumatized person's long-term construction of their self-awareness and self-perception. Compassion satisfaction and compassion fatigue speak to the "here and now" perceptions of one's work with trauma victims, something that can be compared to taking one's blood pressure, pulse, and temperature to establish a current state of wellness. Alternately, VT is more aligned with an overall examination of one's health and wellness across time. Another metaphor would be VT as a vessel and CS/CF as a snapshot of what is in the vessel.

What follows is a discussion of the various concepts based on the most current theory and research of the above constructs. The advances in the theory and constructs are based on research and on continuing theoretical work. All of the concepts are related to helping those who have been hurt and experienced extremely stressful events that could be traumatizing.

Table 7.1 summarizes core concepts of the negative and positive aspects of caring for people who have been traumatized. This table is simplistic but helps convey an image

TABLE 7.1 Synthesizing and Integrating Compassion Satisfaction and Compassion Fatigue with Vicarious Trauma and Vicarious Transformation

| | Positive Aspects | | Negative Aspects | | |
Characteristic	Compassion Satisfaction	Vicarious Transformation	Burnout	Secondary Trauma	Vicarious Trauma
Current, here and now state of relationship to helping those who have been hurt	X		X	X	
Long-term state of relationship to helping those who have been hurt		X			X
Schemas, world view		X			X

(continued)

TABLE 7.1 (Continued)

Characteristic	Positive Aspects		Negative Aspects		
	Compassion Satisfaction	Vicarious Transformation	Burnout	Secondary Trauma	Vicarious Trauma
Beliefs and values about one's self	X	X	X	X	X
Day-to-day perception of ability to do work	X		X		X
Sense of altruism	X	X	X	X	X
Ego resources			X		X
Ability to keep up with resources, changes, and skills in one's field	X		X		X
Feeling helpless about being able to provide care			X		X
Feeling alone and unsupported			X	X	X
Being frightened for self or loved ones by work or by something related to work				X	X
Ability to manage strong affect					X
Decision-making ability			X	X	X
Ability to foresee consequences	X		X	X	X
Ability to establish & maintain boundaries			X		X
Symptoms of depression			X	X	X
Symptoms of traumatic stress				X	
Feelings of hope	X	X	X	X	X
Ability to maintain sense of self		X			X
Transcendence/spirituality		X	X		X
Desire to continue work as a helper for those who have experienced trauma	X	X	X	X	X
Feelings of being supported by coworkers and colleagues	X	X	X	X	X

of how the parts fit together. Many characteristics are affect-neutral such as "day to day perception of ability to do one's work." There can be both positive and negative aspects in care provision impacts. For example, burnout may reduce one's perception of ability while compassion satisfaction may increase it. Thus, X's in columns are associated with a positive or negative side of the characteristic.

Vicarious Traumatization and Vicarious Transformation

Both vicarious traumatization and vicarious transformation are change processes (McCann & Pearlman, 1990; Pearlman & Caringi, 2009). Vicarious traumatization and transformation are changes in psychological needs-based beliefs, self-capacities, ego resources, and frame of reference that can occur across time when providing assistance in response to others' suffering and need. Beliefs, also known as schemas, are inner working models (Bowlby, 1969) by which a person defines and understands himself or herself in relation to others. Self-capacities, a less studied part of VT, are also sensitive to the impact of trauma work (Saakvitne, Gamble, Pearlman, & Lev, 2000). Self-capacities are used to regulate the internal world. They include sense of self-worth, inner connection with others, and affect tolerance (Pearlman, 1998). Finally, frame of reference refers to the big picture: people's identity, world view, and spirituality. Experiencing others' suffering and trauma can challenge a person's belief system and lead to negative outcomes for that person, including negative changes in all three of these realms: beliefs, self-capacities, and frame of reference. Engaging and responding directly to the challenges of VT can lead to positive changes in these realms, known as vicarious transformation (Pearlman & Caringi, 2009).

Vicarious Traumatization (VT)

One aspect of VT is evident when an individual's schemas have been disturbed by experiences that are not consistent with one's previous understandings. Those schemas that are sensitive to the effects of direct and indirect trauma include safety, trust, esteem, intimacy, and control (Pearlman, 2003). For example, a person may believe that humanitarian workers are all altruistic and good. This belief could be challenged if there were evidence that a humanitarian worker was stealing donated food and selling it for profit. Challenges to beliefs can result in negative changes in relationships.

Self-capacities affect the manner in which people relate to themselves. Self-capacities incorporate the ability to manage strong affect, maintain a sense of self-worth, and maintain an inner connection with others. Ego resources are abilities that affect the management of the interpersonal world, such as judgment, decision making, and the abilities to foresee consequences and to establish and maintain boundaries. Frame of reference, the big-picture ways people experience and make sense of the world, includes spirituality, which is also potentially affected by both vicarious trauma and transformation. Within Pearlman's framework, spirituality is people's experience of meaning and hope and awareness of all aspects of life, including non-tangible and non-material aspects, transcendence, and dimensions of experience related to something greater than the individual.

Professional Quality of Life: Compassion Satisfaction and Compassion Fatigue

Professional quality of life (ProQOL) is how one feels in relation to his or her work as a helper. Both the positive and negative aspects of doing one's job influence one's ProQOL. Thus ProQOL incorporates two aspects, the positive (compassion satisfaction, CS) and the negative (compassion fatigue, CF). CF breaks into two parts. The first part concerns things such as such as exhaustion, frustration, anger, and depression typical of burnout (BO). The second part, Secondary traumatic stress (STS), is a negative feeling driven by fear and work-related trauma.

Compassion satisfaction is about the pleasure one derives from being able to do their work well. People may find positive feelings and pleasure because they can help others. People can experience CS in relation to their ability to interact with their colleagues and make meaningful contributions to their work environment or even the greater good of society. As noted above, compassion fatigue is composed of two parts: (a) burnout, being worn down and overwhelmed by work, and (b) secondary traumatic stress—that is, experiencing fear and from work-related traumatic stress exposure. Most people have an intuitive idea of what burnout is. From the research perspective, burnout is associated with feelings of hopelessness and difficulties in dealing with work or in doing your job effectively. These negative feelings usually have a gradual onset. People may feel that

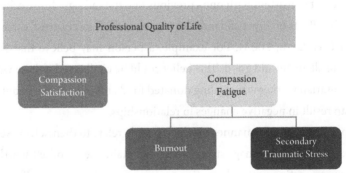

FIGURE 7.1 Professional Quality of Life with Positive and Negative Aspects of Working with Traumatized People.

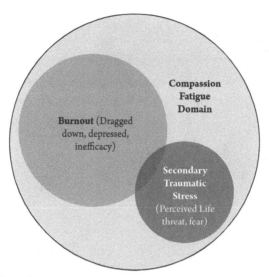

FIGURE 7.2 Compassion Fatigue Domain Containing Burnout and Secondary Traumatic Stress.

their efforts make no difference, or burnout can be associated with a very high workload or a non-supportive work environment. Some work-related trauma comes from helping those who have experienced extremely stressful events and suffering. Other work-related trauma arises from direct (primary) trauma. For example, a physician who attends service men and women who have been hurt by an IED (improvised explosive device) deal with the physical, psychological, and social results of the service person's injury. They may be haunted by the gruesome nature of the person's wounds or their terror of loud sounds. This haunting can begin to follow the physician in their overall life coloring or even adding trauma to their interpretation of their own experiences. This can be conceptualized as secondary trauma. Physicians may experience direct work-related trauma. A physician in an emergency department may be trapped between fighting parties while he or she tries to provide care for a person wounded in the conflict. This would be direct trauma. It could be that this same physician who is in the line of fire in this conflict is also dealing with gruesome injuries and terror with other patients.

The Interrelationships between Compassion Satisfaction and Compassion Fatigue

There are multiple spheres in which CS and CF occur. For physicians, the work environment itself is the usual ground for the entire process. The work environment contains influences that can be protective and resiliency promoting, such as supportive supervision. It can also contain negative influences as simple as not being able to find a parking place. These negative influences can pile on top of each other, effectively wearing away at a person's resiliency and their ego resources and making them vulnerable to other

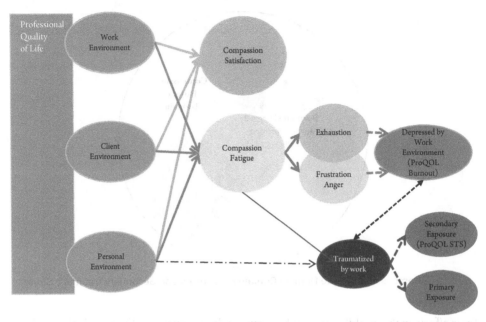

FIGURE 7.3 Theoretical Path Analysis of Positive and Negative Outcomes of Helping Those Who Have Experienced Traumatic Stress.

work-related negative stressors. The client environment is at the center of STS and a powerful part of CS and BO. If the client is traumatized and conveys his or her deep wounds to others, the helper may be affected by those wounds, even to the point of developing traumatic stress symptoms similar to those of the person they help. Alternately, the patient may be traumatized but is making great and encouraging strides toward health. This is a contributor to the physician's compassion satisfaction and resiliency.

A physician's personal environment underlies his or her professional self. The physician's life experiences and overall health may be protective, helping the physician to be resilient. Alternately, the physician may have a trauma history of their own. They may have family problems, or health problems, or financial problems. While none of these leads directly to work-related traumatic stress, they do leave a person vulnerable.

Figure 7.3 shows a theoretical pathway for the interaction between environments and their relationship with CS and CF.

MEASUREMENT OF THE POSITIVE AND NEGATIVE ASPECTS OF HELPING

Vicarious Traumatization

There are multiple measures that contribute to a good understanding of a person's VT. Most people have concentrated on schema alterations, not on self-capacities. A more complete picture of VT includes measures of self-capacities, ego resources, frame of reference (identity, world view, and spirituality), psychological needs, and trauma symptoms (McCann & Pearlman, 1990; Pearlman, 2001; Saakvitne et al., 2000). Two core aspects of VT are psychological needs (measured by the Trauma and Attachment Belief scale; Pearlman, 2003) and self-capacities (measured by the Inner Experience Questionnaire; Brock, Pearlman, & Varra, 2006).

Psychological Needs: Trauma and Attachment Belief Scale

The Trauma and Attachment Belief scale (TABS; Pearlman, 2003) is an 84-item self-report, paper-and-pencil test that assesses beliefs on a 6-point Likert scale with 1 = Disagree Strongly to 6 = Agree Strongly. It measures beliefs about self and others in relation to five human needs commonly affected by traumatic experience. The five needs are safety, trust, esteem, intimacy, and control. The scoring results in 11 scores: one score each for the *self* and *other* dimensions of the five need areas, and a total score.

The TABS subscales have reliability coefficients ranging from 0.79 to 0.92. There are established adult (over 18) and youth (age 9–18) norms. Adult norms are based on a heterogeneous sample of 1,743 individuals ages 18 and older. Youth norms are derived from a sample of 1,242 students, 9 to 18 years of age, from public schools throughout the United States.

Self-capacities: Inner Experience Questionnaire

The Inner Experience Questionnaire (IEQ, Brock et al., 2006) is a 24-item questionnaire assessing three self-capacities: (1) the ability to tolerate, manage, and integrate affective experience; (2) the ability to maintain a sense of self as viable and positive; and (3) the ability to maintain a sense of inner connection with others.

The IEQ has been reported to have reliability coefficients between 0.90 and 0.93 in a study examining the psychometric properties of this measure (Brock et al., 2006). This study reported a range of IEQ scores for young adults of between 1.00 and 4.50.

Professional Quality of Life Scale: Compassion Satisfaction and Compassion Fatigue (ProQOL)

The ProQOL (Stamm, 2009; www.proqol.org) is a 30-item measure with three scales of 10 items each. The three scales are Compassion Satisfaction, Burnout and Secondary Traumatic Stress. Items are rated on a 5-point Likert scale with 1 being "never" and 5 being "very often." The measure can be administered using paper and pencil or with an electronic version (Stamm, 2009). The mean for each scale is set at 50 and the standard deviation at 10, which allows direct comparisons to be made across the scales and across multiple studies. The average Compassion Fatigue score is 50 ($SD = 10$; $SEM = 0.29$; alpha scale reliability .88). The average score on Burnout scale is 50 ($SD = 10$; $SEM = 0.29$; alpha scale reliability .75). The average score on this scale is 50 ($SD = 10$; SEM; alpha scale reliability .81). Since 1990, over 3,000 cases have been collected or contributed to the ProQOL data bank. Normative data are based on a databank of 1,754 adult cases.

The measure demonstrates good construct validity with over two hundred papers published on the construct. Convergent and discriminant validity tests show that the three scales measure separate constructs. The Compassion Satisfaction scale is entirely distinct from the Compassion Fatigue scales. The inter-scale correlations show 2% shared variance ($r = -.23$; co-$\sigma = 5\%$; $n = 1187$) with Secondary Traumatic Stress and 5% shared variance ($r = -.14$; co-$\sigma = 2\%$; $n = 1187$) with Burnout. The compassion fatigue scales do share variance but measure different constructs with the shared variance likely reflecting the distress that is common to both conditions. The shared variance between these two scales is 34% ($r = .58$; co-$\sigma = 34\%$; $n = 1187$). The scales both measure negative affect but are clearly different; the BO scale does not address fear while the STS scale does.

There are two versions of the ProQOL: the full score and the simplified score. The full score is more specific but takes longer to score. It is best for research or organizational use. The simplified scoring is less specific but can be completed quickly and can be intuitively understood as scores are grouped as high, normal, and low. The self-scoring version is particularly good for training situations.

THE POSITIVE AND NEGATIVE ASPECTS OF PHYSICIANS PROVIDING CARE

Coping and Support

A very small number of studies have examined the effects on physicians of caring for patients. Benson and Magraith's paper (2005) discussed various supportive and preventive processes for mitigating the effects of compassion fatigue. Their main suggestion involved the use of Balint Groups as a means for doctors to explore the emotional challenges of their work. Balint Groups are small groups of six to eight doctors who meet with one or two facilitators to discuss clinical material from their practices, with a focus on the doctor-patient relationship. Using semi-structured interviews, Elder, Ricer, and Tobias (2006) studied ways in which family physicians identify, manage, and cope with difficult patient encounters. Although they did not measure compassion fatigue, these authors postulated that compassion fatigue develops when tensions occur between patient behaviors and physician traits. Huggard (2003a, 2003b) wrote two review articles examining the construct of compassion fatigue in physicians and offering some explanation as to the processes involved in its development and strategies for its management. Tehrani (2007) examined the construct of secondary traumatization from the perspective of identifying sources of support and coping methods. This study, which surveyed workers—including a small number of doctors—who assisted distressed and traumatized individuals, did not measure compassion fatigue. Rather, the author postulated that trauma workers were at risk of compassion fatigue should their fundamental assumptions, beliefs, and values be challenged.

Presence of Compassion Fatigue and Burnout in Physicians

Other than a study by Huggard (2009, 2011), the only study we identified that focused specifically on compassion fatigue in physicians was recently carried out by the Doctors-in-Training section of the Australian Medical Association. This survey, coordinated by Dr. Alex Markwell and reported in the *Medical Journal of Australia* (Markwell & Wainer, 2009), included the ProQOL III and surveyed work conditions and potential stressors in a group of approximately 1,000 resident doctors. In this study, a majority of participants met well-established criteria for low job satisfaction, high burnout, and high compassion fatigue. Another finding was that these resident doctors were concerned for their own health (71%) and for the health of a colleague (63%).

The study by Huggard (2009) surveyed a group of resident physicians working in hospitals located in four different District Health Boards in New Zealand. Participation in the survey was voluntary and anonymity of results was maintained throughout the study. Twenty-three percent (n = 253) of the total number of 1,100 invited participants completed the survey. Although this response rate is very low, some demographic data of the non-responders are known, such as that non-responders did not differ demographically from responders, thus enabling some conclusions to be made. The survey instrument for this study included measures of compassion fatigue, burnout, compassion satisfaction, the ProQOL III (Stamm, 2005); resilience, using the Connor Davidson Scale of Resilience (Connor & Davidson, 2003); empathy, using the Jefferson Scale of Physician Empathy (Hojat et al., 2001); spirituality, including religiosity, using the spirituality measures from Ryff's Scale of Psychological Well-being (van Dierendonck, 2005); and emotionality, using a scale developed by Huggard (2009). This latter measure included an eight-item measure identifying participants' sources of support. In additional to completing these measures, all participants had the opportunity to include any qualitative comments. A small number of resident doctors who had not participated in the survey were interviewed. They responded to the results of the survey and provided insight as to what changes in support or what additional support might have been useful in their undergraduate medical training as well as their sources of support in residency. Measures of resilience, empathy, spirituality, and emotionality were included in this study as an attempt to identify possible supportive processes and those that might at least mitigate the effects of compassion fatigue.

The results from this study were almost identical to results for compassion fatigue and burnout previously reported by Stamm (2005) in that approximately 25% of the participants scored high to very high on the measures of these two constructs. The number of participants scoring highly for burnout is similar to results found in another New Zealand study that examined the level of burnout, and the benefits of peer support, in a group of 50 specialist physicians (Bruce, Conaglen, & Conaglen, 2005). Although Bruce et al. used a different measure of burnout—the Maslach Burnout Inventory (Maslach & Jackson, 1986)—results were similar to the Huggard (2009) study in that 28% of their participants were at the greatest risk of burnout. The reported level of burnout in Huggard's study is of concern and indicates the need for effective strategies for managing the emotional and psychological demands that result from exposure to and engagement with the suffering of others. Years spent as a junior doctor have previously been reported to be extremely stressful (Deckard, Meterko, & Field, 1994; Kam, 1998; Riley, 2004). Many doctors are working as a senior resident doctor in their specialty, generally for long hours, and with the need to undertake considerable study in order to be successful in their final examinations that qualify them for specialist or consultant status. Also, at the more junior stage, physicians are likely to be faced with considerable financial burden as they seek to repay student loans, as well as establish themselves in relationships with a spouse or partner, and possibly start a family.

The absence of any main effects for the demographic or contextual variables in Huggard's (2009) study indicated that, over a large range of clinical specialties, in different locations, and with varying degrees of experience of support, compassion fatigue is still present in these physicians to a similar extent as in other health professionals previously surveyed (Stamm, 2005).

Compassion Satisfaction in Physicians

Scores in Huggard's (2009) study for compassion satisfaction were low, with many more participants than expected scoring below the 25th quartile, as compared with those previously reported (Stamm, 2005). This is of concern in that it may indicate significantly reduced capacity on the part of individuals to receive enjoyment, pleasure, and satisfaction from their work. The consequences of reduced satisfaction in one's medical practice have previously been linked to ill health (Leigh, Kravitz, Schembri, Samuels, & Mobley, 2002). Interestingly, results from Huggard's study are different than those found in a New Zealand survey of 593 physicians (Grant, 2004). Using a different measure— the Warr, Cook, and Wall scale (1979)—findings indicated that the level of job satisfaction was high in these physicians. There are several possible reasons for such a difference. Grant's sample had different characteristics from Huggard's study in that his sample was not restricted to resident doctors but included hospital-based consultant physicians and surgeons. In addition, the Warr et al. (1979) job satisfaction measure was developed from a sample of blue-collar workers. There may be inherent difficulties in attempting to compare results from studies that have used different instruments, developed with different populations, to measure similar constructs. Results reported in these studies represent those obtained at one point in time. Differences in the timing of sampling may also account for differences between studies.

Resilience and Emotional Competency

Huggard (2009) found significant negative relationships among compassion fatigue, resilience, and emotionality; and among burnout, resilience, empathy, and emotionality. Statistically significant positive relationships were identified between compassion satisfaction, and resilience, empathy, spirituality, and emotionality. Although there has been much written about the benefits of resilience, particularly in a context of focusing on resilience building rather than risk prevention (Kumpfer, 1999), this study appears to be the first that has attempted to measure resilience in a group of physicians for the purpose of relating resilience to the effects of compassion fatigue.

A key component of Huggard's (2009) study was the examination of the physicians' beliefs about their emotional competence—emotionality—and that a reduced level of emotional competence may contribute to the development of compassion fatigue. The research suggested that both resilience and emotionality impact on the prediction of compassion fatigue, and it supports the development of therapeutic interventions aimed at developing these two factors as a means of mitigating the effects of compassion fatigue. As well as this understanding, there should be a realization and acceptance that certain emotional responses are normal and are to be expected when working in a clinical therapeutic relationship. Such therapeutic interventions should aim to enhance intrapersonal characteristics and behaviors relating to resilience, boundary-setting in clinical and collegial relationships, spiritual connection, seeking supportive professional and personal relationships, and emotional competence—all factors that may develop and enhance supportive frameworks that serve to prevent the development of compassion fatigue.

All health professionals, in particular physicians, adopt the role of caring for individuals and populations by assisting them to achieve better health and quality of life. In contrast, the population receiving comparatively little attention about their own health and well-being is the physicians themselves. Attempts to understand the nature of compassion fatigue in physicians have been largely ignored despite the possibility of it being present at all times. This is the nature of clinical work—clinicians are exposed to the suffering of their patients and clients. However, unless meaning is made of this suffering and clinicians develop ways of integrating these experiences into their lives as well as developing and maintaining useful supportive behaviors, the potential exists for them to become vicariously traumatized and experience compassion fatigue. Strategies that provide necessary support at an organizational, work-team, and personal level need to be in place and integrated into the daily existence of doctors as a way of assisting doctors to understand and manage the exposure to and effects of compassion fatigue, as well as providing support to other colleagues.

The "conversations" in relation to compassion fatigue and physicians are relatively new and not commonly held—there is a need for a greater voice in discussing this important component of clinical practice.

REFERENCES

American Psychiatric Association. (1994). *Diagnostic and statistical manual of mental disorders* (4th ed.). Washington, DC: American Psychiatric Association.

Arnold, D., Calhoun, R.G., Tedeschi, R., & Cann, A. (2005). Vicarious posttraumatic growth in psychotherapy. *Journal of Humanistic Psychology, 45*(2), 239–263.

Australian Medical Association (2008). *AMA Survey Report on Junior Doctor Health and Wellbeing.* Sydney, Australia: Australian Medical Association.

Balch, C.M., Freischlag, J.A. & Shanafelt, T.D. (2009). Stress and burnout among surgeons: Understanding and managing the syndrome and avoiding the adverse consequences. *Archives of Surgery, 144*(4), 371–376.

Benson, J., & Magraith, K. (2005). Compassion fatigue and burnout: the role of Balint groups. *Australian Family Physician, 34*(6), 497–498.

Bowlby, J. (1969). *Attachment and loss.* London: Hogarth.

Brock, K.J., Pearlman, L.A. & Varra, E.M. (2006). Child maltreatment, self capacities, and trauma symptoms: Psychometric properties of the inner experience questionnaire. *Journal of Emotional Abuse, 6*(1), 103–125.

Baird, K., & Kracen, A. C. (2006). Vicarious traumatization and secondary traumatic stress: A research synthesis. *Counselling Psychology Quarterly, 19*(2), 181–188.

Bruce, S.M., Conaglen, H.M., & Conaglen, J.V. (2005). Burnout in physicians: a case for peer-support. *Internal Medicine Journal, 35,* 272–278.

Center, C., Davis, M., Thomas, D., Ford, D.E., Hansbrough, W., Herndin, . . . Silverman, M.M. (2003). Confronting depression and suicide in physicians: A consensus statement. *JAMA* 289:3161–3166.

Collins English Dictionary (1986). *Collins Dictionary of the English Language.* London: William Collins Sons & Co. Ltd.

Connor, K. M., & Davidson, J. R. T. (2003). Development of a new resilience scales: the Connor-Davidson Resilience scale (CD-RISC). *Depression and Anxiety, 18,* 76–82.

Cooper, C. L., Rout, U., & Faragher, B. (1989). Mental health, job satisfaction, and job stress among general practitioners. *British Medical Journal, 298*(6670), 366–370.

Deckard, G., Meterko, M., & Field, D. (1994). Physician burnout: an examination of personal, professional, and organizational relationships. *Medical Care, 32*(7), 745–754.

Dowell, A. C., Hamilton, S., & McLeod, D. K. (2000). Job satisfaction, psychological morbidity and job stress among New Zealand general practitioners. *New Zealand Medial Journal, 113*(1113), 269–272.

Dowell, A. C., Westcott, T., McLeod, D. K., & Hamilton, S. (2001). A survey of job satisfaction, sources of stress, and psychological symptoms among New Zealand health professionals. *New Zealand Medical Journal, 114*(1145), 540–543.

Elder, N., Ricer, R., & Tobias, B. (2006). How respected family physicians manage difficult patient encounters. *Journal of the American Board of Family Medicine, 19*(6), 533–541.

Figley, C.R. (Ed.) (1995). *Compassion fatigue: Secondary traumatic stress disorders from treating the traumatized.* New York: Brunner/Mazel.

Figley, C. F., & Stamm, B. H. (1996). Psychometric review of compassion fatigue self-test. In B. H. Stamm (Ed.), *Measurement of stress, trauma, and adaptation* (pp. 127–130). Lutherville, MD: Sidran Press.

Garelick, A. L., Gross, S. R., Richardson, I. von der Tann, M., Bland, J., & Hale, R. (2007). Which doctors and with what problems contact a specialist service for doctors? A cross sectional investigation. *BMC Medicine, 5:* 26.

Grant, P. (2004). Physician job satisfaction in New Zealand versus the United Kingdom. *New Zealand Medical Journal, 117*(1204). Accessed October 3, 2008, http://www.nzma.org.nz/journal/117-1204/1123/content.pdf

Hatem, C. (2006). Renewal in the practice of medicine. *Patient Education and Counseling, 62,* 299–301.

Hernández, P., Gangsei, D., & Engstrom, D. (2007). Vicarious resilience: A new concept in work with those who survive trauma. *Family Process, 46*(2), 229–241.

Hojat, M., Mangione, S., Nasca, T. J., Cohen, M. J. M., Gonnella, J. S., Erdmann, J. B., Veloski, J., & Magee, M. (2001). The Jefferson Scale of Physician Empathy: development and preliminary psychometric data. *Educational and Psychological Measurement, 61*(2), 349–365.

Huggard, P. K. (2003a). Compassion fatigue: How much can I give? *Medical Education, 37*(2), 163–164.

Huggard, P. K. (2003b). Secondary traumatic stress: Doctors at risk. *New Ethicals Journal, 6*(9), 9–14.

Huggard, P. K. (2009). Managing compassion fatigue: implications for medical education. Unpublished doctoral dissertation, The University of Auckland, New Zealand.

Huggard, P. & Dixon, R. (2011). "Tired of Caring": the Impact of Caring on Resident Doctors. Australasian Journal of Disaster and Trauma Studies, 2011(3), 105–112.

Kam, K. (1998). Finding balance: If not now, when? *Hippocrates, 12*(1), 1–7

Kay, M. P., Mitchell, G. K., & Del Mar, C. B. (2004). Doctors do not adequately look after their own physical health. *Medical Journal of Australia, 181*(7), 368–370.

King, M. B., Cockcroft, A., & Cooch, C. (1992). Emotional distress in doctors: Sources, effects and help sought. *Journal of the Royal Society of Medicine, 85* (10), 605–608.

Kumpfer, K.L. (1999). Factors and processes contributing to resilience: The resilience framework. In M. D. Glantz and J. L. Johnson (Eds.), *Resilience and Development: Positive Life Adaptations* (pp. 179–224). New York, NY: Kluwer Academics/Plenum Publishers.

Leigh, J. P., Kravitz, R. L., Schembri, M., Samuels, S. J., & Mobley, S. (2002). Physician career satisfaction across specialties. *Archives of Internal Medicine, 62,* 1577–1584.

Markwell, A. L. & Wainer, Z. (2009) The health and wellbeing of junior doctors: Insights from a national survey. *Medical Journal of Australia, 191*(8), 441–444.

Maslach, C. & Jackson, S.E. (1986). *Maslach Burnout Inventory Manual* (2nd Ed.). Palo Alto, CA: Consulting Psychologists Press Inc.

McCann, I. L., & Pearlman, L.A. (1990). Vicarious traumatization: A framework for understanding the psychological effects of working with victims. *Journal of Traumatic Stress*, 3(1), 131–149.

Novack, D. H., Suchmam, A. L., Clark, W., Epstein, R. M., Najberg, E., & Kaplan, C. (1997). Calibrating the physician: Personal awareness and effective patient care. *Journal of the American Medical Association*, 278(6), 502–509.

Pearlman, L. A. (1998). Trauma and the self: A theoretical and clinical perspective. *Journal of Emotional Abuse*, 1, 7–25.

Pearlman, L. A. (2003). *Trauma and attachment belief scale manual*. Los Angeles, CA: Western Psychological Services.

Pearlman, L.A., & Caringi, J. (2009). Living and working self-reflectively to address vicarious trauma. In C.A. Courtois & J.D. Ford (Eds.), *Treating complex traumatic stress disorders: An evidence-based guide* (pp. 202–224). New York, NY: Guilford Press.

Pearlman, L.A. (2001). The treatment of persons with complex PTSD and other trauma-related disruptions of the self. In J.P. Wilson, M.J. Friedman, & J.D. Lindy (Eds.), *Treating psychological trauma & PTSD*, pp. 205–236. New York, NY: Guilford Press.

Pearlman, L. A., & Saakvitne, K. W. (1995). *Trauma and the therapist: Countertransference and vicarious traumatization in psychotherapy with incest survivors*. New York, NY: Norton.

Petersen, M.R. & Burnett, C.A. (2008). The suicide mortality of working physicians and dentists. *Occupational Medicine*, 58(1), 25–29.

Pines, A. M. (1993). Burnout. In L. Goldberger and S. Breznitz (Eds.), *Handbook of stress: Theoretical and clinical aspects. 2nd edition* (pp. 386–402). New York, NY: Free Press.

Pullen, D., Lonie, C. E., Lyle, D. M., Cam, D. E., & Doughty, M. V. (1995). Medical care of doctors. *Medical Journal of Australia*, 162(9), 481–484.

Ramirez, A. J., Graham, J., Richards, M. A., Cull, A., Gregory, W. M., Leaning, M. S., Snashall, D. C., & Timothy, A. R. (1995). Burnout and psychiatric disorder among cancer clinicians. *British Journal of Cancer*, 71(6), 1263–1269.

Ramirez, A. J., Graham, J., Richards, M. A., Cull, A., Gregory, W. M., (1996). Mental health of hospital consultants: The effects of stress and satisfaction at work. *Lancet*, 347(9003), 724–728.

Richards, J. G. (1999). The health and health practices of doctors and their families. *New Zealand Medical Journal*, 112(1084), 96–99.

Riley, G. J. (2004). Understanding the stresses and strains of being a doctor. *Medical Journal of Australia*, 18(7), 350–353.

Rogers, T. (1998). Barriers to the doctor as patient role: A cultural construct. *Australian Family Physician*, 27(11), 1009–1013.

Saakvitne, K. W., & Pearlman, L. A. (1996). *Transforming the pain: A workbook on vicarious traumatization*. New York, NY: W. W. Norton & Company.

Saakvitne, K. W., Gamble, S., Pearlman, L., & Lev, B. (2000). *Risking connection: A training curriculum for working with survivors of childhood abuse*. Lutherville, MD: Sidran Press.

Saakvitne, K. W., & Pearlman, L. A. (1996). *Transforming the pain: A workbook on vicarious traumatization*. New York, NY: Norton.

Shanafelt, T. D., Bradley, K. A., Wipf, J. E., Back, A. L. (2002). Burnout and self-reported patient care in an internal medicine residency program. *Annals of Internal Medicine 136*, 358–367.

Schernhammer, E. S. & Colditz, G. A. (2004). Suicide rates among physicians: A quantitative and gender assessment (meta-analysis). *American Journal of Psychiatry 161*, 2295–2302.

Snibbe, J. R., Radcliffe, T., Weisberger, C., Richards, M., & Kelly, J. (1989). Burnout among primary care physicians and mental health professionals in a managed health care setting. *Psychological Reports*, 65(3 pt 1), 775–780.

Stamm, B. H. (Ed.) (1999). *Secondary traumatic stress: Self-care issues for clinicians, researchers, and educators, 2nd Edition*. Lutherville, MD: Sidran Press.

Stamm, B. H. (2002). Measuring compassion satisfaction as well as fatigue: Developmental history of the Compassion Fatigue and Satisfaction Test. In C. R. Figley (Ed.), *Treating compassion fatigue* (pp. 107–119). London: Taylor and Francis Ltd.

Stamm, B. H. (2009). *The Concise ProQOL Manual*. Pocatello, ID: ProQOL.org.

Stamm, B. H. (2005). *The ProQOL Manual*. Pocatello, ID: Idaho State University.

Sutherland, V. J., & Cooper, C. L. (1993). Identifying distress among general practitioners: predictors of psychological ill-health and job dissatisfaction. *Social Sciences and Medicine, 37*(5), 575–581.

Tehrani, N. (2007). The cost of caring: The impact of secondary trauma on assumptions, values, and beliefs. *Counselling Psychology Quarterly, 20*(4), 325–339.

van Dierendonck, D. (2005). The construct validity of Ryff's Scales of Psychological Well-being and its extension with spiritual well-being. *Personality and Individual Differences, 36*, 629–643.

Warr, P., Cook, J., & Wall, T. (1979). Scales for measurement of some work attitudes and aspects of psychological well-being. *Journal of Occupational Psychology, 52*, 129–148.

Wilson, J. P., & Lindy, J. D. (1994). *Countertransference in the treatment of PTSD*. New York: Guilford Press.

Wilson, J. P. & Thomas, R. B. (2004). *Empathy in the treatment of trauma and PTSD*. New York: Brunner-Routledge Publications.

/// 8 /// # THE MEDICO-LEGAL ENVIRONMENT AND HOW MEDICO-LEGAL MATTERS IMPACT THE DOCTOR

Research Findings from an Australian Study

LOUISE NASH, MICHELE DALY,
ELIZABETH VAN EKERT, AND PATRICK KELLY

A BACKGROUND TO THE MEDICO-LEGAL ENVIRONMENT

Many patients who are injured by negligent care are not compensated, whereas some of those who do receive compensation have not received negligent care (Localio et al., 1991; Brennan, Sox, & Burstin, 1996; Runciman, Merry, & Tito, 2003; Studdert et al., 2000). Compounding this is the high financial cost of litigation and the defensive medicine that it promotes (Berstein, MacCoour, & Abramson, 2008; Helland & Showalter, 2009). Furthermore, the tort system of law promotes a climate of blame and discourages the reporting of errors, which is a prerequisite to learning from them (Donaldson, 2003). Finally, the law can turn patients and doctors into adversaries (Rowe, 2004).

Australia, other commonwealth countries, and the United States of America (USA) inherited medical negligence as part of tort law from the United Kingdom (UK), where compensation for medical harm is dealt with by the tort of medical negligence. A tort is an act or omission that causes harm. Claims against medical practitioners relate to personal injury and death, and are lodged against a doctor due to a breach, or perceived breach, of care in the treatment of a patient. There are other systems for resolving negligence. In Taiwan, medical negligence is dealt with by criminal law (Lin, 2009). Between 2000 and 2004 one doctor was found guilty every 3 months of the crimes of delayed or missed diagnoses or surgical complications. This is the highest criminal rate of doctors in the world (Lin, 2009). A no-fault compensation system occurs in Sweden, Denmark, and New Zealand. The Nordic systems use an avoidability standard, principally defined as injury that would not occur in the hands of the best practitioner (Kachalia, Choudhry, & Studdert, 2005). In New Zealand, compensation is payable for personal injury caused by medical error, where there is a negligence test, or mishap, where the consequence is a rare outcome of treatment (Donaldson, 2003).

There is a natural tension between systems that focus on outcomes for the individual patient, usually against the individual doctor such as in tort law, and the systems for health care improvement that focus on quality improvement. For example, Runciman et al. (Runciman, Merry, & Tito, 2003) described a tendency for the harmed to blame those involved with an adverse outcome, often inappropriately. This is aggravated by the need to attribute blame before compensation can be obtained through tort. Blaming and punishing for errors that are made by well-intentioned people working in health care systems drives the problem of iatrogenic harm underground (Runciman et al., 2003). Similarly, Studdert described a "clash" between the tort law system and the patient safety movement that undermines efforts to improve quality (Studdert, Mello & Brennan, 2004). Likewise, May and Aulisio argue that efforts to prevent error must first address clinicians' fear of litigation, as this is an obstacle to reporting and discussing medical mistakes in an attempt to prevent future mistakes (May & Aulisio, 2001).

Thus the tort law system is problematic for the health care system, in general, and for patients as individuals. How is this process for the doctors?

BACKGROUND TO THE IMPACT OF MEDICO-LEGAL MATTERS ON THE DOCTOR

Medico-legal matters such as complaints, inquiries, and lawsuits are a source of concern and distress for doctors. A current medico-legal matter ranks very highly as a risk for psychiatric morbidity in doctors (Nash et al., 2010), and almost a quarter of doctors who had been sued for medical malpractice in a sample of US doctors identified this as their most stressful life experience ever (Charles, Wibert & Kennedy, 1984).

Doctors identify both physical and psychological sequelae such as depressed mood, suicidal thoughts, insomnia, anxiety, frustration, anger, onset or exacerbation of physical illness, and disturbance of family life (Charles et al., 1984; Schattner & Coman, 1998; Martin, Wilson, Fiebelman, Gurley & Miller, 1991; Cook & Neff, 1994; Mello et al., 2004;

Goldberg, Kuhn, Andrew & Thomas, 2002; Waterman et al., 2007; Zuger, 2004; Charles, Pyskoty & Nelson, 1988; Nash, Curtis, Walton, Willcock & Tennant, 2006).

Significantly greater functional impairment in work, social, and family life measured using the Sheehan's Disability Scale (Leon et al., 1997) were found in Australian General Practitioners (GPs) who had a current medico-legal matter compared to those who did not, and there was an increase in potentially hazardous alcohol use in males with a current medico-legal matter (Nash et al., 2007).

Medico-legal issues not only have an impact on the health of the doctor, but also on their practice of medicine and the care their patients receive. Defensive medicine occurs when clinical judgment is clouded by fear of medico-legal action. Medico-legal concerns can prompt changes such as excessive referrals, inappropriate diagnostic testing, unnecessary prescribing, avoidance of certain procedures or certain patients, and reduction in goodwill toward patients. However, there are also potentially good changes, such as the introduction of audit procedures, which provide better explanations to patients and better record keeping (Charles et al., 1984; Cook & Neff, 1994; Mello et al., 2004; Nash et al., 2006; Nash, Tennant & Walton, 2004; Jain & Ogden, 1999; Summerton, 1995; Harris Interactive, 2002; Weisman, Morlock, Teitelbaum, Klassen & Celentano, 1989; Elmore et al., 2005; Birbeck et al., 2004; Hiyama et al., 2006; Cunningham, 2004; Cunningham & Dovey, 2006; Nash, Walton, Daly & Johnson, 2009).

The frequency of doctors' involvement with medico-legal matters has been shown to vary with gender, age, specialty, hours worked, and country of practice (Mello et al., 2004; Nash et al., 2007; Firth-Cozens, 2008; Cunningham, Crump & Tomlin, 2003; Aasland, & Førde, 2005; Hickson et al., 2002). Doctors who are male (Nash et al., 2007; Firth-Cozens, 2008; Cunningham et al., 2003; Aasland & Førde, 2005; Hickson et al., 2002), work in high-intervention specialties (Mello et al., 2004; Nash et al., 2007; Aasland & Førde, 2005; Hickson et al., 2002), and work long hours (Nash et al., 2007; Hickson et al., 2002) are more likely to be the subject of a medico-legal matter. Internationally, the frequency varies, with the extreme of 86% of interventional specialist doctors in the United States having been named in a malpractice suit at least once (Mello et al., 2004).

In this chapter we report findings from a large and broad sample of Australian doctors comprising specialists, GPs, and trainees. We report and compare with the international literature the perceived changes to medical practice due to concerns about medico-legal matters and the frequency and factors associated with experiencing medico-legal matters. We explore the factors associated with psychiatric morbidity and potentially hazardous alcohol use in doctors. We also report retrospective accounts of the impact on psychological health of a medico-legal matter and what types of support would help if this happened again.

THE STUDY

This was a collaborative research project between the University of Sydney and the Australian medical insurance company Avant (previously United Medical Protection). Eight thousand five hundred doctors were invited to participate in the study, and 140 formally declined the invitation. A questionnaire was mailed to specialists (obstetricians, gynecologists, physicians, surgeons, anesthetists, psychiatrists, pathologists, radiologists, pediatricians, and accident and emergency specialists), registrars, and specialists-in-training, and a sample of GP nonproceduralists who were insured with the collaborating medical insurer. GP proceduralists were not included, as they were part of a GP study the previous year (Nash et al., 2007; Nash et al., 2009) that acted as a pilot for the larger study. The questionnaire consisted of demographic and practice details (age, gender, specialty, hours worked per week, country of medical degree, teaching role, attendance at peer review, holiday or no holiday in last 12 months) and perceived changes to practice due to medico-legal concerns.

Psychiatric morbidity was measured by the General Health Questionnaire (GHQ), a sensitive and well-validated 28-item screening tool used to detect common nonpsychotic psychiatric morbidity that considers symptoms over the past two weeks. It has four subscales: somatic symptoms, anxiety and insomnia, social dysfunction, and depression. The case identification score is reached with a score greater than 4 on the binary scoring system (Goldberg, 1998).

Potential for hazardous alcohol use was measured by the Alcohol Use Disorders Identification Test (AUDIT). This test is sensitive to detecting hazardous and harmful drinking. The AUDIT questions are scored from 0 to 4, with participants who score a total of 8 or more classified as potentially hazardous drinkers (Saunders, Aasland, Babor, de la Fuente & Grant, 1993).

Personality was measured using the Eysenck Personality Questionnaire (EPQ)—Revised Short Scale version (48-item). The EPQ is a valid and reliable self-report questionnaire that measures three major dimensions of personality: extroversion (a low score representing introversion); neuroticism (a high score measuring high emotional sensitivity); and "psychoticism" (a high score representing tough mindedness and, at the extreme, lack of empathy. It does not represent psychotic features) (Eysenck & Eysenck, 1996).

The medico-legal section of the questionnaire asked which of the following medico-legal matters the doctor had experienced: claim for compensation for damages, a complaint to a Health Care Complaints body, a Medical Registration Board inquiry, a disciplinary hearing, a Medicare Australia/Health Insurance Commission (HIC) inquiry, a hospital dispute, a hospital investigation, a pharmaceutical services inquiry, a complaint before an anti-discrimination board, a coronial inquiry, a criminal charge and patient complaint directed at the doctor. There was a retrospective, impact on health, component to the study for doctors who had experienced a medico-legal matter. They were asked to consider their most recent matter for the following items: anxiety, depression, anti-depressant use, alcohol use, benzodiazepine use, and other medical problems. Doctors were also asked if they sought treatment for these items (items listed in Table 8.1). They were also asked what support services they would find useful if they experienced another matter (items listed in Table 8.2).

STATISTICAL METHODS

Data were analyzed using SAS software, version 9.1 (SAS Institute, Cary, NC, USA). Response categories were dichotomized for the change in practice questions. Differences between respondents who had experienced medico-legal matters and those who had not were assessed using Pearson's chi-square tests. Pearson's chi squared test was also used to test for association between involvement in a current medico-legal matter and individual categorical variables. Multivariate logistic regression analysis was conducted on the outcome of being involved in a current medico-legal matter. Multivariate logistic regression models were also fitted to outcome measures of both GHQ case identification for psychiatric morbidity and AUDIT case identification for potentially hazardous drinking.

RESULTS

Demographic and Medico-Legal Characteristics of Respondents

Out of 8360 surveys sent, 2999 responded, representing a 36% (2999/8360) response rate to survey. Seventy-one percent of respondents were male, and 85% were married or in a de facto relationship. Thirteen percent of the cohort had not taken a holiday in the previous year. The mean number of hours of attendance at formal education programs (such as conferences) in the previous year for the total cohort was 53.3 (SD, 40.0). Peer review meetings were attended by 70% of respondents (range 36% [GPs] to 97% [psychiatrists]), with a mean of 12.3 sessions per year (SD, 13.9). Ninety-six percent of the cohort were meeting their Continuing Medical Education (CME) requirements. The mean hours worked per week was 44.8 ($SD = 15.1$), with mean hours for males 48.0 ($SD = 14.2$) and for females 37.1 ($SD = 14.3$). Mean weeks worked per year was 46.0 ($SD = 6.0$).

Medico-legal matters had been experienced at some time by 65% of respondents, with 14% having a current matter. The frequency of occurrence of medico-legal matters within each specialty group is reported already (Nash, Kelly et al., 2009) The most common medico-legal matters for the cohort were claims for compensation (31%) and complaints to a health care complaints body (30%). The groups with the highest proportion who had experienced any kind of medico-legal matters were obstetricians and gynecologists (91%) and surgeons (86%). The group with the lowest was specialists-in-training (45%).

The proportion of respondents who had been involved in one or more matters was as follows: one matter (22%), two matters (16%), three matters (9%), four matters (6%), five matters (4%), and six or more matters (7%).

Respondents Versus Nonrespondents

There were minor differences between respondents and nonrespondents in age (51.7 vs. 50.3 years) and sex (71% vs. 74% male) ($P < 0.05$). Based on data from the Avant database, respondents were slightly more likely than nonrespondents to have been involved in claims for compensation (28.0% vs. 23.0%), complaints to a health care complaints body (20.6% vs. 17.1%), and coronial inquiries (4.7% vs. 3.3%) ($P < 0.05$ for all three comparisons). There was no difference between respondents and nonrespondents with respect to involvement in the other nine categories of medico-legal matter ($P > 0.05$) listed in the medico-legal section of the questionnaire described previously.

Change in Practice Due to Medico-Legal Concerns

Perceived changes in medical practice due to medico-legal concerns have been reported extensively elsewhere (Nash, Walton et al., 2010). The major findings were that some behaviors were either increased (e.g. test ordering) or avoided (e.g. certain procedures) that could have either positive or negative outcomes, for example, 43% referred their patients to specialists more than usual, 11% prescribed more medication than usual, 55% of the cohort reported that they ordered more tests than usual, 40% avoided a particular invasive procedure more than usual, and 34% of the total cohort reported that they would avoid a particular type of obstetric procedure more than usual due to medico-legal concerns (these last three items were significantly more for those who had experienced a medico-legal matter compared with those who had not).

There was also a tendency to improve checking systems for some doctors, with 48% of the total cohort putting systems in place to track test results; 39% putting systems in place to identify nonattenders, and 66% of the total cohort providing communication of risk to patients more than usual due to medico-legal concerns. The latter two items were statistically significantly more for those doctors who had experienced a medico-legal matter compared with than those who had not.

Perceived Influence of Medico-Legal Issues on Career Choices

Concerns about medico-legal issues led 33% of the respondents to contemplate giving up medicine, 32% considered reducing their hours of work, and 32% considered retiring early. These figures were all significantly greater for doctors who had experienced a medico-legal matter compared with those who had not (Nash, Walton et al., 2010).

Relating to Patients

Respondents report that concern about medico-legal issues influenced how they relate to patients. Those who had experienced a medico-legal matter were more likely to have changed how they relate to patients, compared to those with no experience of a medico-legal matter (p < 0.001). Eighteen percent of the sample felt more emotionally distant from patients due to medico-legal concerns (significantly more for those doctors who had experienced a medico-legal matter) (Nash and Walton et al., 2010).

Factors Associated with Being Involved in a Current Medico-Legal Matter

A multivariate analysis (logistic regression) was performed of factors associated with being involved in a current medico-legal matter. The factors included in the analysis were medical specialty, sex, age, marital status, country of medical degree, solo or non-solo practice, hours worked per week, attendance at peer review meetings in the last 12 months, meeting continuing medical education requirements in the past 12 months, having a teaching role, having an AUDIT case identification for potentially hazardous drinking, and having a GHQ case identification for psychiatric morbidity. Of these, statistically significant factors were medical specialty, with obstetricians and gynecologists having the highest risk, followed by surgeons; males higher risk compared with females; divorced and separated doctors higher risk compared with single doctors and married doctors; more than 40 hours worked per week; and GHQ case identification were all associated with higher risk of being involved in a current medico-legal matter. Potentially hazardous alcohol use measured by the AUDIT case identification was approaching significance (p = 0.05) (Nash, Kelly et al., 2009).

A Closer Look at Psychiatric Morbidity and Potentially Hazardous Alcohol Use in the Sample

Potential for psychiatric morbidity: GHQ case identification for psychiatric morbidity for the total cohort was 28% (31% for women, 26% for men). A multivariate logistic regression analyses for psychiatric morbidity found that the significant variables associated with increased risk of psychiatric morbidity were having a current medico-legal matter (odds ratio [OR], 1.96 [95% CI, 1.52–2.54]); not having had a holiday in the previous year (OR, 1.92 [95% CI, 1.47–2.50]); and working long hours per week (OR, 1.65 [95% CI, 1.20–2.26] for 60 hours compared with < 40 hours). Doctors 60 years of age or older had a lower likelihood of psychiatric morbidity than doctors under 40 years of age (OR, 0.58 [95% CI, 0.39–0.84]). Solo practitioners had a lower risk of psychiatric morbidity than non-solo practitioners (OR, 0.78 [95% CI, 0.61–0.99]). The personality trait of neuroticism (defined as having a neuroticism score greater than the median) was the highest risk factor for psychiatric morbidity (OR, 4.65 [95% CI, 3.82–5.65]). Introversion was also a statistically significant risk factor for psychiatric morbidity ($p = 0.04$) (Nash, Daly et al., 2010).

Potential for hazardous alcohol use: AUDIT case identification for potential for hazardous alcohol use for the total cohort was 15% (8% for women, 17% for men). The results of the multivariate logistic regression analyses for potentially hazardous alcohol use found the demographic and work-related variables associated with increased risk of potentially hazardous drinking were being male (OR, 2.55 [95% CI, 1.83–3.55]); being aged 40–49 years compared with under 40 years (OR, 1.86 [95% CI, 1.22–2.83]); not having met CME requirements (OR, 1.72 [95% CI, 1.04–2.87]); and being a solo practitioner rather than a non-solo practitioner (OR, 1.33 [95% CI, 1.01–1.75]). Neuroticism (OR, 2.20 [95% CI, 1.74–2.78]), extroversion (OR, 1.62 [95% CI, 1.28–2.04]), and psychoticism (meaning high scores for tough mindedness) (OR, 1.27 [95% CI, 1.01–1.60]) were all associated with potential for hazardous alcohol use. Doctors were at less risk of hazardous alcohol use if they trained overseas rather than in Australia (OR, 0.56 [95% CI, 0.39–0.81]); worked more than 60 hours a week compared with less than 40 hours a week (OR, 0.67 [95% CI, 0.45–0.99]); and had not taken a holiday in more than a year (OR, 0.63 [95% CI, 0.43–0.93]) (Nash, Daly et al., 2010).

Impact on health of Most Recent Medico-Legal Matter—Retrospective Account

Respondents were asked to recall how their most recent medico-legal matter had impacted on their health (see Table 8.1). No time frame was recorded, simply their most recent matter, which could have been a current matter or one many years ago.

TABLE 8.1 Recall of the Impact on Doctor's Health of Most Recent Medico-Legal Matter

Did you:	% who replied "more than usual" N = 1902	% who sought professional help for this problem N = 1902
Become anxious	73	9
Become depressed	44	8
Require anti-depressant meds	5	5
Drink alcohol	14	3
Use benzodiazepines	5	3
Have other medical problems	13	7

Nearly three quarters of doctors reported becoming more anxious than usual, nearly half said they became more depressed than usual, 14% reported increasing their alcohol intake, 5% reported taking benzodiazepines more than usual, and 13% reported having other medical problems more than usual. Only a minority of these doctors sought professional help for these problems.

What Would Be Helpful If the Respondent Experienced Another Medico-Legal Matter?

As reported in Table 8.2, a significant proportion of respondents wanted access to support, for example, someone from their medical defense organization to attend court with them or to be a contact person for them. Many wanted access to a peer support program, and others wanted access to an independent counseling service. Such services are available to doctors in Australia, although these results suggest that many are unaware of them. A majority also required more information about medico-legal processes and about what support services are available.

TABLE 8.2 Support Services That Would Be Useful for a Future Medico-Legal Matter

1 Useful Services	2 Agree (%)
More information about the medico legal process	76.5
More information on services available	78.3
MDO* contact to discuss concerns	81.8
MDO* person to attend Court	88.3
Formal peer support programmed	75.6
Contact with DHAS^	47.5
Access to independent counselling	73.4

*Medical Defense Organization

^ Doctors Health Advisory Service

DISCUSSION

Involvement in medico-legal processes is a stressful part of life for many professions. Doctors may be more affected by such processes because of the nature of their relationship with patients, their commitment to healing and care that underpins this relationship, and for some doctors, their personality style. Difficulty relaxing, reluctance to take vacations from work, problems allocating time to family, chronic feelings of not doing enough, difficulty setting limits, and guilt feelings that interfere with the healthy pursuit of pleasures are not uncommon in doctors (Gabbard, 1985).

Some medico-legal processes may be minimal, but others such as being the subject of a claim or complaint can be more confronting. Most of these cases, however, will not result in severe disciplinary procedures or litigation, but the stress of the process can be unnerving and long-term. Education to inform doctors about the legal processes, the psychological sequelae, possible supports available, and the potential impact on practice are important steps for educators to take.

The doctors in our study sample report significant perceived changes to their practice, as in international studies. These Australian doctors report an increase in referrals in 44% due to medico-legal concerns, compared with 50% in a UK GP study (Summerton, 1995) and 74% in the US Common Good study (Harris Interactive, 2002). The costly issue of test ordering more than usual due to medico-legal concerns by 55% of our sample is similar to the UK GP study of 50% (Summerton, 1995) and 79% in the US Common Good study (Harris Interactive, 2002). The trend toward prescribing medication more than usual due to medico-legal concerns was only reported by 11% of our sample, which compares favorably with the US Common good study, where 41% reported prescribing more medication for fear of litigation. Recent Australian campaigns for safe prescribing may have impacted on this (NSW Therapeutic Advisory Group Inc, 2009). Providing more information to patients and being more attentive to patients, as reported by this cohort, are changes that can promote better relationships and understanding.

The perceived changes in career choice by this cohort of Australian doctors is concerning. It is likely that changes such as leaving medicine are contemplated in the immediate period during and after being involved in a medico-legal process and that these intentions are not acted upon in the long-term. Nevertheless, it is worrying that doctors who has no doubt successfully treated thousands of patients over their career would consider giving up because of the expressed dissatisfaction of one or two. There is need for support to assist these doctors to restore their confidence and satisfaction in their work when involved in a medico-legal matter.

Concerning relating to patients, 18% of the sample felt more emotionally distant from patients due to medico-legal concerns (significantly more for those doctors who had experienced a medico-legal matter). This is similar to the New Zealand finding in which doctors who had received a medical complaint reported feeling reduced trust and goodwill toward patients (Cunningham, 2004). On the one hand, being more distant from patients may interfere with the therapeutic relationship and building of trust. On the other hand, being more distant from certain patients is a way of establishing boundaries that may have previously been ambiguous, especially if this was the source of the complaint.

As with international studies, our study found that male doctors, those working long hours, and in high intervention areas of medicine (surgery and O & G) were associated with experiencing a medico-legal matter. Doctors who have a current medico-legal matter have significantly higher rates of psychiatric morbidity.

Considering work-related factors associated with psychiatric morbidity in doctors, our study found that a current medico-legal matter was the factor most associated with psychiatric morbidity, followed by not taking a holiday in the previous year and working long hours. However, the personality trait of neuroticism carried the highest risk for psychiatric morbidity. As this was a cross-sectional study, associations can be made, but not the direction of causality. A longitudinal study is required for that. However, the findings from the retrospective component of the study indicate that the Australian cohort recall an increase in psychological distress at the time of the matter.

With regard to what support doctors would like when facing a medico-legal matter, they want to be better informed and would seek support if it were available or if they knew about it. A recent initiative of a counseling service for stressed New Zealand doctors found that this program was effective and well received, but there was insufficient awareness of its availability (Cunningham & Cookson, 2009). Clearly, doctors who are the subject of complaints and claims also need to be offered support services in addition to receiving legal advice.

Doctors need to be educated about medico-legal processes and the support available to them, and to understand how the experience may affect them, their health, their work, and their loved ones both during the process and into the future. This education can be undertaken by undergraduate and postgraduate programs, medical colleges, and medical defense organizations. Stressful life events need to be actively managed by doctors as they would advise their own patients to do. The doctor and his or her employer and colleagues need to be mindful of positive coping strategies such as stress reduction techniques, regular exercise, good sleep and diet, seeking support, considering reducing hours of work in times of stress, and avoidance of negative coping strategies such as seeking refuge in alcohol or self-medication.

CONCLUSION

In conclusion, as a doctor, there are five particular issues to be mindful of if you are the subject of a medico-legal matter:

1. Understand that this will occur at some stage to the majority of doctors, but it is still a rare event in the life of a doctor.

2. Try to learn from the process to minimize the chance of this happening again.

3. Be mindful of the personal impact on the doctor—either as the subject of a medico-legal matter yourself or as a colleague.

4. Seek advice from legal experts and be informed about what to expect, and tell advisers how you are feeling.

5. Seek early advice from your own doctor or other professional support if the process is causing distress in order to maintain your own good health and ameliorate distress and anxiety. This will help you regain a sense of competence and confidence to be able to perform your work and manage family life to the best of your ability.

REFERENCES

Aasland, O.G., & Førde, R. (2005). Impact of feeling responsible for adverse events on doctors' personal and professional lives: The importance of being open to criticism from colleagues. *Quality and Safety in Health Care; 14*(1), 13–17.

Berstein, J., MacCoour, D., & Abramson, B. (2008). Topics in Medical Economics: Medical Malpractice. *Journal of Bone and Joint Surgery, 90*(8), 1777–1782.

Birbeck, G., Gifford, D., Song, J., Belin, T., Mittman, B., & Vickrey, B. (2004). Do malpractice concerns, payment mechanisms, and attitudes influence test-ordering decisions? *Neurology, 62,* 119–121.

Brennan, T., Leape, L., Laird, N., Herbert, L., Localio, R., Lawthers, A., Hiatt, H.H. (1991). Incidence of adverse events and negligence in hospitalized patients. Results of the Harvard Medical Practice study I. *The New England Journal of Medicine, 324*(6), 370–376.

Brennan, T.A., Sox, C.M., & Burstin, H.R. (1996). Relation between negligent adverse events and the outcomes of medical-malpractice litigation: *New England Journal of Medicine, 335,* 1963–1967.

Charles, S., Wibert, J., & Kennedy, E. (1984). Physicians self-reports to reactions to malpractice litigation. *American Journal of Psychiatry, 41,* 563–565.

Charles, S., Pyskoty, M., & Nelson, A. (1988). Physicians on trial: Self reported reactions to malpractice trials. *Western Journal of Medicine, 148*(3), 358–360.

Cook, R., & Neff, C. (1994). Attitudes of physicians in northern Ontario to medical malpractice litigation. *Canadian Family Physician, 40,* 689–698.

Cunningham, W., Crump, R., & Tomlin, A. (2003). The characteristics of doctors receiving medical complaints: A cross-sectional survey of doctors in New Zealand. *New Zealand Medical Journal, 116*(1183), U625.

Cunningham, W. (2004). The immediate and long-term impact on New Zealand doctors who receive patient complaints. *New Zealand Medical Journal, 117* (1198), U972.

Cunningham, W., & Dovey, S. (2006). Defensive changes in medical practice and the complaints process: A qualitative study of New Zealand doctors *New Zealand Medical Journal, 119* (1244).

Cunningham, W., & Cookson, T. (2009). Addressing stress related impairment in doctors. A survey of providers' and doctors' experience of a funded counselling service in New Zealand. *New Zealand Medical Journal, 122*(1300), 19–28.

Donaldson, L. (2003). Chief Medical Officer Department of Health UK. Making Amends. A consultation paper setting out proposals for reforming the approach to clinical negligence in the NHS. Retrieved June 7, 2011, from http://www.dh.gov.uk/prod_consum_dh/groups/dh_digitalassets/@dh/@en/documents/digitalasset/dh_4060945.pdf

Elmore, J., Taplin, S., Barlow, W., Cutter, G., D'Orsi, C., Hendrick, R., Abraham,L., Fosse, J., & Carney, P. (2005). Does litigation influence medical practice? The influence of community radiologists' medical malpractice perceptions and experience on screening mammography, *Radiology, 236*, 37–46.

Eysenck, H.J., & Eysenck S.B.G. (1996). *Manual of the Eysenck Personality Scales (EPS Adult)*. UK: Hodder and Stoughton.

Firth-Cozens, J. (2008). Doctors with difficulties: why so few women? *Postgrad Med J, 84*, 318–320.

Gabbard, G. (1985). The role of compulsiveness in the Normal Physician. *JAMA, 254*(20): 2926–2929.

Goldberg, R., Kuhn, G., Andrew, L., & Thomas, H. (2002). Coping with medical mistakes and errors in judgment, *Ann Emerg Med. 39*(3), 287–292.

Goldberg, D.P. (1998). *Manual of the General Health Questionnaire*, London, UK: NFER.

Harris Interactive (2002). Fear of litigation study: The impact on medicine. Retrieved November 24, 2004' from http://cgood.org/healthcare-reading-cgpubs-polls-6.

Health Care Complaints Commission. (2009). Annual Report data 2008–09: Report on complaints about medical practitioners 2008–09. Retrieved June 8, 2011, from www.hccc.nsw.gov.au/Publications/Annual-Reports/Default/default.aspx

Helland, E., & Showalter, M. H. (2009). The impact of liability on the physician labor market. *Journal of Law and Economics, 52*, 635–663.

Hickson, G., Federspiel, C., Pichert, J., Miller, C.S., Gaild-Jaeger, J., & Bost, P. (2002) Patient complaints and malpractice risk. *JAMA, 287*(22), 2951–2956.

Hiyama, T., Yoshihara, M., Tanaka, S., Urabe, Y., Ikegami, Y., Fukuhara, T., & Chayama, K. (2006). Defensive medicine practices among gastroenterologists in Japan. *World Journal of Gastroenterology, 12*(47), 7671–7675.

Jain, A., & Ogden, J. (1999). General practitioners' experience of patients' complaints: A qualitative study. *British Medical Journal, 318*, 1596–1599.

Kachalia, A., Choudhry, N.K., & Studdert, D.M. (2005). Physician responses to the malpractice crisis: From defence to offense. *Journal of Law Medicine & Ethics, 33*(3), 416–428.

Kessler, D., Summerton, N., & Graham, J. (2006). Effects of the medical liability system in Australia, the UK, and the USA. *The Lancet, 68*, 240–246.

Leon AC, Olfsen M, Portera L, Farber L, Sheehan DV. (1997). Assessing psychiatric impairment in primary care with the Sheehan Disability Scale. *International Journal of Psychiatry and Medicine, 27*, 93–105.

Localio, A., Lawthers, A., Brennan, T., Laird, N., Herbert, L., Peterson, L. & Hiatt H. (1991). Relation between Malpractice claims and adverse events due to negligence. Results of the Harvard Medical Practice Study III. *New England Journal, 325*, 245–251.

Leape, L.L. (1994). Error in Medicine, *Journal of the American Medical Association, 272*(33), 1851–1857.

Lin, P.J. (2009). Criminal judgments to medical malpractice in Taiwan. *Legal Medicine. 11*(Suppl 1), S376–S378.

Martin, C., Wilson, J., Fiebelman, N., Gurley, D., & Miller, T., (1991). Physicians' psychological reactions to malpractice litigation, *Southern Medical Journal, 84*, 1300–1304.

May, T., & Aulisio, M. (2001). Medical malpractice, mistake prevention and compensation. *Kennedy Institute of Ethics Journal, 11*(2), 135–146.

Mello, M., Studdert, D., & DesRoches, C., Peugh, J., Zapert, K., Brennan, T.A., & Sage, W.M. (2004). Caring for Patients in a malpractice crisis: Physician satisfaction and quality of care. *Health Affairs (Millwood), 23*(4), 42–53.

Nash, L., Tennant, C., & Walton, M. (2004). The psychological impact of complaints and negligence suits on doctors. *Australasian Psychiatry, 12*(3), 278–281.

Nash, L., Curtis, B., Walton, M., Willcock, S., & Tennant, C. (2006). The response of doctors to a formal complaint. *Australasian Psychiatry, 14*(3), 246–250.

Nash, L., Daly, M., Johnson, M., Walter, G., Walton, M., Willcock, S., Tennant C. (2007). Psychological morbidity in Australian doctors who have and have not experienced a medico-legal matter: a cross sectional survey. *Australian New Zealand Journal of Psychiatry, 41*(11), 917–925.

Nash, L., Walton, M., Daly, M., Johnson, M. (2009). GPs' concerns about medico-legal issues—How it affects their practice. *Australian Family Physician. 38*(1/2), 66–70.

Nash, L., Daly, M., Johnson, M., Coulston, C., Tennant, C., van Ekert, E. & Walton, M. (2009). Personality, gender and medicolegal matters in medical practice. *Australasian Psychiatry,17*(1),19–24.

Nash, L., Kelly, P., Daly, M., Walter, G., van Ekert, E., Walton, M., Tennant, C.(2009). Australian doctors' involvement in medicolegal matters: a cross-sectional self-report study. *Medical Journal of Australia, 191*(8), 436–440.

Nash, L., Walton, M., Daly, M., Kelly, P., Walter, G., van Ekert, E., et al. (2010). Perceived practice change in Australian doctors due to medico-legal concerns, *Medical Journal of Australia, 193*(10), 579–583.

Nash, L., Daly, M., Kelly, P., van Ekert, E., Walter, G., Walton, M., Willcock, S., Tennant C. (2010). Factors associated with psychiatric morbidity and hazardous alcohol use in Australian doctors *Medical Journal of Australia, 193*(3):161–166.

NSW Therapeutic Advisory Group Inc (2009). Safe Prescribing. Retrieved May 31, 2009, from http://www.ciap.health.nsw.gov.au/nswtag/.

Rowe, M. (2004). Doctors' responses to medical errors. *Critical Reviews in Oncology/Haematology. 52*(3), 147–163.

Runciman, W., Merry, A., & Tito, F. (2003). Error, blame, and the law in health care—An ANTIPODEAN PERSPECTIVE. *Annals of Internal Medicine, 138,* 974–979

Saunders, J., Aasland, O.G., Babor, T.F., de la Fuente J.R., & Grant, M. (1993). Development of the Alcohol Use Disorders Identification Test (AUDIT): WHO collaborative project on early detection of persons with harmful alcoholic consumption, II, *Addiction, 88* (6), 791–804.

Studdert, D., Thomas, E., Burstin, H., Bar, B., Or, E., & Brennan T. (2000). Negligent care and malpractice claiming behavior in Utah and Colorado. *Medical Care. 38*(3), 250–260.

Studdert, D., Mello, M., Sage, W., Desroches, C., Peugh, J., Zapert, K., & Brennan, T. (2005). Defensive medicine among high-risk specialist physicians in a volatile malpractice environment. *Journal of the American Medical Association, 293*(21), 2609–2617.

Studdert, D., Mello, M., & Brennan, T. (2004). Medical malpractice. *The New England Journal of Medicine, 350,* 283–202.

Schattner, P.L., & Coman, G.J. (1998). The stress of metropolitan general practice. *Medical Journal of Australia, 169,* 133–137.

Summerton, N. (1995). Positive and negative factors in defensive medicine: A questionnaire study of general practitioners. *British Medical Journal, 310,* 27–29.

Waterman, A., Garbutt, J., Hazel, E., Dunagan, W., Levinson, W., Fraser, V., & Gallagher, T. (2007). The Emotional impact of medical errors on practicing physicians in the United States and Canada. *The Joints Commission Journal of Quality and Patient Safety, 33*(8), 467–476.

Weisman, C., Morlock, L., Teitelbaum, M., Klassen, A., & Celentano, D. (1989). Practice changes in response to the malpractice litigation climate. Results of a Maryland physician survey. *Medical Care. 27,* 16–24.

Wilson, R., Runciman, W., Gibberd, R., Harrison, B., Newby, L., & Hamilton, J.(1995). The Quality in Australian Health Care Study. *Medical Journal of Australia, 163*(9), 458–471.

Wu, A.W. (2000). Medical error: The second victim. The doctor who makes the mistake needs help too. *British Medical Journal, 320,* 726–727.

Vincent, C., Neale, G., & Woloshynowych, M. (2001). Adverse events in British hospital: Preliminary retrospective record review. *British Medical Journal, 322,* 517–519.

Zuger, A. (2004). Dissatisfaction with Medical Practice. *The New England Journal of Medicine, 350,* 69–75.

///9/// THE IMPAIRED PHYSICIAN

FRASER C. TODD

HOW DO DOCTORS BECOME ILL AND WHY DON'T THEY PRESENT LIKE OTHER PEOPLE?

There needs to be a justification for writing a chapter about how doctors become patients. Why not a chapter on how lawyers become patients? First it is not because doctors are sicker than other professionals (the evidence is contradictory) but having medical knowledge and working in healthcare can distort the normal presentation of illness. Second it is hard for doctors and others to recognize when a doctor transitions from the role of healer to patient, and third, doctors may also self-treat (Davidson & Schattner, 2003).

MEDICAL KNOWLEDGE AND WORKING IN HEALTH CARE CAN DISTORT THE NORMAL PRESENTATION OF ILLNESS

There is some empirical evidence that working in health care changes how professionals present with illness. McKevitt's study surveyed doctors (family and hospital doctors) and a comparison group of senior managers working outside health care (McKevitt, Morgan, Dundas, & Holland, 1997). They found that although self-reported health status was the same for both groups, doctors were significantly less likely to take short periods of sick leave. Doctors cited the difficulty of arranging cover and, in response to a question about whether they would take time off work due to a cold, were far more likely to say "definitely not" compared to the managers. (Family doctors odds ratio [OR]16.2, 95% confidence interval [CI] 10.8–24.3; hospital doctors OR 2.9, 95% CI 1.9–4.4). Hospital doctors quoted the absence of backup as the main reason for being at work when sick while family doctors cited unfairness to colleagues as the principal reason with both groups unwilling to accept a patient role. Studies now recognize that "presenteeism," attendance at work when sick, is as much as a problem as "absenteeism" (Aronsson & Gustafsson, 2005). It has also led to suggestions that physician wellness become a quality indicator in health care systems (Wallace, Lemaire, & Ghali, 2009).

There is other evidence that doctors distort the normal presentation of illness by not taking care of themselves as others would do. For example, they delay getting medical treatment, as shown in a Canadian study of physicians that found that of the 1 in 6 doctors who identified as depressed only a quarter considered getting help and only 2% sought treatment (Canadian Medical Association, 2003). A systematic review of doctors' health care access and the barriers they experience found a wide range, from 21% to 100%, of doctors who registered with a family doctor (Kay, Mitchell, Clavarino, & Doust, 2008). The wide range reflects different national health systems but it was clear that many physicians do not choose a family doctor who is independent. The studies in the review found a quarter of doctors registered with a partner, a third registered with a family doctor they considered a friend, and one in ten registered with a member of their family or a spouse.

The barriers to seeking health care by doctors are, with few exceptions, similar to the general population (Kay et al., 2008). They include embarrassment (including fear that their self-diagnosis may be wrong) particularly around mental health disorders, concerns about confidentiality, a culture in which doctors are expected to be healthy, and a tendency to self-treat because it is not culturally acceptable within the medical profession to recognize illness in a peer. Having medical knowledge means it is easy to justify symptoms as insignificant, to be aware of the limits of medical care, to know about the difficulty in getting future insurance, and to recognize the potential implications of the burden on colleagues and patients. A qualitative study of family doctors in Northern Ireland found that they felt a need to portray a healthy image to others, which was stressful and created a barrier to self-care. Additionally the working arrangements of the family doctors, for example long hours and having to be "strong" to manage distress in others, reinforced a culture in which distress was overlooked (Thompson, Cupples, Sibbett, Skan, & Bradley, 2001).

Doctors also have different rules for treating themselves compared to their patients. Primary care physicians in the United States were randomized to one of two scenarios and asked to choose a treatment depending on whether they were the patient or were recommending the treatment to a patient. For both scenarios the physicians recommended treatments with a higher mortality rate and lower frequency of adverse events for themselves compared to patients (Ubel, Angott, & Zikmund-Fisher, 2011).

PATIENTS MAKE DOCTORS SICK

There are several specific stresses in the role of doctor that contribute towards doctors becoming sick. Long work hours and burnout are also a factor. Medical practice means working with dying patients, people in pain, and people who are diseased, which can cause anxiety about coping with daily reminders of mortality and the limits of what we can offer. This results in several predictable psychological defenses such as denial where doctors deny that they are experiencing anxiety or stress. The evidence for denial includes the findings of Rosvold and Bjertness (2002) who found that about a quarter of doctors hide their illness from colleagues. This may be motivated by how disclosure will affect them professionally, as well as the need to present an image of success (Stoudemire & Rhoads, 1983). There is also a culture of corridor or coffee consultations that is accepted practice and encourages self-prescribing. Other defenses include hypomania or over-work, in which the doctor works ever harder to avoid feeling tension, intellectualization or the medicalization of distress, identification with patients' symptoms through some form of hypochondria or somatoform presentation, and acting out distress directly by self-destructive acts such as taking drugs and suicide attempts or indirectly through eating disorders or depression.

SELF-PRESCRIBING

Another way in which doctors distort the normal presentation of illness is that they treat themselves, present with partially treated syndromes and the adverse effects of medication, and present later in the course of illness than do other professionals. In an Australian study of 358 doctors (40% response rate) more participants believed it was acceptable to self-treat acute conditions (315/351; 90%) than to self-treat chronic conditions (88/350; 25%) (Davidson & Schattner, 2003). Nine percent (30/351) of participants believed it was acceptable to self-prescribe psychotropic medication. The systematic review of Kay, et al. (2008) found that between a third and nearly all doctors had provided self-treatment, with family doctors more likely to do this than specialists. Other barriers to seeking health care identified in this review included patient factors around embarrassment, time, cost, an awareness of the implications of the disorder, and medical knowledge leading to a justification of the symptoms as insignificant. Systemic issues included concerns about confidentiality, the quality of care provided, the culture of doctors' needing to be "healthy," and structural difficulties around the lack of available medical cover, long hours, and lack of training about seeking medical help as a doctor. A qualitative study of doctors seeking help for psychiatric problems confirmed these barriers but also suggested that non-medical friends and family may be good at identifying problems but had difficulties enabling the doctors' access to care (Stanton & Randal, 2011). The potential of doctor's non-medical network to encourage care has yet to be fully examined.

THE DIFFICULTY OF RECOGNIZING WHEN A DOCTOR BECOMES A PATIENT

Why are doctors not recognized as impaired? Their impairment may be covered up by junior doctors and forgiven by their senior colleagues. Also, recognizing that a doctor may be unwell may cause problems for colleagues, and may adversely affect working relationships, have a negative impact on the impaired doctor's career, or result in a complaint about the doctor reporting on his or her colleague's illness. However, there is a duty to recognize when a colleague is unwell, especially if this is causing impairment. A doctor's primary duty is to put patients' interests first and there is some legal protection for recognition of doctor impairment. For example, in New Zealand, legislation makes it compulsory for doctors and organizations that provide health services to tell the Medical Council if they believe a doctor may be unable to perform the functions required to practice medicine because of a physical or mental condition. Also, failure to act may be considered misconduct in some jurisdictions and result in convictions for negligence (Laing, 2007). Doctors might feel uncomfortable in the role of patient, and fear that others will interpret their need for help as a sign of their inability to cope. This is similar to the discussion on the "overcoper" in Chapter 12. The effect of professional factors on wellness is exacerbated by the professional culture of ignoring signals of distress. This is important in substance abuse disorders where professional knowledge and denial make it easier to hide signs and symptoms of abuse (Baldisseri, 2007). For doctors, problems at work often mark the last signs of substance abuse (Vaillant et al., 1983). Farber et al. (2005) presented hypothetical scenarios to doctors and showed that most of them described themselves as more likely to report a physician with a substance-abuse disorder than one who is emotionally or cognitively impaired. Doctors who had a broader public health view were more likely to report colleagues to physician-health programs. It was also found that if a doctor knew about guidelines on reporting impaired colleagues they were more likely to take action than doctors who did not know about such guidance.

WHAT DO DOCTORS PRESENT WITH?

Surveys of doctors referred to various treatment programs give some idea of the type of problems faced. However the problems are usually broadly described as stress or as a medical diagnosis. Nor do the studies, which are usually small, indicate what proportion of doctors presented with work problems or what the behavior of concern was. For example, Garelick et al. (2007) describes a cross sectional study of self-referred doctors (n = 121) to the London MedNet service for doctors. The most prevalent problems were depression, anxiety/stress, interpersonal problems, self-esteem problems, and work problems. Three-quarters of clients were dealing with work-related difficulties with the most common being workload and work relationships.

When doctors present with ill health it is usually from psychiatric conditions and substance abuse. The problem is they do not usually present by saying "I feel depressed" or "I have a drinking problem." What they present with is someone smelling alcohol on their breath, irritability, or a change of work habits, such as turning up late, a fear of making a mistake, or working longer hours. In doctors with substance abuse problems the change of work habits may include frequent absences from work without reasonable explanations, missed appointments with patients, inaccessibility to patients and staff, ward rounds at odd hours, and forgotten verbal orders (Baldisseri, 2007). Certain problems may present at different times in a doctor's career so that junior doctors present with anxiety, depression, alcohol or substance abuse; mid-career doctors with depression, alcohol or substance abuse, marital problems, and inappropriate behavior in clinical settings; while mature doctors present with the effects of physical and cognitive decline, sexual indiscretion, and impaired performance. Doctors may also have idiosyncratic reactions to patient deaths—for example, ignoring what happened, or the reverse—overidentifying with the death. The problem is having the difficult conversation with your colleague that results in their recognizing and accepting treatment.

WHAT TO DO ABOUT IT?

In a national survey on professionalism, Campbell et al. (2007) found that 96% of respondents agreed that impaired or incompetent colleagues should be reported to the relevant authorities. However 45% of respondents who had encountered such colleagues had not reported them. In a similar survey of psychologists, 69% had known of colleagues who they thought were experiencing personal or emotional problems but only 36% reported having approached the colleague (VandonBos & Duthie, 1986). The same applied to alcohol abuse in which 33% of the psychologists surveyed reported knowing of colleagues experiencing alcohol problems but only 12% of whom reported attempting to help them. What can be done about the gap between recognition of the problem and action? First, organizations can try to put screening systems in place. For example, as part of the Physician's Achievement Review by the College of Physicians and Surgeons in Alberta, Canada, there is a screen for cognitive problems, although the value of such programs has not been demonstrated.

Second, work-hour regulations such as those from the European Union (Working Time Directive 2003/88/EC) or the US Accreditation Council for Graduate Medical Education are specific examples of measures to prevent burnout, fatigue, and sleep deprivation early in the physician's career. Third, there are attempts to change the culture so that the prevention and detection of health problems in physicians is made acceptable. In the United States, educational programs on the impact of sleep deprivation on performance and burnout are now required in residency. Also the Joint Commission on Accreditation of Health Care Organizations Medical Staff Standard MS 11.01.01 specifically references "physician wellness" as being a required focus of hospital medical staff activity, which has led to an increase in physician wellness committees in US hospitals ("Design Physician Wellness," 2010). Another example of culture change is a Norwegian center for doctors suffering from burnout that provides counseling aimed at the reflection and acknowledgment of needs. The outcomes of doctors attending this center were reported in an observational study that showed that after the intervention doctors had reduced emotional exhaustion, reduced working hours, and less time on full-time sick leave (Isaksson Ro, Gude, Tyssen, & Aasland, 2008). However this was not a randomized, controlled trial and it is unclear if these changes would have happened without the intervention. In the UK, the Department of Health implemented the recommendations of a working group to improve the care of doctors with mental disorders and to improve accessibility of care (Department of Health, 2008). This document noted the need for access to information for doctors seeking health care, designated care pathways and services, and the need for confidentiality and privacy as well as the need to promote mental health and well-being in doctors. Also, as noted above, legislation that makes it clear where doctors' duties lie and the penalties for nonreporting create an environment that encourages recognition and action. Professional bodies such as the Australian Medical Association (http://ama.com.au/node/655) and the American Medical Association very clearly state that doctors have an ethical duty to report impaired colleagues:

> Physicians' responsibilities to colleagues who are impaired by a condition that interferes with their ability to engage safely in professional activities include timely intervention to ensure that these colleagues cease practicing and receive appropriate assistance from a physician-health program. Ethically and legally, it may be necessary to report an impaired physician who continues to practice despite reasonable offers of assistance and referral to a hospital or state physician-health program. The duty to report under such circumstances, which stems from physicians' obligation to protect patients against harm, may entail reporting to the licensing authority (American Medical Association Opinion E-9.031 December 2003).

In the United States, the majority of states have Physician Recovery Networks or Physician Diversion programs that encourage reporting of impaired physicians. Once evaluated and in such a program, the physician's license to practice is preserved. Several residential evaluation and treatment centers have developed to assist impaired and disruptive physicians that frequently work with the State Boards of Medicine (Federation of State Physician Health Programs, 2012).

So how do you have a difficult conversation with a doctor when you have concerns about their health? This partly depends on the relationship. If you are a supervisor of a junior doctor then simply stating what you have observed (a behavior) and then asking "Is this normal for you?" may be sufficient to start the conversation. At other times when the potentially sick doctor is more senior, more preparation needs to go into the encounter including consultation with senior colleagues. The American Psychological Association has guidelines on confronting impaired colleagues (VandonBos & Duthie, 1986) that can be usefully adapted for sick doctors and are described below.

1. *Investigation*. Collect information about what is causing concern. Preferably this should describe observable behaviors or events rather than feelings or thoughts. So, for example record turning up late, errors in procedures, or irritable behavior rather than "I'm worried about your attitude." This information should be documented. Preferably the behaviors should be those that you have directly observed rather than those that have been reported to you by others as you may find yourself in the difficult position of having to protect confidentiality, and consequently you may sound less compelling. The result of this initial problem list may mean that you have to gather more information or clarify events before meeting with the potentially sick doctor.

2. *Intervention—Who should be in the room?* There needs to be a consideration of who else needs to be at a meeting with the sick doctor. Considerations are the roles played by each individual, their relationship with the sick doctor, their role in providing support (friends for example), and whether there needs to be a series of meetings with individuals or a more formal meeting with several people in the room. So, for example, for a junior doctor who has attended work smelling of alcohol it may be appropriate to have several people present in the meeting: the clinical director of the service who represents the concerns of the employer (especially around patient safety), the training director who may be aware of issues elsewhere in the teaching rotation and will be able to give advice on the implications for training, and a senior psychiatrist from the organization whose role would be to provide advice about treatment options, the process of denial, and assess the risk to the doctor of confronting them with these concerns.

3. Intervention—Setting the agenda and how to run the meeting. There is a need to put into words at the start of the meeting that you have a dual role. You are there to let the doctor know of concerns about their behavior, to support and help, but you also have an obligation to report doctors whose behavior causes concern about their ability to practice. You may also want to have a conversation about the limits of confidentiality and the role of any written records. This sets the rules for the meeting and prevents the doctor from being surprised that concerns about performance may be referred elsewhere. It is important to keep written records of any such meetings.

4. Open with a brief statement of your concerns that is accurate and supportive. This should not take longer than a two or three minutes (or 250 to 350 words). It is wise and normal to expect denial and anger. If you don't prepare you may find yourself "struggling to defend your concerns, prove the accuracy of your data, and justify your interpretation of events." If possible, select issues you think are the most critical and the behaviors that support them. Identify what you think would be a good outcome from the meeting and try to steer the meeting toward this. It is useful to have thought ahead about what support or help the doctor may access. It is also important to recognize the strong feelings in the room and the dual role that you may have.

5. Intervention—Speak, listen, and discuss. During the meeting try to be brief, stick to specifics, and use simple language. All participants should agree on a plan to follow the meeting. A good plan is specific, measurable, achievable, relevant, and time limited (SMART). So a specific plan involves behaviors. For example, "I will make an appointment with my family doctor by the end of the week." This is measurable; you either do it or not. It is achievable, it is relevant to managing the sick doctor, and it is time limited (i.e. "the end of the week"). A poor plan would be "I will improve my attitude." It is hard to know how this would be observed or measured, whether it is achievable or relevant, or when this change will happen.

6. Evaluation, recovery, and monitoring. The meeting needs to be documented, including any agreements that have been reached. Be clear about the timing of follow-up plans and who is responsible for them and set limits if behaviors have not changed.

In the United States there is precedent, especially for doctors with substance abuse problems, for physicians acting with the Boards of Medicine, to confront the doctor with a treatment plan already formulated. This may include presenting the physician with only one option to return to practice, which includes a prearranged plane flight to an in-patient evaluation and treatment center where comorbid psychiatry disorders are evaluated and addressed alongside the addiction. The physician then has a reentry into practice under strict guidance and urine monitoring, counseling, and treatment programs usually lasting for a five-year period.

OTHER CONSIDERATIONS WHEN YOU HAVE CONCERNS ABOUT ANOTHER PHYSICIAN'S HEALTH

Confidentiality

Confidentiality is not absolute. Behaviors that may harm patients that are revealed in the meeting may be reported to the proper regulatory bodies, whereas details about the doctor's personal health are generally confidential. The legal framework around confidentiality varies in different countries, and different states within countries. For these reasons it is wise to be familiar with legal opinion in this area and to seek legal advice if unclear.

Risk

There are risks to patients, risks to the impaired doctor, risks to colleagues, and risks to the Organization. All these need to be recognized and managed. Risks to patients may be so severe—for example, if the impaired doctor is a hypomanic surgeon—that immediate action is called for. Risks to the impaired doctor may involve suicide, whose management should be included in any SMART plan. Risks to the Organization may involve bad press or threat of legal action, which again will involve talking with others to manage.

Consultation

Deciding to intervene with an impaired colleague is a difficult decision and like all difficult decisions there is rarely a correct answer. However there is a correct process, which nearly always involves appropriate consultation with others who may be colleagues, supervisors, or legal experts. These consultations should be documented and done early in the process.

Strong Feelings and Power

Power differentials between the impaired doctor and the "whistleblower" that brought the doctor to attention can cause difficult problems and the risk of the abuse of power. The conversation with the impaired doctor should be done by someone of at least equal seniority. The strong feelings of the impaired doctor may include feelings of anger, of being attacked, loss, panic and shock, and possibly relief. There may also be strong feelings, from the doctor's colleagues and those involved in difficult conversations, such as judgment and anger or a wish to protect someone from themselves. These conversations may also involve conflicts of interest—for example, not wanting to lose another doctor from the team—or competitive, narcissistic feelings of being "better" than the potentially sick doctor.

Case histories of sick doctors that illustrate the problem of transitioning from doctor to patient:

There are several case histories written by doctors or by those that survive them that have described the difficulties and barriers that doctors have in becoming patients (Jones, 2005; McKall, 2001). One of the more high profile cases that resulted in a major inquiry was the death of a psychiatrist, Daksha Emson, and her three-month-old baby. "*On 9th October 2000 Daksha stabbed Freya, her 3 month-old baby, stabbed herself, covered both of them in accelerant and set it alight. Freya died of smoke inhalation; Daksha survived for a further three weeks in a burns unit, but died without regaining consciousness. The incident, which should be regarded as a single act of suicide, took place during a psychotic episode.*" The inquiry highlighted major deficiencies in the way mental health care in doctors is managed (http://www.simplypsychiatry.co.uk/sitebuildercontent/sitebuilderfiles/deinquiryreport.pdf). "*The relationship between [her psychiatrist] and Daksha had the characteristics of many doctor-to-doctor relationships. She was not formally a patient of the Community Mental Health Team at her own request, in order to protect her anonymity in the NHS.*" "*Throughout Daksha's post-graduate training she went to considerable lengths to conceal her illness from her supervisors with one exception late on in her training, and was seemingly aided in this by National Health Service staff who shared her fear that the widespread stigma against mental illness in the NHS would damage her career prospects. She did not conceal her mental illness history from Occupational Health Services but received no help, support, or advice from them.*"

REFERENCES

American Medical Association (2011). *Policies related to physician health.* Chicago, IL: American Medical Association, Department of Physician Health & Health Care Disparities.

American Medical Association Opinion (2003) http://www.ama-assn.org/ama/pub/physician-resources/medical-ethics/code-medical-ethics/opinion9031.Page issued March 1992 based on the report "Reporting impaired, incompetent, or unethical colleagues," adopted December 1991 (*J Miss St Med Assoc.*1992;33:176–177); updated June 1994; updated June 1996; and updated June 2004, based on the report "Physician health and wellness," adopted December 2003.

Aronsson, G., & Gustafsson, K. (2005). Sickness presenteeism: Prevalence, attendance-pressure factors, and an outline of a model for research. *Journal of Occupational and Environmental Medicine, 47,* 958–966.

Baldisseri, M. R. (2007). Impaired healthcare professional. *Critical Care Medicine, 35*(Supplement), S106–S116.

Campbell, E. G., Regan, S., Gruen, R. L., Ferris, T. G., Rao, S. R., Cleary, P. D., et al. (2007). Professionalism in Medicine: Results of a National Survey of Physicians. *Annals of Internal Medicine, 147*(11), 795–802.

Canadian Medical Association, (2003). *CMA guide to physician health and well-being.* Ottawa: Canadian Medical Association.

Davidson, S. K., & Schattner, P. L. (2003). Doctor's health-seeking behaviour: A questionnaire survey. *The Medical Journal of Australia, 179*(6), 302–305.

Department of Health (2008). Mental health and ill health in doctors. Accessed on August 14 from (http://www.dh.gov.uk/prod_consum_dh/groups/dh_digitalassets/@dh/@en/documents/digitalasset/dh_083090.pdf).

Design physician wellness activities around health not discipline (2010). Accessed August 10, 2012 from http://www.healthleadersmedia.com/content/PHY-251054/Design-Physician-Wellness-Activities-Around-Health-Not-Discipline.

Federation of State Physician Health Programs (2012) http://www.fsphp.org/

Farber, N. J., Gilibert, S. G., Aboff, B. M., Collier, V. U., Weiner, J., & Boyer, E. G. (2005). Physicians' willingness to report impaired colleagues. *Social Science and Medicine, 61*(8), 1772–1775.

Garelick, A. I., Gross, S. R., Richardson, I., von der Tann, M., Bland, J., & Hale, R. (2007). Which doctors and with what problems contact a specialist service for doctors? A cross sectional investigation. *BMC Medicine, 5,* 26.

Isaksson Ro, K. E., Gude, T., Tyssen, R., & Aasland, O. G. (2008). Counselling for burnout in Norwegian doctors: One year cohort study. *BMJ, 337*(2004a doi:10.1136/bmj.a2004).

Jones, P. (2005). *Doctors as patients.* Oxford: Radcliffe Publishing Ltd.

Kay, M., Mitchell, G., Clavarino, A., & Doust, J. (2008). Doctors as patients: A systematic review of doctors' health access and the barriers they experience. *British Journal of General Practice, 58,* 501–508.

Laing, B. A. (2007). To tell the truth: Potential liability for concealing physician impairment. *Journal of Clinical Anesthesia, 19,* 638–641.

McKall, K. (2001). An insider's guide to depression. *BMJ, 323*(doi: 10.1136/bmj.323.7319.1011).

McKevitt, C., Morgan, M., Dundas, R., & Holland, W. W. (1997). Sickness absence and "working through" illness: A comparison of two professional groups. *Journal of Public Health Medicine, 19*(3), 295–300.

Rosvold, E. O., & Bjertness, E. (2002). Illness behavior among Norwegian physicians. *Scandinavian Journal of Public Health, 30*(2), 125–132.

Stanton, J., & Randal, P. (2011). Doctors accessing mental-health services: An exploratory study. *BMJ Open, doi: 10.1136/bmjopen*-2010-000017.

Stoudemire, A., & Rhoads, J. M. (1983). When the doctor needs a doctor: Special considerations for the physician-patient. *Annals of Internal Medicine, 98*(Part 1), 654–659.

Thompson, W. T., Cupples, M. E., Sibbett, C. H., Skan, D. I., & Bradley, T. (2001). Challenge of culture, conscience, and contract to general practitioners' care of their own health: Qualitative study. *BMJ, 323*(7315), 728–731. doi:10.1136/bmj.323.7315.728

Ubel, P. A., Angott, A. M., & Zikmund-Fisher, B. J. (2011). Physicians recommend different treatments for patients than they would choose for themselves. *Archives of Internal Medicine, 171*(7), 630–634.

Vaillant, G. E., Clark, W., Cyrus, C., Milofsky, E. S., Kopp, J., Wulsin, V. W., et al. (1983). Prospective study of alcoholism treatment: Eight year follow-up. *The American Medical Journal, 75*(3), 455–463.

VandonBos, G. R., & Duthie, R. F. (1986). Confronting and supporting colleagues in distress. In R. R. Kilburg, P. E. Nathan & R. W. Thoreson (Eds.), *Professionals in distress: Issues, syndromes, and solutions in psychology* Washington, DC: American Psychological Association.

Wallace, J. E., Lemaire, J. B., & Ghali, W. A. (2009). Physician wellness: a missing quality indicator. *Lancet, 374*(9702), 1714–1721.

/// 10 /// HOW DOCTORS BECOME PATIENTS

SIMON HATCHER

INTRODUCTION

While the health of physicians and its impact on their ability to practice adequately has been recognized as an important personal and public health issue for over 150 years (Baldisseri, 2007), it has become an increasing concern over the past three decades for several reasons. First, because of the nature of their work, an impaired physician presents a significant health risk to the general public. Second, physicians with some disorders such as substance use problems may respond particularly well to treatment when compared to the general public. Third, doctors often do not attend to their own health with the same care as they do to their patients. They may present late for help if they present at all, leading to worsened outcomes for the physician in terms of both health and ability to continue practicing. Finally, impaired physicians cause ongoing risk to patients, as sub-optimal and unsafe practice continues unchecked.

A range of strategies have been developed to help doctors overcome some of these difficulties. In the United States, most states have developed specific health programs for impaired physicians with the aim of removing a number of traditional barriers to treatment. Similar programs exist in a number of other countries including the United Kingdom, Australia, and New Zealand. Mandatory reporting of physicians when there are concerns about their health impacting significantly on their practice has been introduced in many places. The evidence regarding the nature of impairing health problems, their prevalence, and how they might best be treated is developing. However there is a lot that is still unknown. Much of the research involves impaired physicians who have come to the attention of their organizations and disciplinary bodies. This group is likely to be a small subgroup of the sum of impaired physicians in practice. Much of the literature is also anecdotal especially when dealing with treatment approaches. This chapter provides an overview of physician impairment focusing particularly on its prevalence, the underlying health problems that lead to it, and its detection, treatment, and prevention.

DEFINITIONS

The definition of impairment has varied over time, initially describing those who, for whatever reason, were unable to attend work regularly and has developed over recent decades to acknowledge that impaired physicians may appear to work normally on the face of it while actually being unable to develop safe and competent care (Baldisseri, 2007). Many definitions describe impairment as a degree of suboptimal practice that is unsafe for patients (Baldisseri, 2007; Westermeyer, 1991) and often narrow the focus to impairment that this is due to substance use problems or mental illness (Boisaubin & Levine, 2001). More recently, the concept has extended to include disability or health conditions that detrimentally affect the capacity to practice regardless of whether practice is impaired to the point of being unsafe (Peisah & Wilhelm, 2007; Peisah, Adler & Williams, 2007; Taub, Morin, Goldrich, Ray & Benjamin, 2006). Other definitions include the concept that the conditions are enduring if not treated, up to the point that the doctor is unable to deliver competent care (Carinci & Christo, 2009).

Australia, New Zealand, and the United Kingdom have moved to incorporate the concept of impairment into the broader one of fitness to practice, in which practice is more broadly defined as involving the provision of good clinical care, the maintenance of professional standards, and the development and maintenance of good relationships with patients and with colleagues. (New South Wales Medical Board, n.d.; General Medical Council (United Kingdom), n.d.; Medical Council of New Zealand, n.d.). These definitions have in common the concept that physicians suffer health problems that impair their clinical practice so that patient care suffers. However, the definitions are limited in a number of ways. They appear to preclude acute problems such as intoxication due to alcohol abuse, which although may be repeated, is not necessarily enduring without treatment, and also to exclude difficulties that lead to a doctor delivering suboptimal, yet safe, care. It seems reasonable to further expand the definition of impairment to include such situations. Some also specify certain health conditions, particularly mental health and substance use problems. These may be the most common problems that come to the attention of physician-health programs and disciplinary bodies but there are likely to be a number of other conditions, especially those leading to fatigue and cognitive impairment that are also important (Taub, Morin, Goldrich, Ray & Benjamin, 2006). An example of this is burnout (see also Chapter 7), which has received considerable attention in terms of physician health but which may well impair practice in its own right and which warrants consideration in the context of impaired practice (Brown, Goske, & Johnson, 2009).

One difficulty in this area is the definition of impairment itself. As mentioned, some definitions specify that impairment occurs when patient safety is compromised. However, this definition is inadequate in that it does not recognize safe but sub-optimal practice that must also be of concern. But it is unclear how to quantify impairment and therefore uncertain at what point action should be taken to help physicians whose health is compromising their practice. There are also problems with the way diagnostic terms are used (Baldisseri, 2007). Depression may represent a symptom of temporary lowered mood in response to life crises. A major depressive episode is a more serious condition and much more likely to lead to impaired practice. Psychoactive substance use, problematic use, abuse, and dependence are also terms that are used loosely. Alcohol and drug use does not necessarily lead to impaired practice, and nor does problematic use or abuse. Dependence is more likely to, especially if it is severe. The term abuse is also often used simply to indicate patterns of substance use that the person making the statement does not like. As with major depressive episode and disorder, substance abuse and substance dependence are specific diagnostic terms clearly described in DSM-IV (American Psychiatric Association, 1994) and ICD-10 (World Health Organization, 2004).

When used in this chapter, these terms will represent the DSM-IV diagnosis, the criteria for which are outlined in Tables 10.1 to 10.3.

EPIDEMIOLOGY

There are no reliable data on the prevalence of impaired practice in physicians due to health problems though estimates are in the range of 7–12% of all physicians (Wilson et al., 2009). It is likely that those referred to physician health programs or disciplinary bodies represent a small proportion of impaired physicians. Most estimates rely on the

TABLE 10.1 DSM-IV Diagnostic Criteria for Substance Abuse

A. A maladaptive pattern of substance use leading to clinically significant impairment or distress as manifested by one (or more) of the following:
  (1) recurrent substance use resulting in a failure to fulfill major role obligations at work, school, or home
  (2) recurrent substance use in situations in which it is physically hazardous
  (3) recurrent substance-related legal problems
  (4) continued substance use despite having persistent or recurrent social or interpersonal problems caused or exacerbated by the effects of the substance
B. The symptoms have never met the criteria for substance dependence for this class of substance.

TABLE 10.2 DSM-IV Diagnostic Criteria for Substance Dependence

A. A maladaptive pattern of substance use leading to clinically significant impairment or distress as manifested by three (or more) of the following, occurring at any time in the same 12-month period:

    (1) tolerance, as defined by either of the following

        a) a need for markedly increased amounts of the substance to achieve intoxication or desired effect

        b) markedly diminished effect with continued use of the same amount of the substance

    (2) withdrawal as manifested by either of the following

        a) the characteristic withdrawal syndrome for the substance

        b) the same (or closely related substance) is taken to avoid withdrawal symptoms

    (3) the substance is often taken in larger amounts or over a longer period than was intended

    (4) there is a persistent desire or unsuccessful efforts to cut down or control substance use

    (5) a great deal of time is spent in activities necessary to obtain the substance (e.g. visiting multiple doctors or driving long distances), use the substance (e.g. chain-smoking) or recover from its effects

    (6) important social, occupational, or recreational activities are given up or reduced because of substance use

    (7) the substance use is continued despite knowledge of having a persistent or recurrent physical or psychological problem that is likely to have been caused or exacerbated by the substance (current cocaine use despite recognition of cocaine-induced depression or continued drinking despite recognition that an ulcer was made worse by alcohol consumption).

Specify if:

with physiological dependence

without physiological dependence

TABLE 10.3 Key Elements of the DSM-IV Diagnostic Criteria for a Major Depressive Episode

Five (or more) of the following symptoms have been present during the same 2-week period and represent a change from previous functioning. At least one of the symptoms is either 1) depressed mood or 2) loss of interest or pleasure:

    1. depressed mood most of the day, nearly every day, as indicated by either subjective report (e.g. feels sad or empty) or observation made by others (e.g. appears tearful). Note: in children and adolescents, can be irritable mood.

    2. markedly diminished interest or pleasure in all, or almost all, activities most of the day, nearly every day (as indicated by either subjective account or observation made by others)

    3. significant weight loss when not dieting or weight gain (e.g. a change of more than 5% of body weight in a month) or decrease or increase in appetite nearly every day. Note: in children, consider failure to make expected weight gains

    4. insomnia or hypersomnia nearly every day

    5. psychomotor agitation or retardation nearly every day (observable by others, not merely subjective feelings of restlessness or being slowed down)

    6. fatigue or loss of energy nearly every day

    7. feelings of worthlessness or excessive or inappropriate guilt (which may be delusional) nearly every day (not merely self-reproach or guilt about being sick)

    8. diminished ability to think or concentrate, or indecisiveness, nearly every day (either by subjective account or as observed by others)

    9. recurrent thoughts of death (not just fear of dying), recurrent suicidal ideation without a specific plan, or a suicide attempt or a specific plan for committing suicide

prevalence of those health problems that may lead to impairment, but this provides unreliable information, assuming that they frequently do impair practice. This is by no means certain. However, with the lack of other forms of data, the prevalence rates of these problems are relevant.

Substance use problems underlie over half of referrals to physician-health programs (Wilson et al., 2009). It should be noted however that impairment due to substance use problems is more likely to be reported to the relevant authorities than impairment due to other conditions such as major depression or dementia (Farber, Gilbert, Aboff, Collier, Weiner & Boyer, 2005). Physicians appear to use psychoactive substances at similar rates as the general population, though rates of alcohol, opioid, and benzodiazepine use are higher, and rates of other drugs such as cannabis, amphetamines and cocaine are lower than those of the general population (Epstein & Eubanks, 1984; Holtman, 2007). Rates of problematic substance use are also similar to those in the general population with various studies suggesting that 10–15% of physicians experience alcohol use disorders and 6–8% experience drug use disorders in their lifetime (Baldisseri, 2007). Certain specialty areas have higher rates of substance use problems than others. Emergency medicine specialists used more illicit drugs overall, closely followed by psychiatrists who also have the highest rates of benzodiazepine use, while anaesthetists have the highest rates of opioid use. Availability is likely to influence different specialists' choice of drug (Hughes, Storr, Brandenburgh, Baldwin, Anthony & Sheehan, 1999; Marshall, 2008).

Rates of depression in medical students, junior doctors, and physicians are similar to those in the general population (Center et al., 2003; Urbach, Levenson & Harbison, 1989; Hurwitz, Beiser, Nichol, Patrick & Kozack, 1987) and higher in female than male physicians (Frank & Dingle, 1999). This suggests that between 12–20% of physicians are likely to suffer depression. However, rates may be significantly higher, especially in some subgroups of physicians. For example, 31% of family practitioners in British Columbia reported scores suggestive of major depression on the Beck Depression Inventory, a widely used rating scale for depression, and 55% scored positively on a widely used scale for burnout, the Maslach Burnout Inventory (Thommasen, Lavanchy, Connelly, Berkowitz & Grybowski, 2001). Suicide rates are approximately twice that of the general population for male and four times the general population in female physicians (Miller, McGowen & Quillen, 2000). However, it should be noted that most cases of depression do not lead to impairment to the extent that practice is seriously affected. Other mental health problems such as psychosis and bipolar disorder may lead to impairment but are much less common, while personality disorders, though arguably more frequent, tend to result in disruptive behaviors rather than impairment (Wilhelm & Reid, 2004).

Cognitive impairment due to dementia and physical illnesses such as multiple sclerosis, diabetes mellitus, Parkinson's Disease, cerebro-vascular accidents, and epilepsy, which that can impair cognition and also lead to impairment through general malaise, are also an issue, but have received much less attention (Wilhelm & Reid, 2004). These usually present close to retirement age and may not be easy to detect when mild but are more likely to lead to the termination of practice when they begin to affect clinical practice (Harrison, 2008).

ETIOLOGY

The etiology of physician impairment is important for many reasons, arguably the most important being that it allows identification of dynamic factors that may be changed. This identification helps us prevent or minimize the impact of these problems and enhances the chances of successful recovery. When considering the etiology of impairment in physicians, we are considering the illnesses that commonly lead to impairment, and the factors that cause these illnesses and that influence their severity. The etiology of most of these problems is multifactorial and complex. Factors that influence severity and therefore the likelihood of leading to impaired practice include the natural history of the disorders in particular individuals, factors that influence help seeking, whether or not treatment is accessed before impairment occurs, and compliance with treatment plans.

The etiology of addiction in physicians includes genetic vulnerability (Lutsky, Hopwood, Abram, Cerletty, Hoffman, Kampine, 1994), depression and anxiety, psychological stress both in their work and family lives, preexisting vulnerable personality styles (Brooke, Edwards & Andrews, 1993), such as perfectionism and obsessionality, high levels of self-control and a strong sense of independence (Vaillant, Brighton & McArthur,1970; Vaillant, Brighton & McArthur,1972; Merlo & Gold, 2008), a belief in the effectiveness of medication (Kleber, 1984), and a tendency to treat themselves with medication (Forsythe, Calnan & Wall, 1999), which is facilitated by the easy availability of abusable drugs (Marshall, 2008).

Major depression is associated with impairments in neural networks involving the prefrontal cortex and subcortical and temporal lobe areas involved in executive control, memory, affective processing, and feedback sensitivity. Such impairments present as poor memory and concentration and indecisiveness. Affect processing that is associated with negative thinking and feedback sensitivity associated with more intense responses to negative feedback are particularly amenable to treatment with serotonergic medications such as the selective serotonin reuptake inhibitors (Clark, Chamberlain & Sahakian, 2009). These cognitive deficits may be worse in women and memory impairment may be more severe in older people with depression, and may not resolve completely with treatment of depression (Marazziti, Consoli, Picchetti, Carlini & Faravelli, 2010). Sleep disturbance is also a hallmark of major depression, and, coupled with the irregular sleep patterns necessitated by the demands of being a doctor, it is likely to play some role in impaired performance (Pandi-Perumal et al., 2009; Srinivasan et al., 2009). Circadian disturbances such as those caused by on-call and shift work may cause or exacerbate a subgroup of depressed patients (Moneteleone & Maj, 2008).

Cognitive impairment can arise from multiple causes including neurological illnesses associated with dementia, depression, and alcohol and other substance-related brain damage. Key impairments that are likely to impact on clinical practice include problems with executive functioning involved in problem-solving, mental flexibility, and reasoning (Turnbull, Cunnington, Unsal, Norman & Ferguson, 2006). Standard clinical cognitive screening tests such as the Mini Mental State Examination seldom pick up on the extent of the cognitive impairment and more detailed neuropsychological testing may be necessary to detect subtle abnormalities (Peisah, Adler & Williams, 2007).

Similar etiological factors therefore underpin the cause of both substance use disorders and mood and anxiety disorders. Each has a significant genetic predisposition interacting with early environmental and family influences, personality variables, coping and problem solving skills, social and relationship skills, support networks, and environmental stressors (Kohnke, 2008; aan het Rot, Mathew, Charney, 2009). It is not surprising therefore that there are high levels of comorbidity between these illnesses (Adamson, Todd, Sellman, Huriwai & Porter, 2006; Todd, 2010). Stress, burnout, and disturbed sleep patterns are etiological factors that may also directly lead to impairment in their own right. However, they appear to be amenable to change (Taub, Morin, Goldrich, Ray, & Benjamin, 2006). While there has been considerable interest in the issue of burnout in physicians and its impact on patient care, it has only recently been recognized as a direct contributor to impairment (Brown, Goske, & Johnson, 2009). Burnout is a response to the experience of high levels of stress that can lead to a range of harms including emotional exhaustion, inefficiency, depersonalization, and cynicism—including negative thoughts toward patients and low job satisfaction (Maslach, Schaufeli & Leiter, 2001). While personal coping styles such as denial and avoidance are thought to contribute to the symptoms of burnout, there is a large component attributed to organizational factors (Kisa, Kisa & Younis, 2009), especially when there are significant differences between the physician and the organization within which they work in terms of expected workload, the degree of control over work practices, rewards, and values (Maslach et al., 2001). Organizations that stress cooperation between staff, that enable effective communication, emphasize the need for training, and allow clinicians high levels of self-direction in their work tend to be associated with significantly lower levels of stress (Firth-Cozens, 2001; Wall, Bolden, Borrill, 1997). However, sleep deprivation and substance misuse also appear to play a role in stress and burnout, as does the presence or absence of protective factors such as having hobbies (Sargent, Sotile, Sotile, Rubash & Barrack, 2009). Of considerable concern is that burnout may affect between 35% and 67% of physicians, more commonly younger physicians and those working in specialties (Shanafelt, Sloan & Habermann, 2003), and appears to be associated with less than optimal care (Shanafelt, Bradley, Wipf & Back, 2002; Williams, Manwell, Konrad & Linzer, 2007).

A number of common factors also appear to delay the presentation of these disorders. Examples include the stigma physicians feel toward disability in general and mental health and substance use problems in particular, a strong personal investment in being a physician in terms of personal identity and the fear of loss of status, identity, and income that they believe is associated with impairment (Harrison, 2008) (see also Chapters 8 and 10). Contact with psychoactive drugs within the workplace may be particularly important for older physicians. McAuliffe proposes two subtypes of substance dependence in physicians. The first is usually found in trainees and younger physicians due to exposure to others who use drugs recreationally, and the second is found in older physicians due mainly to the availability of and contact with prescribed drugs in the workplace (McAuliffe et al., 1987).

There are a number of factors that are likely to play a role in the development of the health problems underpinning impairment and that may be amenable to intervention. Of particular interest are personal experiences of workplace stress and burnout, coping styles and personal resilience, and organizational characteristics such as styles of communication, workload, role clarity, and self-determination. These will be discussed further below in the section on prevention.

IDENTIFICATION AND DIAGNOSIS

As mentioned, it is likely that a significant number of impaired physicians are not being identified. Unfortunately, impairment usually comes to light after there are complaints from patients or there is a serious lapse in patient treatment (Khong, Sim & Hulse, 2002). In one study of doctors in a physician health program, opioid users were shown to have been using opioids for two years before detection (Cadman & Bell, 1988). Other studies suggest that alcohol use problems have been present for up to six years before the physician seeks help (Marshall, 2008).

Many reasons have been suggested for the failure to identify impairment and for the late presentation of the illnesses associated with it: The signs and symptoms of impairment in the physician are often subtle (Berge, Seppala & Schipper, 2009), when exactly a physician becomes impaired is uncertain, colleagues are reluctant to report impairment in a physician, those with health problems are even more reluctant to acknowledge them (Pesiah, Adler, & Williams, 2007), and physicians who are impaired are very good at denying it and finding ways to avoid detection (Rosen et al., 2009). Physicians are used to practicing more independently than many other professionals. The fear of loss of independence, of the financial consequences of loss of income from impairment (Pesiah, Adler, & Williams, 2007), and the loss status and what is often a core part of their identity, may drive this reluctance (Baldisseri, 2007), as may having a negative and potentially terrifying awareness of the process and consequences of serious illness. A perfectionist personality, a feeling of indispensability to their patients, and the stigma toward mental health and alcohol and drug problems within the profession are further factors that (Baldisseri, 2007) undermine reporting and acknowledgement of impairment (Baldisseri, 2007).

Early identification of impairment and of associated health conditions is important in terms of the outcome of these conditions and the protection of the general public. Waiting for clear evidence of impairment may delay access to help and in doing so increase the risk to patients and to the physician (Berge et al., 2009).

A number of authors have described signs and symptoms that may suggest impairment is present and indicate the need for further investigation (Marshall, 2008; Baldisseri, 2007; Peisah & Wilhelm, 2007; Khong, et al., 2002; Berge, et al., 2009; Breiner, 1979; Bryson & Silverstein, 2008; Hulse, O'Neil, Hatton & Paech, 2003). With respect to substance use, there are certain signs and behaviors associated with intoxication, withdrawal, and chronic use that should raise concern. Slurred speech, ataxia, dilated or pinpoint pupils, and erratic behavior may suggest intoxication. Irritability, agitation, anxiety, and sweating may point to withdrawal states. A disheveled appearance, repeated lateness or unexplained absences during the day, hidden bottles of alcohol, an increase in prescribing errors, heavy drinking at professional social events, and forgetfulness may be present with chronic alcohol and drug use. Volunteering to work extra shifts, coming into work at unusual hours, and remaining close to sources of drugs may be due to attempts to access drugs. Professional isolation, frequent changes in employment, significant gaps in their employment history, and taking jobs for which they are overqualified may also indicate chronic problems with impairment. Depression may reveal itself as persistent negative attitudes, tiredness and irritability, sadness, poor memory and concentration (i.e. as evidenced by forgetting appointments and meetings), and social withdrawal. Repeated patterns of such behaviors indicate the need for further exploration.

Certain signs are clear indicators of concern and even isolated incidents require further investigation. Smelling of alcohol at work, a conviction for driving under the influence of drink or drugs, and complaints from patients and from colleagues or other staff such as pharmacists, are highly suggestive of significant problems that are no longer able to be hidden and therefore are likely to be impairing.

Improving the identification of impaired physicians is not straightforward. Changes to the culture of medicine in which mental health and addiction problems become less stigmatized, increasing awareness of signs of impairment and the successful outcome for treatment of impairing conditions early in medical careers, and enhancing physicians' sense of responsibility for the wellbeing of colleagues—especially as it relates to patient care—are likely to be beneficial. Mandatory reporting of impaired colleagues may help, though it should be noted that this is currently in force in many places that have well-developed physician health programs but still experience significant underreporting. Some authors have proposed compulsory random screening measures involving random urinary drug screens or hair drug analysis and breath alcohol testing in the work place, monitoring of peer-review performance, and also using disciplinary action against colleagues of impaired doctors who could reasonably have been expected to detect and report the impairment (Avery, Daniel & McCormick, 2000). A three-tiered approach has been proposed in which a selection of all physicians are routinely screened, high-risk groups such as those over a specific age are more intensely scrutinized, and frequent mandatory screening is carried out for those with clear indicators of performance issues such as a history of complaints against them (Peisah et al., 2007). Similar approaches are used in other professional groups with responsibility for public safety and seem logical for physicians, but are likely to meet considerable resistance until there is a change of attitude within the profession about the need to maintain a high level of wellbeing in order to perform adequately in their roles.

TREATMENT

Once a physician has been identified as having problems likely to lead to impairment and in need of further evaluation, the physician should be gently confronted about the problems and assessment and treatment should be initiated as indicated. There is limited research evidence to indicate how this is best done. There are, however, clear indications of best practice from the opinions and experiences of practitioners involved in this process. Much of the literature comes from the United States and, less so, from the United Kingdom and Australia. The differences in practicing environment, resources dedicated to helping impaired physicians, and the legislator framework in which such problems are dealt requires caution in generalizing from this literature.

Many countries now organize services for impaired physicians from a specific body established by or under the registration or disciplinary body. The focus of these physician-health programs is to organize the assessment, treatment, and post-treatment monitoring of these health problems but they also have a responsibility to report ongoing, serious impairment to the registration and disciplinary bodies. Where possible, these health programs maintain a degree of independence from the registration and disciplinary bodies to encourage privacy and entry into treatment (Baldisseri, 2007).

The general approach to assessment and treatment should be to combine specific evidence-based treatments within a highly supportive treatment plan, adapting treatment to take into consideration the special circumstances and needs of the patient group. This latter group includes the features described earlier that make identification and early treatment difficult, such as high levels of denial and a reluctance to engage in treatment, the increased risk of suicide (especially during the early phases of treatment and at times of relapse), issues of confidentiality and privacy that arise when physicians need to get help from the system they work in, use of knowledge of the treatment as an excuse to avoid addressing their problems adequately, the poorer outcomes and higher suicide rates reported for anesthesiologists who misuse opioids, and the issues of public safety that arise from illness and impairment (Rosen et al., 2009).

It is useful to think of treatment as occurring in three stages (Bryson & Silverstein, 2008; DuPont, McLellan, Carr, Gendel & Skipper, 2009):

1. Initial evaluation and assessment
2. Formal treatment
3. Long-term support and monitoring, which includes facilitating a return to work where appropriate.

1. INITIAL EVALUATION AND ASSESSMENT

This involves gently confronting the impaired physician with the concern that they are potentially unwell and that it has become apparent that their practice is impaired, and organizing further assessment and treatment planning.

As mentioned, the body responsible for addressing the physician's health issues should ideally be separate from the body that controls professional registration, disciplinary action, and licensing to practice. Such an arrangement is likely to ensure confidentiality and privacy and to increase the likelihood of referral itself and engagement and compliance with the treatment process. Treatment can then be seen as being dedicated to the health of the physician rather than serving a punitive function and thereby increase the chances of them engaging with treatment, a significant problem when treating physicians (Arana, 1982). There is however a significant overlap in function (Pesiah, Adler, & Williams, 2007); those responsible for attending to the physicians' health concerns need to have clear guidelines and lines of reporting to the registration and disciplinary body and need to be able to use the threat of restrictions on practice to enhance motivation.

The initial interview in which the impaired physician is confronted with the issues regarding their health and its impact on their ability to practice safely is a delicate process. The people conducting the interview need to find a gentle balance between concern and firmness (Marshall, 2008). It should be a formal process with clear documentation (Berge et al., 2009). A detailed outline of the bounds of confidentiality and assurances that this will be maintained should be given, but it should also be made clear who needs to be spoken to and what records need to be accessed with the physician's agreement before the safety of patients can be assured and practice can resume (Taub et al., 2006; Khong, et al., 2002; Bryson & Silverstein, 2008). Depending on the nature of the health problems, the impaired physician usually continues to have a choice about whether or not to be subject to the process, though there should be no doubt about the consequences of not agreeing in terms of the licensing body being informed and ability to practice being suspended (Bryson & Silverstein, 2008; DuPont et al., 2009). Several authors stress the elevated risk of self-harm after the initial interview and recommend immediate placement in a residential treatment facility, especially for those with psychoactive substance-related problems (Carinci & Christo, 2009; Bryson & Silverstein, 2008; DuPont et al., 2009). This may not always be feasible. Regardless, it is important to assess risk at this time, especially the risk of serious self-harm and to manage this appropriately.

Referral for a comprehensive health assessment and treatment plan needs to be made to a specialist in the relevant health area, preferably one who is not a close colleague of the impaired physician (Baldisseri, 2007; Rosen et al., 2009). This assessment needs to cover physical and mental health, substance misuse, and a range of likely stressors, being mindful of the high rates of comorbidity that occur. The assessment also needs to contain a collateral history from family members, colleagues, and relevant managers, and include relevant investigations including urine drug screens or hair analysis for psychoactive substances. It should be noted that urine drug screens only detect use in the previous few days for most drugs likely to be abused except cannabis, with which regular use may be detected several weeks after the last exposure. Hair analysis may detect use in the past few months and therefore may be more useful. Hair for analysis may be obtained from a range of areas on the body (Bryson & Silverstein, 2008). In-depth neuropsychological testing may be indicated where cognitive impairment is an issue.

It is also useful to consider issues of motivation and treatment adherence from the beginning. Motivation for treatment may be enhanced by stressing it by speaking to the physician's values (likely to involve serving patients well, keeping the respect of family, friends, and colleagues, and ensuring status and income), by offering a degree of choice in areas that are negotiable (but not in those that are non-negotiable) (Todd, 2010), and by everyone involved working hard to develop empathy for the impaired physician. It is also important not to give an impression of being permissive and thereby offer hope to the physician that the issue can be avoided or that the physician can get away with being untruthful (Rosen et al., 2009).

2. FORMAL TREATMENT

Formal treatment involves specific interventions targeting the specific health problems the physician suffers from, especially those affecting their ability to practice competently.

Specific issues related to the treatment of physicians include, as mentioned above, their skill at avoiding confronting their problems due to their knowledge of the health system, prejudice against mental health and substance use problems in particular (Brandon, 1997), a high rate of dropout from treatment especially for mental health problems when compared to other population groups, and high rates of suicide (Arana, 1982). It is therefore important that they are treated as patients not as colleagues, that effort is put into maintaining an appropriate doctor-patient relationship, and that they are offered the same range and quality of treatment as all other patients (Rosen et al., 2009). Insight and motivation to change is at the heart of treatment. While the issue of legal and disciplinary action should largely be separated from the health needs of the physician, it cannot be avoided and is an important factor in enhancing motivation. The threat of loss of status, personal esteem, identity, and income is a powerful motivator. It is also a significant factor in the risk of self-harm. It therefore needs to be carefully managed, but the provision of caring and supportive treatment focusing on the health needs of the physician and the expectation that a return to work is likely in most cases, can be useful. Some authors recommend a formal contract be signed specifying what has been agreed to in treatment and during the follow-up phase, with the consequence of significant non-compliance including reporting to the local legal or professional registration bodies (DuPont, McLellan, Carr, Gendel & Skipper, 2009). Older doctors, especially those with cognitive impairment, may find it harder to gain insight into their impairment, may be less likely to return to practice, and therefore may struggle to participate in the treatment process (Pesiah, Adler, & Williams, 2007). In such cases, a managed retirement or retraining into other areas of health care might be a more appropriate goal.

Treatment should involve the delivery of high-quality comprehensive care for the problems at hand. This involves a combination of education, medication and psychotherapy, advocacy, and case management. Motivational interviewing and relapse prevention approaches are especially relevant for physicians with addictions but may also be very useful for a range of other health problems. For substance dependence, 12-step approaches are also helpful and medication such as disulfiram, naltrexone, or acamprosate for alcohol dependence and naltrexone for opioid dependence may also be helpful. Medication compliance may be difficult to ensure; close monitoring is advisable and there is some evidence that naltrexone implants may improve the outcome for opioid dependence (Hulse, O'Neil, Hatton & Paech, 2003). Standard treatment for major depression involves medication and psychotherapy, especially cognitive-behavioral therapy. Regular group sessions with other doctors exploring issues around work-related stress may be helpful in reducing levels of burnout (Rø, Gude, Tyssen & Aasland, 2004). Cognitive impairment from other illnesses such as cerebro-vascular accidents and Parkinson's disease may respond less well to treatment. Highly skilled and aggressive management of these other conditions is essential but in such cases redirecting the patient into other areas of employment or into retirement may be necessary. When residential or inpatient treatment is indicated, consideration should be given to placement out of the area in which the physician practices to maintain confidentiality and privacy and to avoid having physicians in treatment alongside their patients (DuPont et al., 2009). Similarly, group treatments may be useful, and, where possible, groups with other physicians may help in gaining insight and the acceptance of the need for change (Bryson & Silverstein, 2008). Other interventions that are considered standard practice by many include the active screening for and treatment of comorbid problems and the involvement of family members in the treatment process, including specific family therapy when indicated (Berge et al., 2009). Prior to considering a return to work, it is advisable to put considerable effort into anticipating factors that are likely to lead to relapse and to put into place strategies to minimize this risk. Common precipitants of relapse include a lack of insight into and acceptance of the problems, poor coping and social/relationship skills, social and professional isolation, overconfidence, family problems, and a lack of commitment to attending follow-up (Baldisseri, 2007).

3. LONG-TERM SUPPORT AND MONITORING

Long-term support and monitoring follows from the formal treatment phase and focuses on maintaining the gains made, minimizing the risk of relapse, and ensuring a safe and supported return to practice or redeployment, whichever is appropriate.

A return to practice is usually considered once formal treatment has been completed and symptoms have resolved to the point that the physician is likely to be able to practice competently. The time course for this depends on the condition being treated, as does the duration of follow-up and monitoring. This may be reasonably brief in cases of resolved major depression. For substance use problems, with their high risk of precipitous relapse and potential to compromise patient safety, a period of at least five years is often recommended. When close monitoring is felt to be necessary a formal signed contract outlining monitoring requirements and the consequences of relapse can be very useful (Carinci & Christo, 2009; DuPont, McLellan, Carr, Gendel, & Skipper, 2009).

Returning to practice may be assisted by an evaluation of the physician's ability to practice, especially if there has been a prolonged period off work, restricted working hours, restrictions on the type of patients being seen, or limitations on the scope of practice and prescribing rights, especially in specialties such as anesthesiologists where there is ready access to psychoactive substances (Berge, Seppala & Schipper, 2009; Bryson & Silverstein, 2008). For those physicians for whom the use of potentially dangerous drugs such as opioids is possible, there should also be clear education about the risks of overdose, especially with the lowering of tolerance after a period of abstinence.

Specific monitoring for signs of relapse and further impairment of practice again depends on the nature of the health problems, but at a minimum should include regular appointments with the treating physician or case manager and oversight in the workplace by a senior colleague. More specific measures are advisable when the problem involves substance use (Baldisseri, 2007; Berge et al., 2009; Silverstein, Silva & Iberti, 1993). Ongoing attendance at 12-step meetings can be monitored. Regular breath analysis for alcohol prior to starting a shift, regular random urinary drug screening, and less-frequent hair drug analysis may help to ensure the impaired physician does not cover up any relapses. Close monitoring of prescription patterns and drug waste may be useful especially for those with access to addictive substances such as anesthesiologists. Maintaining an ongoing relationship with a supportive significant other is useful.

Relapse prevention and close monitoring should especially target those with a high likelihood of relapse, predictors of which include a family history of substance use problems, a history of problematic opioid use, coexisting substance use and mental health problems, lack of insight, poor coping and social skills, and reluctant engagement with treatment (Carinci & Christo, 2009).

PROGNOSIS

Most of the outcome data on impaired physicians comes from the well-funded and highly organized physician health programs in the United States that provide prolonged and intensive follow-up monitoring. Caution is needed when generalizing the results to other systems. There is good evidence, however, that physicians who enter treatment for impairing health conditions do better than the general public. Many small studies of single programs have been published with successful outcomes ranging from 29–92% (Baldisseri, 2007). The best evidence on prognosis comes from a 5-year follow-up study of physicians with substance misuse problems in 16 physician health programs by McLellan and colleagues (McLellan, Skipper, Campbell & DuPont, 2008), which confirms the high success rates of most of the early studies. Eighty percent of those entering these programs completed treatment and resumed clinical practice. Of those who returned to work, fewer than 20% had positive evidence of further substance use and 78% had continued to remain in practice 5 years after completing initial treatment. These rates are considerably better than those reported for substance use problems in the general population (DuPont et al., 2009).

From the same study, Skipper and colleagues (Skipper, Campbell & DuPont, 2009) reported on outcomes for anesthesiologists who have higher rates of substance misuse than other specialists and are more likely to be misusing opioids than other physicians. Earlier reports raised concern that anesthesiologists, especially those using opioids, may experience worse outcomes and have higher suicide rates than physicians from other specialties using other substances. The study by Skipper and colleagues found that anesthesiologists misusing opioids did no worse than others and that the suicide rates were no higher. They pointed to differing methodologies in the studies and to more intensive follow-up and monitoring in their sample as possible explanations. While these results are reassuring, further research is needed. Another subgroup, older doctors, do appear to have much lower rates of successful return to work. In a study of older doctors from New South Wales, approximately 70% were unable to return to practice (Pesiah, Adler, & Williams, 2007). This group contained a signficiant number of physicians impaired by cognitive decline and physical problems, suggesting that, as would be expected, these conditions have a worse outcome than substance misuse. The information on other conditions such as depression and other mental health problems is sparse and outcomes for these are less clear.

Outcomes reported from other systems such as those in the United Kingdom and Australia appear lower than those from the physician health programs in the United States, being more in the range of 50–60% (Gossop et al., 2001; Pethebridge, 2005). As mentioned, differences in approaches, system organization, and resources may explain these differences.

PREVENTION

Prevention of impairment can occur at the primary (preventing the occurrence of impairing health conditions), secondary (early detection and intervention) and tertiary (preventing the severity of the impact of impairing health conditions) levels. The most attention has been given to primary prevention.

Primary Prevention

Suggested measures to prevent the onset of impairment and those conditions that lead to it include educating physicians early in training about the risks of key etiological factors such as stress and burnout and strategies to minimize these, teaching appropriate coping skills and stress management techniques, and communicating the importance of maintaining a healthy lifestyle including developing interests outside medicine and of developing supportive relationships. Education has not been shown to have a significant impact on health and impairment (Bryson & Silverstein, 2008). Strategies to reduce personal stress levels, including maintaining a healthy diet, spending time with friends and family, being involved in continuing medical education (Lee, Stewart & Brown, 2008; Jensen, Trollope-Kumar, Waters & Everson 2008), specific coping skills and stress management training (Baldisseri, 2007; Firth-Cozens, 2001; Kumar, 2007) and training in time management and practice management (Jensen, 2008) have been shown to reduce the risk of burnout and the subsequent impairment that can result.

Placing controls on access to drugs has been proposed, especially for areas where the misuse of prescription medication is an issue such as with anesthesiologists (Bryson & Silverstein, 2008). Strategies such as careful documentation and monitoring of prescribing and use patterns, the use of computerized dispensing units, and the monitoring of drug waste have been suggested. Other systemic approaches include random screening (as mentioned above), focusing on developing a workplace atmosphere that encourages open communication, training, allowing staff discretion in their work practices, and limiting the burden of paperwork and service-orientated documentation (Wall, Bolden, & Borrill, 1997; Kumar, 2007).

Secondary Prevention

Strategies to encourage early identification and intervention for health conditions focus on changing attitudes among physicians to overcome the barriers to reporting. Mandatory reporting on legal grounds has been implemented with questionable success as mentioned above (Pesiah, Adler, & Williams, 2007; Avery, Daniel, & McCormick, 2000). A culture change in which physicians come to accept that they have a responsibility to both colleagues and patients to maintain their own health and that of other physicians, supported by a stronger emphasis on the ethical imperative to address impairment in self and others may be necessary, but will require concerted efforts over time to achieve. A change in the stigmas physicians often have for substance use and mental health disorders is also needed (Baldisseri, 2007; Harrison, 2008).

Tertiary Prevention

Prevention of the impact of impairing health conditions on physicians and their patients involves those strategies already mentioned in the section on treatment, specifically, the suspension of practice when necessary until fitness can be demonstrated, active treatment of the health conditions, and close monitoring after return to the workplace to ensure that treatment gains are maintained.

CONCLUSIONS

There have been significant developments in the treatment of impaired physicians in the past three decades. The establishment of physician health programs where the focus is on health more than punishment, the increasing base of evidence on the epidemiology of impairment, and the recognition of several key etiological factors such as coping styles and stress that are amenable to intervention and may help prevent impairment, all promise to improve the health of both physicians and their patients. There remain significant areas of difficulty, however. Physicians are still reluctant to admit certain health conditions and to help colleagues with problems access treatment. Programs to improve coping skills and stress management are uncommon. There continues to be a lack of knowledge about the prevalence, impact on practice, and best treatment options for important health conditions associated with impairment such as major depression and conditions associated with cognitive impairment. The role of organizational style and change on impairment warrants attention. The extent of the impact of lifestyle issues such as lack of sleep and burnout continues to be under-appreciated.

At the heart of the changes needed to improve the health of impaired physicians and their patients is a change in culture and attitude within the profession. Physicians need to take responsibility for their own health and the health of colleagues and to change attitudes that stigmatize mental health and substance use problems. They need to embrace strategies that reduce stress and coping to help prevent ill-health and subsequent impaired practice. Health organizations need to consider more closely the style of management and the impact it has on physician well-being. Awareness of these issues has been increasing steadily but many challenges still remain.

REFERENCES

aan het Rot, M., Mathew, S.J., & Charney, D.S. (2009). Neurobiological mechanisms in major depressive disorder. *Canadian Medical Association Journal, 180*(3), 305–313.

Adamson, S.J., Todd, F.C., Sellman, J.D., Huriwai, T., & Porter, J. (2006). Coexisting psychiatric disorders in a New Zealand outpatient alcohol and other drug clinical population. *Australian and New Zealand Journal of Psychiatry, 40*(2),164–170.

American Psychiatric Association. (1994). *Diagnostic and statistical manual of mental disorders, fourth edition.* Washington, D.C.: Author.

Arana, G.W. (1982). The impaired physician: a medical and social dilemma. *General Hospital Psychiatry, 4*(2), 147–154.

Avery, D.M., Daniel, W.D., & McCormick, M.B. (2000). The impaired physician. *Primary Care Update for OB/GYNS, 7*(4), 154–160.

Baldisseri, M.R. (2007). Impaired healthcare professional. *Critical Care Medicine, 35*(2 Suppl.), S106–S116.

Berge, K.H., Seppala, M.D., & Schipper, A.M. (2009). Chemical dependency and the physician. *Mayo Clinic Proceedings. 84*(7), 652–631.

Boisaubin, E.V., & Levine, R.E. (2001). Identifying and assisting the impaired physician. *American Journal of Medical Sciences., 322*(1), 31–36.

Brandon, S. (1997). Persuading the sick or impaired doctor to seek treatment. *Advances in Psychiatric Treatment, 3,* 305–311.

Breiner, S.J. (1979). The impaired physician. *Journal of Medical Education, 54*(8), 673.

Brooke, D., Edwards, G., & Andrews, T. (1993). Doctors and substance misuse: types of doctors, types of problems. *Addiction, 88*(5), 655–663.

Brown, S.D., Goske, M.J.,& Johnson, C.M. (2009) Beyond substance abuse: stress, burnout and depression as causes of physician impairment and disruptive behavior. *JACR Journal of the American College of Radiology, 6*(7), 479–485.

Bryson, E. O., & Silverstein, J.H. (2008). Addiction and substance abuse in anesthesiology. *Anesthesiology, 109*(5), 905–917.

Cadman, M., & Bell, J. (1998). Doctors detected self-administering opioids in New South Wales 1985–1994. Characteristics and outcomes. *Medical Journal of Australia, 169,* 419–421.

Carinci, A.J., & Christo, P.J. (2009). Physician impairment: is recovery feasible? *Pain Physician, 12*(3), 487–491.

Center, C., Davis, M.,Detre, T., Ford, D., Hansborough, W., Hendin, H., (...) Silverman, M. (2003). Confronting suicide and depression in physicians: a consensus statement. *Journal of the American Medical Association. 289*(23), 3161–3166.

Clark, L., Chamberlain, S.R., & Sahakian, B.J. (2009). Neurocognitive mechanisms in depression: implications for treatment. *Annual Review of Neuroscience, 32,* 57–74.

DuPont, R.L., McLellan, A.T., Carr, G., Gendel, M., & Skipper, G.E. (2009). How are addicted physicians treated? A national survey of physician health programs. *Journal of Substance Abuse Treatment, 37*(1), (1–7).

Epstein, R., & Eubanks, E.E. (1984). Drug use among medical students. *New England Journal of Medicine. 311*(14), 923.

Farber, N.J., Gilbert, S.G., Aboff, B.M., Collier, V.U., Weiner, J., & Boyer, E.G. (2005). Physicians' willingness to report impaired colleagues. *Social Science & Medicine, 61*(8), 1772–1775.

Firth-Cozens, J. (2001). Interventions to improve physicians' well-being and patient care. *Social Science & Medicine. 52*(2), 215–222.

Forsythe, M., Calnan, M., & Wall, B. (1999). Doctors as patients: a postal survey examining consultants and general practitioners adherence to guidelines. *British Medical Journal, 319*(7210), 605–608.

Frank, E., & Dingle, A. (1999). Self-reported depression and suicide attempts among US women physicians. *American Journal of Psychiatry, 156*(12),1887–1894.

General Medical Council (United Kingdom). (n.d). The meaning of fitness to practise. Retrieved June 7, 2011, from, http://www.gmc-uk.org/the_meaning_of_fitness_to_practise.pdf_25416562.pdf

Gossop, M., Stephens, S., Stewart, D., Marshall, J., Bearn, J., & Strang, J. (2001). Health care professionals referred for treatment of alcohol and drug problems. *Alcohol & Alcoholism, 36*(2), 160–164.

Harrison, J. (2008). Doctor's health and fitness to practice: the need for a bespoke model of assessment. *Occupational Medicine, 58*(5), 323–327.

Holtman, M.C. (2007). Disciplinary careers of drug-impaired physicians. *Social Science & Medicine. 64*(3), 543–553.

Hughes, P.H., Storr, C.L., Brandenburgh, N.A., Baldwin, D.C.J., Anthony, J.C., & Sheehan, D.V. (1999). Physician substance abuse by medical specialty. *Journal of Addictive Disorders, 18*(2), 23–37.

Hulse, G.K., O'Neil, G., Hatton, M., Paech, M.J. (2003). Use of oral and implantable naltrexone in the management of the opioid impaired physician. *Anaesth Intensive Care. 31*(2), 196–201.

Hurwitz, T.A., Beiser, M., Nichol, H., Patrick, L.,& Kozack, J. (1987). Impaired interns and residents. *Canadian Journal of Psychiatry, 32*(3),165–169.

Jensen, P.M.(2008). Building physician resilience. *Canadian Family Physician 54*(5), 722–729.

Jensen, P.M., Trollope-Kumar, K., Waters, H., & Everson, J. (2008). Building physician resilience. *Canadian Family Physician, 54*(5), 722–729.

Khong, E., Sim, M.G., & Hulse, G. (2002). The identification and management of the drug impaired doctor. *Australasian Family Physician, 31*(12), 1097–1100.

Kisa, S., Kisa, A., & Younis, M.Z. (2009). A discussion of job dissatisfaction and burnout among public hospital physicians. *International Journal of Health Promotion and Education. 47*(4), 104–111.

Kleber, H.D. (1984). The impaired physician: changes from the traditional view. *J Subst Abuse Treat, 1*(2):137–140.

Kohnke, M.D. (2008). Approach to the genetics of alcoholism: a review based on pathophysiology. *Biochemical Pharmacology, 75*(1),160–177.

Kumar, S. (2007). Burnout in psychiatrists. *World Psychiatry. 6*(3), 183–189.

Lee, F.J., Stewart, M., & Brown, J.B. (2008). Stress, burnout and strategies for reducing them. What's the situation among Canadian family physicians? *Canadian Family Physician, 54*(2), 234–235.

Lutsky, I., Hopwood, M., Abram, S.E., Cerletty, J.M., Hoffman, R.G., & Kampine J.P. (1994). Use of psychoactive substances in three medical specialities: aneasthesia, medicine, surgery. *Canadian Journal of Anesthesia. 41*(7), 561–567.

McAuliffe, W.E., Santangelo, S., Magnuson, E., Sobol, A., Rohman, M., & Weissman, J. (1987). Risk factors of drug impairment in random samples of physicians and medical students *Substance Use & Misuse, 22*(9), 825–841.

McLellan, T.A., Skipper, G.S., Campbell, M., & DuPont, R.L. (2008). Five year outcomes in a cohort study of physicians treated for substance use disorder in the United States, *British Medical Journal, 337*, 1154–1158.

Marazziti, D., Consoli, G., Picchetti, M., Carlini, M., & Faravelli, L. (2010). Cognitive impairment in major depression. *European Journal of Pharmacology, 626*(1), 83–86.

Marshall, E.J. (2008). Doctors' health and fitness to practise: treating addicted doctors. *Occupational Medicine, 58*(5), 334–340.

Maslach, C., Schaufeli, W.B., & Leiter, M.P.(2001). Job Burnout. *Annual Review of Psychology. 52*, 397–422.

Medical Council of New Zealand. (n.d). Good medical practice: a guide for doctors. Retrieved June 7, 2011, from, pdf
http://www.mcnz.org.nz/news-and-publications/good-medical-practice/

Merlo, J.L., & Gold, M.S. (2008). Prescription opioid abuse and dependence among physicians. *Harvard Review of Psychiatry. 16*(3),181–194.

Miller, M., McGowen, K., & Quillen, J. (2000). The painful truth: physicians are not invincible. *Southern Medical Journal, 93*(10), 966–972.

Moneteleone, P., & Maj, M. (2008). The circadian basis of mood disorders: recent developments and treatment implications. *European Neuropsychopharmacology, 18*(10),701–711.

New South Wales Medical Board. (n.d). Fitness to practice. Retrieved June 7, 2011, from,http://www.medicalboard.gov.au/

Pandi-Perumal, S.R., Moscovitch, A., Srinivasan, V., Spence, D.W., Cardinali D.P., Brown, G.M. (2009). Bidirectional communication between sleep and circadian rhythms and its implications for depression: Lessons from agomelatine. *Progress in Neurobiology, 88*(4), 264–271.

Peisah, C., & Wilhelm, K. (2007). Physician don't heal thyself: A descriptive study of impaired older doctors. *International Psychogeriatrics. 19*(5), 974–984.

Pesiah, C., Adler, R.G., & Williams, B.W. (2007). Australian pathways and solutions for dealing with older impaired doctors: A prevention model. *Internal Medicine Journal, 37*(12), 826–831.

Pethebridge, A. (2005). *Rehabilitation of the impaired doctor by the New South Wales Medical Board. Thesis submitted for Master of Medicine by Research.* Sydney, Australia: University of New South Wales.

Rø, K.E.I., Gude, T., Tyssen, R., & Aasland, O.G. (2004). Counselling for burnout in Norwegian doctors: One year cohort study. *British Medical Journal, 337,* 1146–1149.

Rosen, A., Wilson, A., Randal, P., Petheridge, A., Codyre, D., Barton, D. & Rose, L. (2009). Psychiatrically impaired medical practitioners: Better care to reduce harm and life impact, with special reference to impaired psychiatrists. *Australasian Psychiatry, 17*(1), 11–18.

Sargent, M.C., Sotile, W., Sotile, M,O., Rubash, H., & Barrack, R.L. (2009). Quality of life during orthopaedic training and academic practice. Part 1:Orthopaedic surgery residents and faculty. *The Journal of Bone and Joint Surgery. 91*(10), 2395–2405.

Shanafelt, T.D., Bradley, K.A., Wipf, J.E., & Back, A.L. (2002). Burnout and self-reported patient care in an internal medicine residency program. *Annals of Internal Medicine, 136*(5), 358–367.

Shanafelt, T.D., Sloan, J.A., & Habermann, T.M. (2003). The well-being of physicians. *The American Journal of Medicine, 114*(6), 513–519.

Silverstein, J.H., Silva, D.A., & Iberti,, T.J. (1993). Opioid addiction in anesthesiology. *Anesthesiology. 79*(2), 354–375.

Skipper, G.E., Campbell, M.D., & DuPont, R.L. (2009). Anesthesiologists with substance use disorders: A 5-year outcome study from 16 state physician health programs. *Anesthesia & Analgesia, 109*(3), 891–896.

Srinivasan, V., Pandi-Perumal, S.R., Trakht I, Spence, D.W., Hardeland, R., Poeggeler,B., & Cardinali, D.(2009). Pathophysiology of depression: Role of sleep and the melatonergic system. *Psychiatry Research, 165*(3), 201–214.

Taub, S., Morin, K., Goldrich, M. S., Ray, P., & Benjamin, R. (2006). Physician health and wellness. *Occupational Medicine (London). 56*(2), 77–82.

Thommasen, H.V., Lavanchy, M., Connelly, I., Berkowitz, J., & Grybowski, S. (2001). Mental health, job satisfaction, and intention to relocate. Opinions of physicians in rural British Columbia. *Canadian Family Physician. 47*(4), 737–744.

Todd, F.C. (2010). *Te Ariari o te Oranga: The assessment and management of people with co-existing mental health and substance use problems.* Ministry of Health, Wellington.

Turnbull, J., Cunnington, J., Unsa, A., Norman, G., & Ferguson, B. (2006). Competence and cognitive difficulty in physicians: A follow-up study. *Academic Medicine, 81*(10), 915–918.

Urbach, J.R., Levenson, J.L., & Harbison, J.W. (1989). Perceptions of housestaff stress and dysfunction within the academic medical center. *Psychiatric Quarterly, 60*(4), 283–295.

Vaillant, G., Brighton, J., & McArthur, C. (1970). Physicians' use of mood-altering drugs. A 20-year follow-up report. *New England Journal of Medicine. 282*(7), 365–370.

Vaillant, G., Sobowale, N., & McArthur, C. (1972). Some psychological vulnerabilities of physicians. *New England Journal of Medicine. 287*(8), 372–375.

Wall, T.D., Bolden, R.I., & Borrill, C.S. (1997). Minor psychiatric disorders in NHS trust staff: Occupational and gender differences. *British Journal of Psychiatry. 171,* 519–523.

Westermeyer, J. (1991). Substance use rates among medical students and resident physicians, *Journal of the American Medical Association, 265*(16), 2110–2111.

World Health Organization. (2004).*The international classifications of diseases and health related problems: Tenth revision (2nd ed.).* Geneva.

Wilhelm, K.A., & Reid, A.M. (2004). Critical decision points in the management of impaired doctors: The New South Wales Medical Board program. *Medical Journal of Australia, 181*(7), 372–375.

Williams, E.S., Manwell, L.B., Konrad, T.R., Linzer, M. (2007) The relationship of organizational culture, stress, satisfaction, and burnout with physician-reported error and suboptimal patient care: Results from the MEMO study. *Health Care Management Review, 32*(3), 203–212.

Wilson, A., Rosen, A., Randal, P., Pethebridge, A., Codyre, D., Barton, D., (…)Rose, L. (2009). Psychiatrically impaired medical practitioners: An overview with special reference to impaired psychiatrists. *Australasian Psychiatry, 17*(1), 6–11.

/// 11 /// HEALTHY DOCS = HEALTHY PATIENTS

Arguably the Most Important Reason to Care about Physician Health

ERICA OBERG, FELIPE LOBELO,
ROBERT SALLIS, AND ERICA FRANK

THE EVIDENCE ON PHYSICAL ACTIVITY-RELATED ASPECTS OF
HEALTHY DOC = HEALTHY PATIENTS

The Healthy Doc = Healthy Patient linkage has evolved over a series of research studies and demonstration projects that have been conducted around the world to help health-care providers (and through them, their patients) adopt healthier personal habits. There are abundant data regarding the relationship between physicians' personal and clinical exercise-related habits. Early evidence came from the national questionnaire-based U.S. Women Physicians' Health Study showing that women physicians complying with physical activity (PA) recommendations (30 minutes/day of moderate-to-vigorous PA at least 5 times/week) were more likely to counsel patients on exercise—and with more confidence (Frank, Schelbert et al., 2003). Additional studies assessing the association between personal and clinical PA practices have also concluded that more physically active physicians are more likely to counsel their patients about the health benefits associated with an active lifestyle and become more credible and motivating role models for the adoption of healthy behaviors, reinforcing the HD = HP data and philosophy (Wells, Lewis et al., 1984; Reed, Jensen et al., 1991; Wee, McCarthy et al., 1999; Abramson, Stein et al., 2000).

An important subsequent study was set forth to investigate how the HD = HP principles are shaped during medical education. A study that included a representative sample of medical students from 16 U.S. schools in the class of 2003 showed that 64% of students met PA recommendations and 79% believed physical activity would be highly relevant to their future medical practices to counsel patients about exercise (Frank, Tong et al., 2008). In fact, those who believed exercise counseling to be highly relevant reported engaging in more vigorous PA than those reporting low relevance for exercise counseling (105±4 min/week v. 87±1 min/week p<0.001). Follow-up data over the next four years showed that PA levels were relatively stable during medical education and were strongly correlated with the frequency of PA counseling offered to their patients. In addition, students who felt more positive about their schools and classmates' attitudes towards exercise promotion were more likely to comply with PA recommendations, emphasizing the importance of role modeling, social support, and the medical school environment for PA participation. However, the relevance students gave to PA counseling decreased significantly as they progressed through their medical education (Frank, Tong et al., 2008).

Yet only 13% of 102 U.S. medical schools in 2002 had some curriculum on PA and health (Garry et al., 2002). An updated survey from 2011 found little progress in the development of exercise curricula of medical schools, concluding that "exercise physiology/fitness was the area receiving the least attention in medical schools" (Torabi, Tao et al., 2011).

These findings signal that more emphasis needs to be given to PA instruction (and practice) in medical training, since PA is critical for the prevention and management of the most prevalent chronic diseases we face today. In addition, interventions focused on improving PA levels among medical students have the potential to improve patient counseling. In fact students who participated in a PA intervention perceived their medical school as a healthier environment and had approximately 50% greater odds of providing extensive counseling on exercise to standardized patients compared to control students ($P = .03$:(Frank, Elon et al., 2007). Collectively, evidence indicates that there is a robust association between personal PA behaviors and PA counseling practices in both practicing doctors and medical students.

However, despite the large amount of information about the health benefits of PA and the effectiveness of physician-prescribed PA, rates of doctors providing exercise counseling remain low and clinical providers indicate several barriers for PA prescription including limited time, lack of reimbursement, and lack of training in prevention (Wee, McCarthy et al., 1999; Abramson, Stein et al., 2000), in addition to patient barriers such as depression. An important initiative launched in 2007 by the American Colleges of

Sports Medicine called "Exercise is Medicine" (www.exerciseismedicine.org) will hopefully help turn this reality around. Exercise is Medicine aims at making PA a vital sign and a standard component of the medical paradigm for disease management and prevention in the US and around the globe—and one of its core objectives is indeed to encourage physicians and health care providers to be active themselves.

In summary, there is ample and compelling evidence showing that clinical providers who act on the advice they give, in this case about the health benefits of regular PA, do a better job at counseling and motivating their patients to adopt such health advice. This association is strong and independent of many demographic, training, and clinical practice factors, is already present at the beginning of medical training, and is responsive to intervention. Strategies aimed at improving the number of physicians adopting and maintaining active lifestyles constitute a powerful strategy to improve the rates and quality of physician-delivered PA counseling, which in turn would have a large impact on the management and prevention of chronic diseases in both developed and developing countries. It seems to be that the personal exercise experiences of doctors really make a difference in our professional lives and in the way we work in collaboration with our patients.

THE EVIDENCE ON NUTRITIONAL ASPECTS OF
HEALTHY DOC = HEALTHY PATIENTS

Additionally, there is copious information on the relationship between physicians' personal dietary practices and the advice they give to patients in clinical practice. In addition to the role dietary factors play in overweight/obesity, specific dietary factors such as excess sodium, low intake of fruits and vegetables, low intake of dietary omega-3 fatty acids, and high dietary trans fatty acids also contribute substantially to underlying causes of mortality (Danaei et al., 2009). Physicians, while healthier than the general population, also have room to improve their nutritional intake. U.S. physicians and medical students consume an average of 3.4 servings of fruits and vegetables per day, as compared with only 22.1% of all U.S. men and 32.2% of U.S. women reporting consumption of >3 servings of fruits and vegetables per day (Frank, Wright et al., 2002; Kilmer, Roberts et al., 2008).

Importantly, healthcare providers who eat well themselves, are more likely to counsel patients about nutrition. One of the predictors of nutritional health-promotion counseling includes being a vegetarian oneself (OR 2.0 [1.3, 2.9]) (Frank, Wright et al., 2002); among medical students, increased fruit and vegetable intake was strongly associated with both perceived relevance and the frequency of delivery of dietary counseling (P< 0.0001) for both (Spencer, Frank et al., 2006). Additionally, healthy nutrition impacts other domains of clinical care. In one study, hospital-based physicians who were provided with regular snacks and water throughout the day scored better on tests of cognitive performance and decision-making (Lemaire et al., 2010).

The implications of these findings are several. Physicians can provide better care by focusing on improving their own health behaviors. This not only reduces their own risk of lifestyle-related chronic disease, but it helps patients as well. Furthermore, physicians who have personal knowledge of the challenges of integrating healthy habits into a busy lifestyle are in a better position to share this knowledge with their patients. Providers who disclose their personal health practices are perceived as more credible and motivating, and these patients become more receptive to health-promotion counseling from physicians who demonstrate healthy behaviors (Swinburn, Walter et al., 1998; Simon, Majumdar et al., 2005). This is important given that less than 20% of medical students feel they have been adequately trained to deliver nutritional counseling (Spencer, Frank et al., 2006). Recently, programs have begun to appear that better address nutritional principles; some include additional training on health promotion counseling and behavioral change skills, clearly important domains of clinical practice.

OTHER HEALTHY DOC = HEALTHY PATIENT LINKS

Links between the nutrition and physical-activity habits of doctors and their patients are especially well-documented. Importantly though, our HD = HP team has examined 14 different counseling and screening practices of medical students and of physicians, in Canada, Columbia, and the United States, and we have consistently found that physicians' physical and mental health clinical practices in relation to their patient care were significantly and positively correlated with their own related health practices (Oberg & Frank, 2009). Of note are data on associations between mental health and clinical care delivery. A recent study of hospital-based physicians and residents found a high prevalence of mental health disorders including burnout. Among Canadian physicians, a 23% incidence of depression was recently measured, which is notable given the reported population incidence of depression is only16% across all Canadians (Compton & Frank, 2011). Hospital-based physicians with high mental health complaints had 4 to 14 times increased odds of reporting impaired work abilities (Ruitenburg, Frings-Dresen et al., 2012). Among Canadian physicians, more than a quarter (26.5%) reported that mental health concerns interfered with their work at least some of the time (Compton & Frank, 2011). While these statistics are concerning, what is reassuring is the growing data suggesting health practices such as physical activity are critical and effective in preventing and managing mental health stressors and depression (Carek, Laibstain et al., 2011; Mata, Thompson et al., 2012).

These data of physicians' personal health practices and the relationship to their clinical practice and the health of their patients, provide compelling evidence for physicians to maintain as healthy a lifestyle as possible. Physicians, while healthier than the general population, are at risk themselves (Frank, Biola & Burnett, 2000; Pattison, 2006) and health providers report difficulty counseling patients on behaviors that they struggle with themselves (Vickers, Kiercher, Smith, Petersen & Rasmussen 2007). Interventions that promote provider health improve not only the health of the physician but the rates of health promotion counseling as well. Those interested in promoting physician health would do well to consider the additional, patient-related reason for physician health promotion as it elevates such health promotion efforts from merely helping a typically privileged cohort to improving the health of whole populations—to us, this is the most critical reason to promote physician health.

REFERENCES

Abramson, S., Stein, J., Schaufele, M., Frates, E., & Rogan, S. (2000). Personal exercise habits and counseling practices of primary care physicians: A national survey. *Clinical Journal of Sports Medicine, 10*, 40–48.

Carek, P. J., Laibstain, S.E., Carek, S.M. (2011). Exercise for the treatment of depression and anxiety. *International Journal of Psychiatry and Medicine 41*(1), 15–28.

Chiuve, S. E., McCullough, M. L., Sacks, F. M., & Rimm, E. B. (2006). Healthy lifestyle factors in the primary prevention of coronary heart disease among men: benefits among users and nonusers of lipid-lowering and antihypertensive medications. *Circulation, 114*(2), 160–167.

Compton, M. T. & Frank, E. (2011). Mental health concerns among Canadian physicians: results from the 2007-2008 Canadian Physician Health Study. *Comprehensive Psychiatry 52*(5), 542–547.

Danaei, G., Ding, E. L., Mozaffarian, D., Taylor, B., Rehm, J., Murray, C. J., et al. (2009). The preventable causes of death in the United States: Comparative risk assessment of dietary, lifestyle, and metabolic risk factors. *PLoS Med, 6*(4), e1000058.

Frank, E., Biola, H. & Burnett, C. A. (2000). Mortality rates and causes among U.S. physicians. *American Journal of Preventative Medicine 19*(3), 155–159.

Frank, E., Wright, E. H., Serdula, M. K., Elon, L. K., & Baldwin, G. (2002). Personal and professional nutrition-related practices of US female physicians. *American Journal of Clinical Nutrition, 75*(2), 326–332.

Frank, E., Schelbert, K. B., & Elon, L. (2003). Exercise counseling and personal exercise habits of US women physicians. *Journal of the American Medical Women's Association, 58*, 178–184.

Frank, E. (2004). Physician health and patient care. *JAMA 291*(5), 637.

Frank, E., Elon, L., & Hertzberg, V. (2007). A quantitative assessment of a 4-year intervention that improved patient counseling through improving medical student health. *Medscape General Medicine, 9*(2), 58.

Frank, E., Tong, E., Lobelo, F., Carrera, J., & Duperly, J. (2008). Physical activity levels and counseling practices of U.S. medical students. *Medicine & Science in Sports & Exercise, 40*(3), 413–421.

Garry J. P., Diamond, J. J., & Whitley, T. W. (2002). Physical activity curricula in medical schools. *Academic Medicine* (77), 818–820.

Kilmer, G., Roberts, H., Hughes, E., Li, Y., Valluru, Fan, A., Giles, W., Ali Mokdad, A., & Jiles, R. (2008). Surveillance of certain health behaviors and conditions among states and selected local areas—Behavioral Risk Factor Surveillance System (BRFSS), United States, 2006. *MMWR Surveillance Summary, 57*(7), 1–188.

Knowler, W. C., Barrett-Connor, E., Fowler, S. E., Hamman, R. F., Lachin, J. M., Walker, E. A., et al. (2002). Reduction in the incidence of type 2 diabetes with lifestyle intervention or metformin. *New England Journal of Medicine, 346*(6), 393–403.

Lemaire, J., Wallace, J. E., Dinsmore, K., Lewin, A. M., Ghali, W. A., & Roberts, D. (2010). Physician nutrition and cognition during work hours: Effect of a nutrition based intervention. *BMC Health Services Research 10*, 241.

Mata, J., Thompson, R.J., Jaeggi, S.M., Buschkuehl, M., Jonides, J., & Gotlib, I.H. (2012). Walk on the bright side: Physical activity and affect in major depressive disorder. *Journal of Abnormal Psychology, 121*(2), 297–308.

Oberg, E., & Frank, E. (2009). Personal Health Practices Efficiently and Effectively Influence Patient Health Practices. *Journal of the Royal College of Physicians of Edinburgh, 39*, 290–291.

Pattison, M. (2006). Finding peace and joy in the practice of medicine. *Health Progress 87*(3), 22–24.

Reed, B. D., Jensen, J. D., & Gorenflo, D. W. (1991). Physicians and exercise promotion. *American Journal of Preventative Medicine, 7*, 410–415.

Ruitenburg, M. M., Frings-Dresen, M.H., & Sluiter, J.K. (2012). The prevalence of common mental disorders among hospital physicians and their association with self-reported work ability: a cross-sectional study. *BMC Health Services Research, 12*(1), 292.

Simon, S. R., Majumdar, S. R., Prosser, L. A., Salem-Schatz, S., Warner, ... Soumerai, S.B. (2005). Group versus individual academic detailing to improve the use of antihypertensive medications in primary care: a cluster-randomized controlled trial. *American Journal of Medicine, 118*(5), 521–528.

Spencer, E. H., Frank, E., Elon, L. K., Hertzberg, V. S., Serdula, M. K., & Galuska, D. A. (2006). Predictors of nutrition counseling behaviors and attitudes in US medical students. *American Journal of Clinical Nutrition, 84*(3), 655–662.

Swinburn, B. A., Walter, L. G., Arroll, B., Tilyard, M. W., & Russell, D. G. (1998). The green prescription study: a randomized controlled trial of written exercise advice provided by general practitioners. *American Journal of Public Health, 88*(2), 288–291.

Torabi, M. R., Tao, R., Jay, S.J., & Olcott, C. (2011). A cross-sectional survey on the inclusion of tobacco prevention/cessation, nutrition/diet, and exercise physiology/fitness education in medical school curricula. *Journal of the National Medical Association 103*(5), 400–406.

Vickers, K. S., Kiercher, K. J., Smith, M. D., Petersen, L. R. & Rasmussen, N. H. (2007). Health behavior counseling in primary care: provider-reported rate and confidence. *Family Medicine 39*(10), 730–735.

Wee, C. C., McCarthy, E. P., Davis, R. B., & Phillips, R. S. (1999). Physician counseling about exercise. *JAMA, 282*, 1583–1588.

Wells, K. B., Lewis, C. E., Leake, B., & Ware, J. E., Jr. (1984). Do physicians preach what they practice? A study of physicians' health habits and counseling practices. *JAMA, 252*, 2846–2848.

World Health Organization (2008). *The global burden of disease: 2004 update*. Geneva: WHO.

Management Of Physician Stress

INTRODUCTION

Charles R. Figley

This section comprises five chapters that, together, identify the sources of stress, stress reactions, and ethical strategies found to be effective in managing stress associated with various roles played by physicians.

In the first chapter of this section, Chapter 12, Overcopers: Medical Doctor Vulnerability to Compassion Fatigue, Anna Baranowsky and Douglas Schmidt note that medical doctors, as skilled professionals, experience many external and internal pressures that are common among highly paid professionals. More important, medical providers such as physicians and nurses must interact with patients who are distressed. Medical providers must constantly and quickly make crucial life-and-death decisions and cope with rapidly changing medical systems, programs, policies, and places of work. Many physicians became interested in medicine initially because of some medical emergency they experienced or was experienced by a loved one. But often these individuals, who chose to study medicine to care for others, neglect their own needs. The training and socialization process for physicians can make it difficult for them to reach out for help or admit vulnerability because of a tendency to engage in self-silencing. These factors can make physicians vulnerable to compassion fatigue. The authors describe these processes, as well as an overview of the Accelerated Recovery Program for alleviating physician compassion fatigue, through two case examples.

In Chapter 13, Stress and Coping: Generational and Gender Similarities and Differences, Jane Lemaire, Jean E. Wallace, and Alyssa Jovanovic point out two significant demographic shifts in medicine that appear to be related to changes in doctors' work experiences and career attitudes: the shifts in generations and an increase in the number of female physicians. They offer a comprehensive overview of how physicians' work-related stress and coping strategies may be similar or different depending on their generation or gender. The literature on this topic demonstrates several key findings: Physicians' work demands and workloads are increasingly stressful; physicians' degree of control over their work may reduce job stress, yet their control is decreasing; female physicians feel more overworked than male physicians, often as a result of balancing work and family responsibilities; and Generation X physicians report more stress and burnout than the Baby Boomer generation. In addition, it is frequently presumed that women and Generation X physicians are less committed to their careers than men and Baby Boomer physicians, though there is no evidence of this.

Emergent findings from a recent large-scale study of physicians allow the authors to further explore the similarities and differences in stress and coping across the two generations and genders of physicians. They present key findings as they relate to physician work and on-call hours and perceived workload and burnout. In addition, they describe work-family issues related to marital status, presence of young children, hours spent in household tasks, and physician's spouse's employment status for both groups of physicians. Finally, they compare coping strategies used at home and at work, types and sources of physicians' support, and attitudes toward medicine across gender and generation.

The Center for Practitioner Renewal (CPR) is dedicated to understanding and helping health care providers by appreciating their special needs (psychological, emotional, and spiritual). In Chapter 14, Treatment and Prevention Work: Center for Practioner Renewal, the Center's founders, David Kuhl, Douglas Cave, Hilary Pearson, and Paul Whitehead, suggest that all medical systems need a practitioner renewal center. They point out the endless challenges faced by providers during and following medical training in the context of present-day health care. Specifically, they address three questions and answer them: How do we sustain health care providers? What is the effect of being in the presence of suffering? What would reparative, healing, or restorative resilience look like in these providers? Much of the chapter is about the formation of the CPR and how its services emerged from the growing needs of providers, including the SIT (safety, inclusion, and trust) program and others. They share other innovations emerging at CPR, including the nine ingredients for an effective treatment team agreement on how to work most effectively. The latter section of the chapter discusses various training tools the team has developed over the years to promote stress resilience, including mindfulness and medication.

In Chapter 16, Ethical Decisions: Stress and Distress in Medicine, Jeffery Spike and Nathan Carlin point out that the House of Medicine contains a combination of applied science and ethics that creates additional stress for physicians. Medical sciences include, of course, both biological and behavioral sciences, with the expectation of writing and carrying out grants and contracts to support the research and write up the results. Physicians are expected to constantly keep up-to-date on the science of medicine or face accusation of practicing at a substandard level. Yet the feeling of fulfillment, success, and peak performance is extremely subjective and can vary greatly from week to week. Spike and Carlin note that most physicians' self-assessment, as well as independent assessments of well-being, are most associated with "the loss of the human connections that they expected when they entered the field, and the loss of their own idealism." Courage is needed on the part of physicians once this reality sets in—courage to reinvigorate their idealism, and; perhaps restore some their initial illusions, and add some sustainable adaptations at midcareer.

12

OVERCOPERS

Medical Doctor Vulnerability to
Compassion Fatigue

ANNA BARANOWSKY AND DOUGLAS SCHMIDT

As highly skilled professionals, medical doctors experience many external and internal pressures. They must interact with patients who are distressed; make crucial life-and-death decisions, and cope with rapidly changing work situations. Primary traumatic stress experienced early in their lives can often motivate these individuals to choose studying medicine to care for others and, ironically, neglect their own needs. The training and socialization process for physicians can make it difficult for them to reach out for help or admit vulnerability because of a tendency to engage in self-silencing. These factors can make physicians vulnerable to compassion fatigue. These processes as well as an overview of the Accelerated Recovery Program for alleviating physician compassion fatigue are described through two case examples.

The following two cases (with names and details altered) from the author's clinical practice illustrate the vulnerability to compassion fatigue that physicians may experience in the course of their professional and personal lives.

Dr. John Fernandez's parents were war survivors and immigrants who struggled for everything they had. Having limited money, they did not take comforts for granted. Although John's parents were loving and kind, they had many anxieties and their aspirations for his success were extremely high. He realized at an early age that his parents expected him to succeed in all he did. The family made many sacrifices to send John to medical school, so he felt that failure was not an option. Once he finished his medical training he started a general family medicine practice. He was overwhelmed to find that he frequently had to make life-and-death decisions, which were sometimes followed by patient illness or death. After making two incorrect diagnoses, the patients complained to his college. His sense of invincibility was shattered and his confidence was uncertain. John was unprepared for how these errors and the subsequent complaints left him shaken. He had thought that once he was a doctor he would feel empowered and protected by his ability to help his patients. Although he recognized the warning signs of depression and heavy drinking in himself, he did not feel he could seek help for his pain and shame. After months passed, he noticed he was not always able to spend as much time with each patient as he might like to and developed an abrupt, confrontational style with patients and colleagues. He began to justify errors in his diagnostic and treatment decisions by telling himself that patients were not being clear about their symptoms, were hypochondriacs, or were "wasting his time."

When Dr. Joanna Kelly was a child she found the violence of her parents' marriage and the chaos of family life stressful and found refuge in books. Because she was socially withdrawn and anxious, she was not popular at school. She felt successful and in control by doing well in school and receiving praise from teachers. Her grades were exemplary and she was at the top of her class, so scholarships for university came easily. Social interactions were not rewarding for her until she entered medical school and was surrounded by bright peers who valued her skills and intelligence. She achieved more than she expected and enjoyed her career as chief oncologist in a prominent hospital. With her career well established, she became more comfortable within herself and enjoyed a newfound sense of connection with co-workers and friends. Many days, however, her great skill could not stop the horrible onslaught of cancer in some patients. After strongly identifying with a bright young patient who reminded her of herself, the patient died, and Joanna was left devastated. Afterward, she felt unable to continue with her work. Feelings of depletion, confusion, sadness, isolation, and agitation became frequent and she found it exceedingly difficult to relate to patients for fear that she would connect with them and again feel a paralyzing sense of loss.

Medical doctors assume a role requiring the responsibility for life-and-death decisions. The pressures of this role can feel overwhelming at times and can strain the resources of even the hardiest individuals. When practitioners feel distressed and uncertain, they are more likely to make unintentional errors (Sloan, Shanafelt & West, 2010). Over time, continued high-performance expectations can lead to a feeling of crushed invincibility. Many physicians feel that it is unacceptable to reach out for help for themselves because it is an indication of even more weakness. This can lead them to be at risk for self-destructive behaviors such as substance abuse, suicide, and self-harm (Sansone & Sansone, 2009). Daily exposure to seriously ill, injured, or traumatized patients combined with a personal history of vulnerability can result in a spiraling sense of strain (Monro, 2009; Pinto, 2002).

In this chapter we reflect on the role of physicians, the pressures they endure, potential negative outcomes, and a promising treatment for encouraging self-awareness and self-care. We conceptualize this process of exhaustion as compassion fatigue, which incorporates burnout and the silencing response, which may lead to negative behaviors such as substance abuse and even suicide. We propose and discuss a new term, *the overcoper,* as an identity that many physicians embody through this process. We emphasize the importance of physicians taking care of themselves and receiving care from others. We also describe the Accelerated Recovery Program for treatment of physicians and other health care professionals who are experiencing compassion fatigue.

PRIMER ON COMPASSION FATIGUE AND RELATED TERMS

The construct of compassion fatigue was developed by Figley (1989, 1995) to explain the potential negative consequences for health care professionals who are working with seriously ill, injured, or traumatized individuals. According to Figley (2002), compassion fatigue is "a state of tension and preoccupation with...traumatized patients [characterized] by re-experiencing traumatic events, avoidance/numbing of reminders, and persistent arousal (e.g., anxiety) associated with the patient" (p. 3). Compassion fatigue was initially recognized as a combination of burnout and secondary traumatic stress. Burnout is typified as perceived demands outweighing perceived resources and is experienced as a cumulative strain that over time results in a depleted reserve of energy to manage life challenges (Cherniss, 1980; Maslach, 1976, 1982). Burnout is a process (rather than a fixed condition) and becomes progressively worse if there is no relief from demands. The process includes (1) gradual exposure to job strain, (2) erosion of idealism, and (3) limited perception of achievements. Figley (1989, 1995) proposed that compassion fatigue includes burnout as well as secondary traumatic stress, a stress response similar to acute stress or posttraumatic stress. These stress reactions are anxiety disorders characterized by hyperarousal (jumpiness associated with the fight or flight response), avoidance (withdrawal from any reminders of the disturbing event), and intrusion (re-experiencing trauma reminders through nightmares, flashbacks, and intrusive thoughts or images).

In addition to burnout and secondary trauma, early traumatic experiences may increase an individual's risk for developing compassion fatigue. Hence, we later conceptualized compassion fatigue as a combination of secondary traumatic stress and burnout, as well as possible preexisting primary traumatic stress caused by earlier experiences (Baranowsky, 2002; Baranowsky & Lauer, 2012). Hyman (2001) and Ghahramanlou & Brodbeck (2000) concluded that severity of earlier experiences of personal trauma was correlated with an increased vulnerability to secondary traumatic stress when exposed to another's pain and suffering. Ironically, for many individuals, early adverse experiences motivate them to help others by pursuing careers in health care and helping professions.

Preliminary research has recently been conducted on the cognitive, behavioral, and emotional response process that occurs when individuals are descending into or are in a state of compassion fatigue. This has been called the silencing response and has been found to be a key characteristic of compassion fatigue (Baranowsky, 2002; Ortlepp, 1998; Ortlepp & Friedman, 2001). The silencing response has been defined as

> The point at which we may notice our ability to listen becomes compromised. It is precisely those times when we feel overwhelmed and in need of skills that we are left most vulnerable to the Silencing Response (SR).... The Silencing Response is a reaction based on a series of assumptions which guide the [individual] to redirect, shutdown, minimize, or neglect the [symptoms and other details that patients attempt to convey to the physician] (Baranowsky, 2002).

Diagnostic acumen often requires close attention to detailed patient explanations, as well as the ability to assist patients with high levels of emotional distress. Health care professionals must often listen to and validate patients when working under time pressure and other stressors. At times the patient's communication of details and distress overwhelm the physician's ability to empathize, take in information, understand, and make decisions. Medical practitioners are most vulnerable to having a silencing response (SR) when it is the only coping response for personal discomfort and uncertainty in the course of patient care.

Dr. John Fernandez reported that he had begun to experience the silencing response after the complaints about his clinical practice. He started to believe that his patients' emotional distress was not as valid as the distress of people like his parents who were war survivors or the distress of high-functioning, hard working professionals like himself. As a result of the silencing response he experienced a great deal of anger and often wanted to tell clients to stop complaining.

After being overwhelmed by the particular patient she had identified so strongly with, Dr. Joanna Kelly noticed that she was using the silencing response. She was unable to listen to and process information about the lives and experiences of clients, as well as coworkers and friends. When hearing the details of a patient's pain or suffering, she felt numb and empty. At other times, she was unable to contain her feelings of sadness and spent time crying silently in her office.

THE OVERCOPER: AN IDENTITY ACCOMPANYING COMPASSION FATIGUE

A new concept we propose here to understand compassion fatigue is that of the *overcoper*. This is the identity that a health care professional with compassion fatigue may assume of "going through the motions" of her or his job and wanting to appear to be coping well without taking care of her or his own emotional and mental health.

We do not see the overcoper as an individual who has a personality problem or disorder. Rather we see him or her as being in a role with a state of high anxiety because of a lack of skills imparted during training, alongside the constraints of the workplace and professional culture. The overcoper, in our view, is a role that involves social isolation and devaluation of oneself. We envision the role of the overcoper as an individual who experiences learned helplessness as described by Martin Seligman (Petersen, Maier, & Seligman, 1995), depletion from "overfunctioning" as described by Murray Bowen in the area of family systems theory and therapy (Bowen, 1990), and reduced self-efficacy as described by social learning theorist Albert Bandura (Bandura, 1997).

Overcopers are people who continue functioning under immense pressure until they are so depleted and burned out that they can no longer deny their emotional and physical state (Shanafelt, Bradley, Wipf, & Back, 2002). They are generally highly dedicated individuals working in a variety of fields who put those they serve ahead of themselves. In some cases, their family role was to care for others or to put aside their personal needs and they take this quality into their professional life. Caring for others is a role they value and has earned them recognition. In many training settings, given the expectations for long hours and putting emotional, social, and recreational needs on hold, physicians may not have role models for self-care. These individuals have a tendency to ignore their own suffering because they pay more attention to taking care of others and the feeling of satisfaction of helping others. Overcopers see themselves first and foremost in their professional capacity for which they will sacrifice everything.

Anecdotal evidence garnered from 10 years of working with professional care providers has helped us identify some common characteristics that are typified by the overcoper. The typical overcoper is intelligent and a skilled problem solver, with abundant energy to accomplish tasks, a high pain threshold, high mental flexibility, high career aspirations, and a tendency to reset the bar higher each time a goal is met. Although the overcoper may have a strong social network, this network may be sacrificed in favor of career success.

Overcopers may regard themselves as high achievers in their careers as a means of establishing a buffer for their lives and job struggles and to ward off, at all costs, their feelings of failure. Frequently overcopers will push beyond pain even when life and work demands have become unmanageable, because of belief that their career identity as viewed by others is more important than their own individual needs. In their world, stopping to rest and reflect is a weakness; high performance at any cost is the expectation.

Dr. John Fernandez acknowledged that he had become an overcoper and his focus became narrowed on his work. He reported that he became cut off from himself and experienced himself as becoming like a machine that did not have needs.

Dr. Joanna Kelly told us that she had become an overcoper even before the silencing response begin to cloud her ability to work with patients. Being an overcoper had become a way for her to feel proud of herself, as she had begun to devalue taking care of her own social, emotional, and physical needs.

COSTS OF OVERCOPING

Clearly there is an extreme cost to this level of work demand. Maintaining this pace is grueling and not sustainable without tremendous life costs. Sometimes in order to maintain this overwhelming level of expectation physicians may drink, misuse prescription or street drugs, and let personal relationships suffer. When life feels exceedingly hopeless they may resort to the ultimate self-sacrifice of suicide rather than show weakness or seek assistance. Diseases of adaptation are common among overcoping individuals, including high blood pressure, heart disease, ulcers, substance abuse, suicidal ideation and risk, as well as emotional and relationship losses.

Myers (2003) outlines a profile of many physicians at great risk for suicide. Variables include the following:

Male or female; age 45+ (female physicians) or 50+ (male physicians) years; white; divorced, separated, or single; alcohol or other drug abuse, workaholic, gambler, risk taker, thrill seeker; psychiatric symptoms of depression and anxiety; physical symptoms of chronic pain or chronic debilitating illness; change in (or threat to) status— autonomy, security, financial stability, recent losses, increased work demands; access to lethal medications; and access to firearms.

Myers (2003) goes on to explain that many physicians are "hard-working and driven perfectionists who don't cut themselves much slack—they are prone to undue guilt, self-recriminations, and despondency."

Hawton, Clements, Sakarovitch, Simkin, and Deeks (2001) conducted a study involving 223 medical practitioners in the United Kingdom's National Health Service and found that the suicide risk of female medical doctors was twice as great and statistically significantly greater than that found in the general female population (12.6% vs. 6.3% per 100,000). The researchers found that male physicians were significantly less likely to commit suicide than males in the general population (14.3% vs. 21% per 100,000). Male *and* female medical practitioners in the fields of anesthesiology, general practice, community health, and psychiatry were at significantly greater risk of suicide than those in internal medicine in a hospital based setting. Amount of time within a medical career and seniority did not appear as an increased risk or protective factor.

The researchers found that gender and type of medical specialty were related to suicide risk. The rates of suicide for male and female physicians appear to be about the same (12.6% to 14.3%) and may not have been statistically significantly different. These findings suggest that overall, being a physician was protective for suicide for males, but that being a physician increased risk of suicide for females. The reasons being a physician was protective for suicide for males was not explained, but it may be related to factors such as increased socioeconomic status, increased knowledge of social and health care supports, or increased knowledge of coping behaviors. For women, however, being a physician may perhaps be associated with added psychological burden because of multiple family care giving roles as mothers and partners, as well as being adult daughters taking care of aging parents.

In addition to having a higher suicide rate (for females and in some specialties), physicians are at risk for having a higher rate of substance abuse. Because of their access to medications, physicians are at significant risk for prescription drug abuse, most commonly benzodiazepines and opiate based medications (Weir, 2000; Aach et al., 1992). Male physicians, although at decreased risk for suicide, when compared to the general male population, are at greater risk of substance use. Compared to the general population, female physicians are at a greater risk of both suicide and substance abuse. These are high costs for individual physicians, their families, and society.

Drinking too much had become a problem for Dr. John Fernandez and he noticed that he was having physical symptoms such as shortness of breath, dizziness, and irritability. In the back of his mind he had thoughts of suicide if the complaints against him went to court.

Dr. Joanna Kelly had recurring thoughts of suicide as she descended into a state of anxiety and depression. She began to avoid work and slept a great deal. Slowly she had begun to depend on sleeping pills and drank more and more coffee to keep going at work, a combination that eventually led to feelings of anxiety.

THE COST OF OVERCOPING: CLINICAL PRACTICE ERRORS

Practice errors are undoubtedly a significant risk factor for physicians developing compassion fatigue and the silencing response (Baranowsky, 2002). Yet Redelmeier (2005) recognizes diagnostic errors as a regular event and one that could be mitigated through an improved awareness of cognitive psychology with a focus on diagnostic reasoning and decision-making processes. Redelmeier explains:

Cognitive psychology is the science that examines how people reason, formulate judgments, and make decisions. The term "science" implies that cognitive errors may be predictable in some situations—not the result of ignorance or the acts of a few bad performers. Instead, some pitfalls are sufficiently systematic that most people repeatedly make them in both routine and extraordinary situations (p. 116).

Through their training and in clinical practice, physicians are repeatedly reminded by regulatory bodies, insurance companies, and research about the legal and professional implications of making practice errors. Accompanying this is the anxiety about revealing weakness and vulnerability.

Redelmeier (2005) cautions against either demonizing physicians or denying that errors are made by physicians, and emphasizes the importance of identifying typical mistakes and making efforts to protect against them. He reflects on the potential errors caused by the use of diagnostic heuristics or shortcuts in decision making and by miscommunication as a result of lack of feedback systems. Clearly when physicians are using the silencing response as a result of feeling overwhelmed, making errors is more likely to occur, further exacerbating their vulnerability, distress, and uncertainty and increasing the likelihood of chronic strain and deterioration.

Skilled physicians, whatever their discipline, have comprehensive training to draw from and are required to apply those skills to the demands of their medical practice. However, medical work exposes practitioners to serious injury, illness, and death on a regular basis whether due to iatrogenic causes (caused or made worse by incorrect treatment) or natural causes. In many cases these regular stressors are compounded by an overwhelming caseload.

The pressures of dealing with a demanding patient caseload, whether in emergency, surgery, general practice, or any specialization, can result in misdiagnoses, poorly formulated conclusions and iatrogenic treatment effects. Patient deterioration can lead to an escalation of demand for treatment, as well as possible serious illness or even patient death. Faced with these consequences, physicians may retreat (i.e., self-medicate, develop compassion fatigue, shut down communication, or even become suicidal) because they may feel that this is their only option.

Dr. John Fernandez was aware that he had made practice errors because of his deteriorating ability to concentrate, empathize, and listen to his clients. Rather than admitting these errors and correcting them, however, he became guarded, mistrustful, and isolated.

Dr. Joanna Kelly did not make practice errors, but she knew that her judgment was deteriorating and that she was at risk for making such errors. As a result, she took a great deal of sick time away from work, although she found that this did not improve her state of functioning and ability to perform her job.

PHYSICIAN COMPASSION FATIGUE PATHWAY

The trajectory from a highly competent and skilled practitioner to a compassion fatigued and depleted individual is common when routinely exposed to injured, ill, and traumatized patients.

ACCELERATED RECOVERY PROGRAM

In 1997, the Accelerated Recovery Program (ARP) for Compassion Fatigue was launched as a five-session individual treatment model for treating professional care-providers who had become overwhelmed by the demands of their work. The treatment model was developed with the recognition that burnout was an insufficient theoretical construct to conceptualize the distressed state of professional care-providers (Rafferty, 1986). There was a need to understand that secondary exposure to the serious illness, injury, or trauma of patients results in a wound in the caregiver that requires special attention.

In addition to the individual care model, we began training professionals nationally and internationally so that skilled practitioners using the ARP could respond to the needs of a broad section of professionals. A large group format was also created to offer a psycho-educational model in bigger venues. The Traumatology Institute (Canada) has provided compassion fatigue care and training to thousands of practitioners, in large groups, online, and individually, both nationally and internationally. We have worked with physicians, psychiatrists, nurses, psychologists, mental health practitioners, emergency responders, funeral home workers, clergy members, Red Cross members, and other professionals in varied fields. In addition to providing training for physicians and other health care professionals with compassion fatigue, we have also provided a train-the-trainer model for professionals who will provide this service (Gentry, Baggerly, & Baranowsky, 2004).

The stages of this treatment process focus on issues such as the therapeutic alliance between clinician and patient, clinicians' quantitative assessment of their own distress, anxiety management skills, the importance of narrative regarding personal and work-related experiences, and issues related to the exposure and resolution of secondary traumatic stress (STS). A key component of this training is cognitive restructuring for self-care and integration of new concepts and skills. In addition, the ARP provides an aftercare resiliency plan emphasizing resiliency skills, self-management and self-care skills, connection with others, skills acquisition, and conflict resolution.

In treatment with the Accelerated Recovery Program, skills that are taught include self-reflection and self-care to establish the skills of displaying a nonanxious presence and self-validated care giving. These skills allow for greater attention to the pitfalls of short-cuts in diagnostic problem solving. Nonanxious presence is the ability to sit comfortably with the emotional strain of exposure to patient distress and remain a compassionate witness. This skill can allow for continued engagement with patients and enable physicians to remain alert and attentive to important diagnostic signs and symptoms they may otherwise miss if overly distressed or feeling rushed. Physicians might otherwise shut down and disengage in an attempt to remove themselves from overly disturbing patient concerns (West et al., 2006). The skill of nonanxious presence is not a skill routinely taught in medical school.

Self-validated care giving requires awareness of and confidence in one's medical knowledge and skills and an understanding that there are factors beyond one's control as a physician that may have a negative impact on patient outcomes. If a physician only uses cure of the patient as the measure of his or her success (an external form of validation), he or she will quite often be a "failure." For some physicians this would require a paradigm shift from being a "hero" to being a "healer."

It is within this "healer" paradigm that maintaining a nonanxious presence can make sense for physicians. Here they can learn that being nonanxious can be healing *in and of itself* to a patient possibly facing the most terrifying time in his or her life. Through this practice physicians may also learn a more spiritual lesson: that healing and being successful as a healer doesn't necessarily mean the cure of the disease. The development of nonanxious presence and self-validated care-giving intervention approaches (Baranowsky & Gentry, 1999b) can act as a buffer to patient demands and may allow physicians to remain engaged and compassionate while assessing and diagnosing.

For those individuals who have significant unresolved primary traumatic stress, treatment would address these symptoms through a cognitive behavioral trauma therapy approach or the utilization of a staged model. The first stage would address compassion fatigue utilizing the ARP approach; the second stage would follow a tri-phasic approach for resolution of primary traumatic stress disorder (PTSD) (Baranowsky & Lauer, 2012).

Both Dr. John Fernandez and Dr. Joanna Kelly benefited from the Accelerated Recovery Program. This allowed each of them to identify their own primary stress, secondary trauma, and silencing response and learn new, alternative ways of coping. Physicians also find the program helpful because they can hear about the overcoper experiences of other physicians.

Dr. John Fernandez learned about how his family's experience of trauma in war had led to primary stress reaction for them and increased his anxiety about survival and success. He also became aware of how, over time, he had experienced compassion fatigue and coped using the silencing response, which then led to practice errors and increased alcohol use.

In the ARP, Dr. Joanna Kelly learned about her own primary stress related to childhood experiences and how her silencing response had led to her vulnerability to deny her own needs and overidentify with her patients.

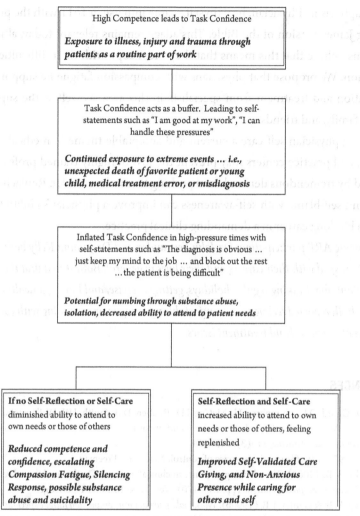

High Competence leads to Task Confidence

Exposure to illness, injury and trauma through patients as a routine part of work

Task Confidence acts as a buffer. Leading to self-statements such as "I am good at my work", "I can handle these pressures"

Continued exposure to extreme events … i.e., unexpected death of favorite patient or young child, medical treatment error, or misdiagnosis

Inflated Task Confidence in high-pressure times with self-statements such as "The diagnosis is obvious … just keep my mind to the job … and block out the rest …the patient is being difficult"

Potential for numbing through substance abuse, isolation, decreased ability to attend to patient needs

If no Self-Reflection or Self-Care
diminished ability to attend to own needs or those of others

Reduced competence and confidence, escalating Compassion Fatigue, Silencing Response, possible substance abuse and suicidality

Self-Reflection and Self-Care
increased ability to attend to own needs or those of others, feeling replenished

Improved Self-Validated Care Giving, and Non-Anxious Presence while caring for others and self

FIGURE 12.1 A Model of Confidence-related Self Reflection and Self Care

CONCLUSIONS

There are few roles that demand so much and are linked so closely with life and death outcomes than that of the medical doctor. Carrying the responsibility for the well-being of others is both a sacred trust and a potentially lethal burden. It's not surprising that physicians frequently succumb to compassion fatigue and associated silencing response, substance abuse, suicide, and practice errors as a result of the demands of their work. With good intentions, the overcoper often pushes himself or herself beyond reasonable and sustainable expectations and thus becomes overburdened to the point of deterioration and difficult recovery.

The aphorism "Physician, heal thyself," came into use in 1611 with the publication of the King James Version of the Bible. This adage remains relevant today, although many physicians believe that this means that they must cope with their difficulties alone and in isolation. We propose that physicians with compassion fatigue be supported through consultation and treatment from specialists in this area, as well as the support of colleagues, family, and friends.

Making physician self-care a current and acceptable theme in medical schools, universities, and practice centers may prevent the loss of highly trained professionals overwhelmed by tremendous demands and pushing themselves harder. Replacing feelings of shame and self-blame with self-awareness can improve a physician's ability to enjoy and sustain a life-long career in a demanding clinical practice.

Following ARP participation, Dr. John Fernandez and Dr. Joanna Kelly both reported feeling more satisfied with their careers and their lives in general. Both stated that they had become more vigilant about taking regular holidays, getting exercise, and having a healthier lifestyle. In addition, both reported feeling more comfortable referring to or consulting with colleagues when uncertain of diagnoses and treatment issues.

REFERENCES

Aach, R.D., Girard, D.E., Humphrey, H., McCue, J.D., Reuben, D.B., Smith, J.W., Wallenstein, L. & Ginsburg, J. (1992). Alcohol and other substance abuse and impairment among physicians in residency training. *Annals of Internal Medicine, 116*(3), 245–254.

Bandura, (1997). Self-efficacy: the exercise of control. New York: Freeman.

Baranowsky, A. B., (2002). The silencing response in clinical practice: On the road to dialogue. In C. Figley, (Ed.), *Treating compassion fatigue* (pp. 155–170). New York: Brunner-Routledge.

Baranowsky, A. B. & Gentry, J. E. (1999b). *Workbook/journal for a compassion fatigue specialist*. Toronto, Ont: Psych Ink Resources. Available FTP: http://www.psychink.com.

Baranowsky, A. B. & Lauer, T. (2012). *What is PTSD?: 3 Steps for healing trauma*. Toronto, Ont: Createspace.

Bowen, M. (1990). *Family therapy in clinical practice*. New York: Aronson.

Cherniss, C. (1980). *Professional burnout in human service organizations*. New York: Praeger.

Figley, C.R. (1989). *Helping traumatized families*. San Francisco: Jossey-Bass.

Figley, C.R. (1995). Compassion fatigue as secondary traumatic stress disorder: An overview. In C. R. Figley (Ed.), *Compassion Fatigue* (pp. 1–20). New York: Brunner/Mazel.

Figley, C.R. (2002). Introduction. In C. R. Figley (Ed.), *Treating compassion fatigue* (pp. 1–14). New York: Brunner/Rutledge.

Gentry, J.E., Baggerly, J., & Baranowsky, A.B. (2004). Training-as-treatment: The effectiveness of the certified compassion fatigue specialist training. *International Journal of Emergency Mental Health, 6* (3), 147–155.

Gentry, J. E., Baranowsky, A. B., & Dunning, K. (2002). ARP: The Accelerated Recovery Program (ARP) for Compassion Fatigue. In C. R. Figley (Ed.), *Treating compassion fatigue* (pp. 123–138). New York: Brunner/Rutledge.

Ghahramanlou, M. & Brodbeck C. (2000). Predictors of secondary trauma in sexual assault trauma counselors. *International Journal of Emergency Mental Health, 2*(4), 229–240.

Hawton, K., Clements, A., Sakarovitch, C., Simkin, S., & Deeks, J. (2001). Suicide in doctors: A study of risk according to gender, seniority and specialty in medical practitioners in England and Wales, 1979–1995. *Journal of Epidemiological Community Health, 55*, 296–300.

Hyman, O. (2001). *Perceived social support and symptoms of secondary traumatic stress in disaster workers.* Unpublished doctoral dissertation, Adelphi University, New York.

Maslach, C. (1976). Burned-out. *Human Behavior, 5*(9), 16–22.

Maslach, C. (1982). *Burnout: The cost of caring.* Englewood Cliffs, NJ: Prentice Hall.

Monroe, J.R. (2009). *Clinical and organizational predictors of burnout and secondary traumatic stress in emergency management professionals [dissertation].* Unpublished doctoral dissertation, University of South Dakota, Vermillion, South Dakota.

Myers M. & Fine, C. (2003). Suicide in physicians: Toward prevention. *Medscape General Medicine: Psychiatry & Mental Health, 5*(4) [Online], Available: http://www.medscape.com/viewarticle/462619.

Ortlepp, K. (1998). *Non-professional trauma debriefers in the workplace: Individual and organizational antecedents and consequences of their experiences.* Unpublished doctoral dissertation, University of Witwatersrand, Johannesburg, South Africa.

Ortlepp, K. & Friedman, M. (2001). The relationship between sense of coherence and indicators of secondary traumatic stress in non-professional trauma counsellors. *South African Journal of Psychology, 31*(2), 38–45.

Petersen, C., Maier, S. F., & Seligman, M. (1995). *Learned helplessness: A theory for the age of personal control.* New York: Oxford University Press.

Pinto, R.M. (2002). *The impact of secondary traumatic stress on novice and expert counselors with and without a history of trauma [dissertation].* Unpublished doctoral dissertation, University of Southern California, Los Angeles, CA

Rafferty, J.P., Lemkau, J.P., Purdy, R.R., Rudisill, J.R. (1986). Validity of the Maslach Burnout Inventory for family practice physicians. *Journal of Clinical Psychology, 42*, 488–492.

Redelmeier DA (2005). Improving patient care. The cognitive psychology of missed diagnoses. Ann Intern Med. 2005 Jan 18;142(2):115-20.

Sansone, R.A., & Sansone, L.A. (2009). Physician suicide: A fleeting moment of despair. *Psychiatry (Edgmont). 6*(1), 18–22.

Shanafelt, T.D., Bradley, K.A., Wipf, J.E. & Back, A.L. (2002). Burnout and self-reported patient care in an internal medicine residency program. *Annals of Internal Medicine, 136*(5), 358–367.

Sloan, J.A., Shanafelt, T.D., & West, C.P. (2010). Resident fatigue, distress and medical errors. *Journal of American Medical Association. 303*(4). 330.

Weir, E. (2000). Substance abuse among physicians. *Canadian Medical Association, 162*(12),1730.

West, C.P., Mashele, M.H., Novotny, B.J., Sloan, J.A., Kolars, J.C., Habermann, T.M., Shanafelt, T.D. (2006). Association of perceived medical errors with resident distress and empathy. *Journal of American Medical Association, 296*(9), 1071–1078.

13

STRESS AND COPING

Generational and Gender Similarities and
Differences

JANE LEMAIRE, JEAN E. WALLACE, AND
ALYSSA JOVANOVIC

INTRODUCTION

The literature clearly shows that physicians around the world are experiencing high
levels of work-related stress (Arnetz, 2001, Visser et al., 2003, Panagopoulou et al.,
2006, Baldisseri, 2007, Umehara et al., 2007, Dunn et al., 2008). In examining the
various types of stressors that physicians face, two significant demographic shifts in
medicine appear related to the changing nature of doctors' work experiences and
career attitudes. One is the entry of new generations of physicians, Millennials and
Generation Xers, and the other is the influx of women into the medical profession
(Jovic et al., 2006). In addition, it is important to recognize that in response to the
diverse stressors and challenges they face, physicians from different generations
and different genders may rely on a wide range of coping strategies (Arnetz, 2001,
Firth-Cozens, 2001, Weiner et al., 2001). The purpose of this chapter is to explore
how physicians' work-related stress and coping strategies may be similar or different
depending on their generation or gender.

This chapter is organized as follows. First, we examine the literature that documents
the impact of the generational and gender shifts on major trends in the medical profession. Next, we present a review of the literature that examines physician work-related
stress with a focus on how the generations and genders are similar or different in their

work experiences and attitudes. Following this, we describe results from a large-scale study of physician well-being to illustrate the similarities and differences between the generations' and genders' experiences of stress, use of coping strategies, and career attitudes. Lastly, we propose a set of learning points developed from the existing literature and research findings.

GENERATIONAL SHIFTS

The generational shift reflects that most doctors practicing medicine are from one of two generations: the Generation Xers (GXs), who were born between 1965 and 1981; and the Baby Boomers (BBs), who were born between 1945 and 1964 and are beginning to retire. More recently, the Millenials, also known as Generation Y (GYs), who were born between 1982 and 2000, are just beginning to enter the medical profession. These generations grew up under different social, economic, and political historical contexts that have helped to shape their work attitudes and work practices (Fay, 1993, O'Neil, 2002, Wallace, 2006). While it is customary to have multiple generations in the workforce at the same time, the BBs and GXers generations in particular appear to differ in their attitudes toward work and emphasis on work, family, and overall life balance. These factors may have implications for the types of work-related stress they face and the kinds of coping strategies they use in response. For example, it has been suggested that the most rigid generational differences between GYs, GXs, and BBs are related to the role that work plays in one's life (Kennedy, 2003, Gursoy, Maier and Chi, 2008). This fundamental difference in how the generations define themselves is often believed to result in both GYs and GXs placing greater emphasis than their BB counterparts on lifestyle choices and making sure they have time for family, friends, and leisure (Kennedy, 2003, Gursoy, Maier and Chi, 2008, Twenge, 2010, Shrestha and Joyce, 2011). Thus, the GYs and GXs are often viewed as less committed to their work, their careers, and their employers than BBs (Carter, 2001, Fong, 2002, Buddeberg-Fischer et al., 2010). It is the perceived erosion of the work ethic and decline in the value and importance of work that has been raised as a critical concern regarding the attitudes and behaviors of the younger generation (Jurkiewicz, 2000, Larson, 2003, Wallace, 2006).

GENDER SHIFTS

The second demographic shift reflects the growing number of women entering medicine. Because women often face different challenges in pursuing a professional career as they try to balance and juggle work and family responsibilities, male and female physicians tend to differ in their work experiences and career paths. This can have important implications related to gender-specific sources of stress and use of coping strategies. For example, women typically work fewer hours per week, see fewer patients (and provide fewer services), take time off to have children, are likely to leave the profession sooner, and are less inclined to join professional organizations compared to men (Heiliger and Hingstman, 2000, Burton and Wong, 2004a, Buddeberg-Fischer et al., 2010). The literature also suggests that women and men tend to enter into different areas of medical specialization (e.g. family practice or predominantly out-patient based specialties of medicine) and types of practice because women tend to select career paths or work arrangements within their profession that best facilitate work-family balance (Levinson and Lurie, 2004, Jovic et al., 2006). As a result, the gender shift is expected to contribute to physicians experiencing different work-related stressors, given the dissimilar work experiences and career paths of female and male physicians.

When considering work-related stress and coping, it is also important to take into account physicians' home lives, where generation and gender become particularly relevant factors. Traditionally, doctors prioritized their professional lives at the expense of their personal or family lives (Dumelow et al., 2000). The literature clearly shows how physicians are increasingly reporting that their work often interferes with their home and family life and how difficult it is to balance their professional and personal lives (Linn et al., 1985, Visser et al., 2003, Shanafelt et al., 2005). In examining the work-family interface, it is essential to recognize that family stage and its associated responsibilities vary considerably depending on physicians' marital status, whether they have children and their age, and the employment status of their spouse, all of which may be linked to their gender or generation. For example, women continue to be responsible for the majority of home and family responsibilities, particularly when the children are young and even when mothers are working in professional careers (Keene and Reynolds, 2005). As well, the younger generation places greater emphasis on intensive parenting and has increased expectations regarding parenthood, where not only young mothers but also young fathers feel pressured to be more involved in their children's lives than parents in the past (Wallace and Young, 2008). As a result, it is also important to acknowledge how the family situations of physicians from different generations and genders vary in order to better understand the broader implications of work-related stress and effective coping strategies.

GENDER AND GENERATIONAL TRENDS IN MEDICINE

It is important to note at the onset that when examining generational and gender shifts, it is sometimes difficult to talk about the two as separate trends, since such a large proportion of women represent the younger generation of doctors in medicine. Data from many countries show that over the last decade, female physicians are more heavily distributed in the younger age categories compared to men (Heiliger and Hingstman, 2000). In addition, with the overall aging of the physician population, more male physicians are represented in the older age groups that are approaching retirement (Kletke et al., 1990, Gjerberg, 2001). For example, in 2007 in Canada, 32% of all female physicians were under age 40 compared to only 17% of male physicians, whereas 27% of male physicians were 60 years of age or older compared to 9% of female physicians (Canadian Institute for Health Information, 2007). Similar patterns have been noted in the United States, United Kingdom, and Australia (McMurray et al., 2002).

GENDER TRENDS

When examining the gender shift in medicine, it is evident how the proportion of men and women earning medical degrees has changed over the last 50 years. In the 1960s, most of the medical graduates were male, and medicine remained a predominately male occupation until the 1990s, when the tables turned and more women than men were graduating from medical school. This pattern has been documented in many countries including, for example, the Netherlands, the United Kingdom, the United States, Australia, and Canada (Heiliger and Hingstman, 2000, McMurray et al., 2002). Although men still predominate in the total number of physicians, about one-third of all practicing physicians in many countries are women (Keizer, 1997, Frank et al., 1999, McMurray et al., 2002). Despite the increasing representation of women in the profession, men still primarily occupy the leadership positions (Levinson and Lurie, 2004, Buddeberg-Fischer et al., 2010). Gjerberg (2001) suggests that, by the year 2015 throughout Europe and North America, about half of the active physicians will be women. This will hold true if the current trend continues in which about half of the newly qualified doctors are women and nearly almost all those who are retiring are men.

Despite the dramatic increase of women entering medicine over the last few decades, women's specialty choices have remained relatively unchanged (McMurray et al., 2002). It has been documented in numerous international studies of physician workforce trends that women choose different areas of medicine than men (Kletke et al., 1990, Gjerberg, 2001, Buddeberg-Fischer et al., 2010). For example, compared to men, women are more likely to choose primary care practices, are equally likely to choose clinical medicine specialties, and are less likely to choose surgical specialties (Kletke et al., 1990, Gjerberg, 2001). Even within these broad categories, there are significant gender differences; for example, within the clinical medicine specialties, women are more likely to enter into the practice of pediatric medicine, geriatric medicine, or psychiatry, and in the surgical specialties they are more likely to enter into the practice of obstetrics and gynecology (Gjerberg, 2001, McMurray et al., 2002, Brotherton et al., 2005). The corollary is also true, where men are more likely to choose other specialties, such as critical care medicine, urology, and orthopedic surgery (McMurray et al., 2002).

In examining these gendered patterns in specialty choices, it is important to note that the work of medical specialists is generally characterized by longer work hours, higher expectations for continuity of care within acute care settings, and less flexible work environments (Heiliger and Hingstman, 2000). Gjerberg's (2001) findings support these ideas. She asked physicians why they chose not to become specialists. Three-quarters of the women said that they believed it is too difficult to combine being a specialist with family responsibilities compared to one-third of their male colleagues. It has also been suggested that those areas of medicine in which the number of women is growing may start to experience significant changes in their practice characteristics, such as shorter work hours and more opportunities for part-time work and leaves of absence, to accommodate women's family responsibilities (Brotherton et al., 2005). Such changes have been documented in pediatrics, which has a large percentage of women, and it is not unreasonable to expect similar changes in other specialties with high percentages of women physicians. Lastly, it should be noted that the areas in which women are most highly represented (e.g., family medicine, pediatrics, psychiatry, and internal medicine) also tend to be among the lowest paid specialties (Swanson et al., 1998).

GENERATIONAL TRENDS

Turning next to generational trends in medicine, there appears to be shifts in the number of medical graduates entering certain specialties that coincides with the entrance of GYs and GXs into the medical profession starting in the mid-1990s. For example, in North America, the number of medical students choosing family medicine has been steadily declining since the mid-1990s (Scott et al., 2007). Several studies have suggested that specialty-related lifestyle has attracted growing numbers of medical students to certain specialties, such as radiology and anesthesiology, and decreasing numbers to others, such as general surgery and family practice (Schwartz et al., 1990, Dorsey et al., 2003, Wright et al., 2004). The idea of a "controllable lifestyle" (e.g., the predictability and number of work hours and the required nights on call) has been found to be an increasingly important determinant of students' specialty selection and to be far more influential than the traditional motivators such as remuneration, prestige, and length of training (Schwartz et al., 1990, Dorsey et al., 2003, Grayson et al., 2011). This trend is consistent with the ideas presented previously, that the younger generation of doctors place greater emphasis on lifestyle balance and having adequate time for leisure, family, and friends. As well, Heiliger and Hingstman (2000) suggest that in the 1990s the centrality of work in the lives of physicians was notably decreasing, which coincides with the entry of GXs. This trend has grown even further with the entry of the newest generation, GYs, who generally are not willing to excel professionally at the expense of personal health and quality family time. They often follow the belief that having a fuller life outside of medicine makes them better doctors (Borges et al., 2006). Thus the growing importance of lifestyle factors in choosing a medical specialty is reflective of both the values and expectations of the younger generation of doctors entering medicine, and the increasing number of women entering medicine who are considering the practicalities of balancing work and family.

At the other end of the age continuum, or the older end of the BBs, the *number* of physicians retiring has almost tripled, mostly due to the increase in the actual physician workforce (Chan, 2002). However, even the *percentage* of physicians retiring, based on the total number of physicians currently in practice, indicates that the retirement rate has almost doubled (Chan, 2002). Historically, physicians have tended to work beyond traditional retirement age, but data show that the average age of retirement is declining as more and more doctors are opting for early retirement as a result of mandatory retirement and retirement incentives (e.g. government buy-outs of physicians' practices) (Chan, 2002). Another contributing factor is that the age distribution of physicians across different specialties varies dramatically. For example, the age distributions in obstetrics, gynecology, and otolaryngology cluster around the older age ranges (e.g., 60–64), and as doctors in these specialties reach retirement age, it can be expected that relatively large numbers of physicians may leave the profession (Ontario Medical Association, 2002). Women physicians have higher retirement rates than men and tend to retire about 10 years earlier than male physicians, a factor that is likely to affect different areas of medicine in different ways (Kletke et al., 1990).

In summary, the key points are that more women than men are graduating from medical school and about one-third of practicing physicians are women. Physicians from the different genders (male and female), and from the different generations (GYs, GXs and BBs), choose dissimilar areas of medical practice. Physician retirement rates are increasing and vary across different areas of medical practice.

REVIEW OF PHYSICIAN WORK STRESS AND COPING STRATEGIES

It is widely perceived that physicians have desirable jobs, even if their work is often complicated, demanding, and stressful. However, researchers are now recognizing that some physicians are dissatisfied with their careers and many experience burnout (Firth-Cozens, 2001, Campolieti et al., 2007). A number of different factors have been correlated with burnout, including excessive work demands and workload, low control and authority, on-call requirements, and fatigue (Firth-Cozens, 2001; Campolieti et al., 2007). The review of the literature begins with an examination of the work-related stress that physicians encounter in their daily work lives, with the focus on how male and female physicians experience and cope with their work stress and how differences may also be observed across the generations.

PHYSICIANS' WORK-RELATED STRESS

Feeling overworked is a psychological state that may affect attitudes, behaviors, social relationships, and health both within and outside of work (Galinsky et al., 2001). Although most physicians spend the majority of their time providing patient care, many also have administrative, teaching, and research responsibilities. Each of these responsibilities carry with them their own unique and competing demands and may be different from day to day, depending on where and what the physicians are working on. Linzer et al. (2002) found that physician stress is increased by a number of specific work demands, including the number of patients they have, being on call, and the complexity of their patient cases (refer also to Section 2).

These demands are not uniform and may differ significantly across specialties and settings. For example, Swanson et al. (1998) found that family physicians report higher stress levels than physicians in many medical specialties. They speculate that the reason for this may be due to more occupational stressors, in terms of the business costs of a medical practice and paperwork. Olkinuora et al. (1990) found that "higher burnout specialties" tend to experience more stress because they deal with gravely or chronically ill patients who have incurable diseases or poor prognoses in contrast to those specialties that deal with patients with less serious life-threatening diseases.

Peeters and Le Blanc (2001) suggest that physicians' work demands are increasing with growing patient expectations and new technological advancements. The aging population and new diseases increases the number of patients and complexity of their health concerns needing medical attention. Although physicians typically enjoy spending more time with patients, these changes in work demands have often meant less physician face-to-face contact, and may constrict this relationship (Hafferty and Light, 1995, Dunstone and Reames, 2001). As a result, physicians often report the doctor-patient relationship is not only one of the most gratifying aspects of work, but it is also one of the most stressful (Arnetz, 2001).

Increasing demands from either the larger organization to work efficiently or patients themselves ultimately adds to the daily workload for physicians. These evolving work demands may present themselves as new challenges, increased stress, and a lowered sense of satisfaction for members of the medical professional.

Gender Differences in Physicians' Work-Related Stress

Although male physicians tend to work longer hours (averaging approximately 10 more per week), female physicians tend to feel more overworked than men (McMurray et al., 2002). Studies have shown that working fewer hours does not necessarily translate into being less productive or taking shortcuts to get the same amount of work done in a shorter period of time. For example, Weisman et al. (1986) found that female physicians' working fewer hours does not necessarily translate into less patient care. Rather women who work fewer hours may use their time more efficiently than those who spend more time at work. McKenzie Leiper's (2006) study of lawyers found that women in law often work a concentrated work day—they may spend fewer hours at the office than their male colleagues but they also avoid socializing with their colleagues at work and often eat lunch at their desk as they work through their lunch time.

In addition, for female physicians, insufficient control over their work environment in combination with high work stress is strongly related to their professional dissatisfaction (Frank et al., 1999). In particular, female physicians report that they want more control over their daily work schedule so that they can spend more time with patients, improve the quality of care they deliver, and have greater flexibility over their work schedule (Frank et al., 1999).

One of the main gender differences in work stress for physicians is how they deal with balancing multiple roles. The demanding nature of medicine means that many physicians will inevitably experience work-family conflict at some point in their career. Physicians' work is characterized as highly demanding and requiring full commitment by placing work responsibilities above all else, including family responsibilities. As a result, many physicians often find that balancing work and family is very difficult and one of the most stressful aspects of work (Firth-Cozens, 2001, Shanafelt et al., 2005). Work-family conflicts are even more pronounced and troublesome for women (Shanafelt et al., 2005). Many female physicians often deal with the stresses and conflicts of being a professional at the same time as being perhaps a wife and a mother. Although male physicians may also be married with children, historically their work and family roles have not appeared to cause as much conflict compared to female physicians (Swanson et al., 1998). Even though many men are now spending more time with their families, it is generally understood that men will work full-time and that their career responsibilities might overshadow the needs of their family (Robinson, 2003). This is evident by the fact that female physicians are responsible for two to three times more of the child care and household responsibilities (Carr et al., 1998), and significantly more female physicians report conflict between their career and family than men (Gross, 1997). For example, a recent national Canadian survey found that female physicians spend an average of 42 hours a week with the primary responsibility for their children, which is almost triple the amount of time reported by male physicians (Martin, 2003).

Interestingly, within a marriage in which at least one spouse works as a physician, wives are more likely to make accommodations in their career than husbands (Izraeli, 1994, Swanson et al., 1998, Swanson and Power, 1999, Sobecks et al., 1999, Katz et al., 2000). The wives either work part-time or quit altogether to become a stay-at-home spouse to address family needs and responsibilities. Often, these women reduce their hours in paid employment so they can focus their efforts on household labor, particularly childcare. The research in this area generally shows that after female physicians have children, they are the ones to reduce their hours to care for the needs of their family (Izraeli, 1994, Swanson et al., 1998, Swanson and Power, 1999, Sobecks et al., 1999, Katz et al., 2000, Sarma, Thind and Chu, 2011). Along the same lines, a study of 419 female Canadian surgeons found that 12% were dissatisfied with role conflict between home and career, and 50% thought that childbearing had slowed their careers (Frank et al., 1999).

Many female physicians often feel strain and guilt between their professional and personal roles. For those who continue to work full-time, many of the daily activities of housework and childcare are still primarily their responsibility (Izraeli, 1994, Sobecks et al., 1999, Katz et al., 2000). For example, one study found that female pediatricians working full-time performed 66% of child care and 63% of their household duties, whereas male pediatricians performed 19% of child care and 26% of their household duties (Fritz and Lantos, 1991). Tesch et al. (1995) reported that 24% of women physicians in their study experienced conflict between their career and family roles as opposed to only 6% of the men.

Recent data from the Canadian Medical Association (CMA) clearly illustrates how male and female physicians differ in the hours they spend in paid (professional) and unpaid (home) activities. They report that the total number of hours per week spent in both paid and unpaid activities is 103 for women versus 78 for men (Martin, 2003). Even though female physicians spend significantly less time in work activities than male physicians (49 vs. 56 hrs/week), they spend almost twice as much time per week (13 vs. 8 hrs) doing housework. Female physicians who are mothers then spend another whole week's worth of work (41 hours) in child care activities compared to 14 hours for the fathers. In the sociology literature, this pattern is referred to as the "second shift," in which women basically start their second full time job when they come home from their paid job (Hochschild, 1989).

Generational Differences in Physicians' Work-Related Stress

Some researchers find that more GYs and GXs tend to prefer part-time hours compared to BBs (McMurray et al., 2002, Weinstein and Wolfe, 2007). Although all three generations may suffer from burnout, GXs have been shown to have higher levels (Sargent et al., 2004). In a study by Campbell et al. (2001) that surveyed 582 practicing surgeons, substantially higher levels of burnout were identified in younger surgeons. Different factors were associated with burnout for GXers and BBs, where, for example, GXs reported longer work hours, greater conflict between work and home life, and a high debt load (Sargent et al., 2004). In contrast, factors associated with burnout for the BBs included greater anxiety with regard to clinical competence, more worries about the future in terms of physician shortages, greater financial concerns, and more concerns with regard to drug and/or alcohol abuse (Sargent et al., 2004).

In summary, the key points are that physicians' work demands and workloads are increasingly stressful. The control over their work may reduce job stress and yet their control is decreasing. Female physicians spend fewer hours in professional paid activities and more hours in home unpaid activities than male physicians and spend the equivalent of another full-time job in home related duties such as child care and housework. They also feel more overworked than male physicians, most likely as a result of balancing work and family responsibilities. GX physicians report more stress and burnout than BBs physicians.

PHYSICIANS' COPING STRATEGIES

Given that physicians work in a very stressful work environment, they likely rely on a variety of different coping strategies. It is important to understand what strategies they use and how effective these strategies are in coping with stress. Some strategies that physicians use at work involve problem-solving and seeking social support (Tattersall et al., 1999, Campolieti et al., 2007). Those used outside of work often involve physical exercise and talking to their spouse (Abramson et al., 2000, Sotile and Sotile, 2001). One common coping resource both within and outside of work is social support. The literature consistently demonstrates that during stressful times, social support, or having people to provide assistance and understanding, is a valuable coping resource (Wallace and Lemaire,

2007). However, physicians often think of themselves as the ultimate healer and, as a result, may not always recognize they need help when dealing with stressful situations (Reilly and Ring, 2007). This makes identifying and examining the coping strategies that physicians use a challenging task.

Gender Differences in Physicians' Coping Strategies

The general literature on coping strategies consistently reports gender differences. This has often been explained by sociological theories of gender socialization. It is argued that the socialization of young children produces gender differences in dispositions, personality characteristics, and ways of communicating (Kessler and McLeod, 1984, Thoits, 1995). Specifically, as children, women are socialized to be more emotional and interpersonal (Kessler and McLeod, 1984, Thoits, 1995). Men instead are socialized to control their emotions and to be engaged in problem-solving efforts (Kessler and McLeod, 1984, Thoits, 1995). Men more often report controlling their emotions, accepting the problem, not thinking about the situation, and engaging in problem-solving efforts, whereas women more often report seeking social support, distracting themselves, and letting out their feelings (Thoits, 1995, Ryan-Wenger et al., 2005).

Studies that examine gender differences in the effects of social support tend to report a significantly greater beneficial effect of social support for women compared to men (Flaherty and Richman, 1989). Women also either receive, or make use of, more social supports than men (Thoits, 1995, Fuhrer and Stansfeld, 2002). Women in general, including female physicians, are known to have more extensive and closer social relations than men and as a result, report that they receive more social support from a greater number of different sources such as coworkers, relatives, and friends (Campolieti et al., 2007). Men, on the other hand, have been found to have more limited social groups (Thoits, 1995). Findings suggest that men in general, including male physicians, often mention their wives as their primary and sometimes only source of support (Umberson et al., 1996, Okun and Keith, 1998, Smith et al., 2002, Janning, 2006). Research suggests that wives not only receive less support from their husbands but also that providing support to their husbands can be an additional source of stress for them (Ross and Mirowsky, 1989).

Generational Differences in Physicians' Coping Strategies

There is a noticeable lack of research examining how the different generations of physicians cope with the stresses of their work. However, one study found both similarities and differences for BBs and GXs. In terms of self-care (i.e., regular exercise, adequate sleep, healthy diet, avoiding harmful substances, and relaxation techniques) both GXs and BBs scored similarly. However, they found that BBs tend to report they receive less social support than GXs. Individuals in the BB generation are often seen as mentors and rather than having others available for social support, they report that their friends, family, and coworkers tend to lean on them for support (Santos et al., 2003).

In summary, the key points are that male and female physicians use different coping strategies and BB physicians tend to receive less social support than GXs.

PHYSICIANS' CAREER ATTITUDES AND GENDER AND GENERATIONAL DIFFERENCES

The medical profession is known for its norms and beliefs that physicians should be endlessly available to work long hours and provide patient care and similar assumptions from the public and health care systems contribute to these expectations. The "service ethic" of medicine encourages physicians to work long hours and place their patients' welfare above all else (Grant et al., 1990). These attitudes are often equated with commitment and worth, where working longer hours means a more dedicated doctor who provides better quality and continuity of care (Heiliger and Hingstman, 2000). As noted above, the literature clearly shows that female physicians work fewer hours and are far more likely than male physicians to work part-time, often in order to juggle their work and family responsibilities (Uhlenberg and Cooney, 1990, McMurray et al., 2002, Burton and Wong, 2004b). As a result, the general perception is that women, particularly those who are mothers, are less committed to their careers than men (Jovic et al., 2006). As well, the importance that GYs and GXs place on life balance and lifestyle, which is often correlated with shorter work hours, is viewed as evidence of their lack of commitment to their medical career (Kennedy, 2003, Phelan, 2010). Despite these assumptions in the literature regarding gender and generational differences in attitudes toward one's career, little empirical evidence supports these claims (Jovic et al., 2006).

In summary, the key point is that female, GY, and GX physicians are often *assumed* to be less committed to their careers than male and BB physicians.

EMERGENT FINDINGS FROM AUTHORS' RESEARCH

Study Background

The results presented below are from a multi-stage, mixed-methods study initiated in the fall of 2006, designed to examine the positive and negative determinants of physician well-being in a sample of physicians registered in a single, large health region in Alberta Canada. The initial qualitative stage of the study (Wallace and Lemaire, 2008) entailed semi-structured interviews with a quota sample of the physicians and the second quantitative stage (Wallace and Lemaire, 2009) comprised a mail-out survey consisting mostly of close-ended questions from established scales in the literature. In addition, we constructed scales based on the qualitative results of the earlier stage of the study to measure variables of interest that were not previously examined in the literature. All physicians in the health region were invited to complete the survey. We received 1178 surveys from an eligible 2957, yielding a 40% response rate. In addition to completing the close-ended questions, over 300 respondents also shared their personal experiences and viewpoints in their own words in the space provided on the survey. Some of the survey findings presented below are accompanied by quotes. Many are from the physicians interviewed in the qualitative stage of this study, but some, identified as such, are from the comments that survey respondents wrote on their questionnaires.

Of the study participants who completed our survey, 58% are men and 42% are women. More than half (61%) are BBs and 39% are GXs. On average, our respondents are 49 years of age and have practiced medicine for about 18 years. Some physicians had just begun their careers in the past year and others had been practicing medicine for more than 50 years. The doctors who responded to our survey represented the same distribution as physicians in the study population (the doctors in the health region) with regards to the different types of practice. 37% were in general or family practice, 50% in clinical medical specialties (e.g., anesthesia, emergency medicine, internal medicine, pediatrics, etc.) and 13% in surgical specialties.

The findings that we present from our study relate to several research questions. In regards to physicians' work related stress, we ask "Do work hours, on call hours, work overload, and burnout vary according to generation and gender?" In terms of physicians' work-family issues, we ask "Do marital status, presence and age of children, responsibility for household tasks, and physicians' spouse's employment status vary according to generation and gender?" We also present findings related to generation and gender on physicians' coping strategies at work and outside of work, and the types and sources of physicians' support. Lastly, we present findings related to generation and gender on physicians' attitudes toward medicine in terms of their job satisfaction, commitment to medicine, patient care attitudes, and work life balance.

Physicians' Work-Related Stress

Physicians' work-related stress can be examined in a number of different ways. In the discussion that follows, we present findings that reflect physicians' workload in terms of their work hours and attitudes toward taking call, as well as their perceptions of work overload and feelings of burnout. Comparisons are made by generation and gender for each of these different work-related stressors.

Workload

Do Work Hours and On Call Hours Vary According to Generation and Gender?

Number of work hours is one of the standard measures used to assess workload. In our study, we demonstrated that there are differences across the three broad types of practices of medicine. Family medicine physicians and general practitioners tend to average shorter work hours than their specialty colleagues, reporting 46 hours per week of patient care duties at work and at home. The medical specialties such as pediatrics and internal medicine reported 52 hours per week and the surgical specialties 54 hours per week. When comparing work hours across the two genders, women work on average fewer hours per week than men in the primary care specialties, with no significant gender differences in work hours for the medical and surgical specialties of medicine. Previous research has shown that there are more women working part time in the primary care specialties and this may partly explain the findings from our research (McMurray et al., 2002). When comparing results across the two generations of physicians, contrary to what might be expected, GXs work significantly longer hours per week than the BBs in the medical specialties (i.e., approximately 56 hours a week on average compared to 50 hours a week excluding call), and both generations report similar hours in general and family practice (i.e., both averaging about 46 hours a week excluding call) and the surgical specialties (i.e., both averaging about 54 hours a week excluding call). Possible explanations for these findings are that younger physicians are more enthusiastic in their attitudes toward their work, less experienced in that it takes them longer to accomplish the work tasks, or motivated to work longer hours by a significant post-educational financial burden (Sargent et al., 2004). The following quote is from a male physician who works on average 65 hours a week:

> And the other thing that I think sets us as physicians apart is we learn to work hard and working hard doesn't just mean working long hours, or taking on an excessive amount of call, it also you know means working efficiently and very effectively in various cases, not just putting in hours. Sixty-five hours seems like a lot to me sometimes because I have a spouse who works full time and I have a family and a lot of other things that I like to try and do and sometimes, there's only so many hours in a day. (Wallace and Lemaire, 2008)

We also explored whether or not on call issues showed evidence of generational and gender variation. Although slightly more GXs take call compared to BBs, about 75% of all physicians take call and this does not differ by gender. It is more likely that being on call is related to the type of medical practice (Wallace and Lemaire, 2009). When exploring attitudes related to on call work, men (24%) are more likely than women (16%) to find their on-call hours excessive often or most of the time, yet there is no gender difference in feeling that on call hours contribute to stress (about 40% for both genders). It may be that the different types of practices chosen by male physicians have greater responsibilities during their on call work hours, such as being on site at the hospital rather than taking phone calls from home, or being associated with more sleep deprivation and emergency situations. The issues of on-call work being excessive or stressful do not differ by generation. The following quote is from a 49 year old physician who explains her feelings about working night shifts:

> I really want to get rid of the night shifts. I'm getting too old to do night shifts...I think that the recognition as you get older that they're much harder for you to do physically, so then your enthusiasm for your clinical care at that time is not as good. (Wallace and Lemaire, 2008)

Another physician in his 60s who answered our survey wrote:

> I no longer take call—after age 62 and being in practice with the same group for 32 years and work 4 d/wk. Without that I would have retired yrs ago. I have said this many times— one does not realize how hard call is on oneself until you stop taking it. (Wallace and Lemaire, 2009)

In summary, the key points are that female physicians work fewer hours on average than male physicians in the area of primary care, but not in other areas of medicine. GX physicians work the same or more hours than BBs depending on their area of practice, and male physicians are more likely than female physicians to find their on-call hours excessive.

Does Work Overload Vary According to Generation and Gender?

Another way to examine workload is to assess the degree to which the demands of the job are perceived to be excessive in terms of work overload. We used a five-item Likert measure of work overload to assess the extent to which physicians report that, in their work, they often feel rushed or overextended, there are too many demands on their time and they do not have enough time to get everything done (Caplan et al., 1975, Marks and MacDermid, 1996).

The GXs did not differ significantly from the BBs in their perceptions of work overload with both generations reporting a mean of 3.8 on a scale from 1 (low workload) to 5 (high workload). However, there were gender differences in that female physicians (mean = 3.9) report statistically significantly higher work overload than male physicians (mean = 3.7). These data may be explained in part by prior research that demonstrated that female physicians are more productive in their workday, and thus may perhaps perceive higher workloads than men because they actually get more work done (Fairchild et al., 2001). Another potential explanation is that the female physicians may also have very demanding home responsibilities in addition to those at work, a dynamic that will be explored further later in this chapter. Because of the greater home responsibilities, female physicians may not necessarily come to work as rested as their male colleagues, which may enhance their perceptions of their workplace workload. The following physician works about 45 hours per week in a part-time position and she feels her workload is excessive:

> I think it's too much because to get it done, to get the work done in some kind of reasonable time frame it means, it's just a hundred miles a minute all day long. No breaks whatsoever really. (Wallace and Lemaire, 2008)

This next physician also describes her perceptions of excessive workload:

> My happiness would be greatly improved if I could actually just spend time with my patients, do the things that they need without rushing, would totally make me happy. Yah, I think it's just a little bit too much of everything. (Wallace and Lemaire, 2008)

In summary, the key points are that GX physicians do not differ significantly from BBs in their perceptions of work overload. Female physicians report significantly greater work overload than male physicians.

Does Burnout Vary According to Generation and Gender?

Physicians deal daily with the chronic strains of working with too many patients and having frequent stressful encounters with patients, their families and other medical staff. These encounters are often tense and emotionally charged and draining, which may lead to feelings of burnout (Barnett et al., 1999). Burnout is defined as feeling emotionally exhausted from one's work (refer also to Section 2). In this study, it was measured by five Likert items from Barnett et al. (1999) that tap how often physicians feel emotionally drained and burned out from their work, used up at the end of the day, tired when facing another day of work and strain from working all day. A higher score reflects more frequently experiencing feelings of burnout where the scores range from 1 (not very often) to 5 (most of the time). Our results show that GXs (mean = 3.0) reported feeling burned out more often than BBs (mean = 2.8) and female physicians (mean = 3.0) reported feeling burned out more often than male physicians (mean = 2.7). This finding of more frequent feelings of burnout in the younger generation and the younger female physicians may relate to their career stage (e.g., less experienced clinicians) as well as greater family responsibilities, another dynamic that will be further explored later in this chapter. The following quote is from a participant who commented on how the paradoxical nature of having strong personal connections with her patients may also contribute to burnout:

> *The best part of my job is the people. I feel lucky to have been allowed to share so much of my patients' lives. Unfortunately, this also contributes to the emotional drain. There does seem to be a fine line between coping and burnout.* (Wallace and Lemaire, 2008)

This next physician describes how feelings of burnout guided a change in his practice patterns:

> *I have made major changes to my career in the last 8 years. I have left my family practice and moved to a walk-in clinic plus doing some surgical assisting. I was on the road to complete burnout prior to making these changes. Physician well being is vital but reducing my hours and stress has resulted in less access for my patients. I still feel guilty about this.* (Wallace and Lemaire, 2008)

In summary, the key points are that GX physicians report feeling burned out more often than BBs and female physicians report feeling burned out more often than male physicians.

Work-Family Issues for Physicians

In the section that follows, we examine a number of work-family issues that physicians with a family may face as they manage their career in medicine. These different factors may help us to better understand the ways in which physicians face different challenges in regards to work-related stress as well as different opportunities for a supportive home life. First, we compare the family situation of physicians from both genders and generations in terms of their marital status and age of their children. Next, we examine the division of household tasks and whether this differs by the physicians' generation and gender.

Lastly, we note the employment status of physicians' spouses, which can be related to both home-based stressors and coping resources.

Does Marital Status, Presence and Age of Children Vary According to Generation and Gender?
Comparing marital status, presence and age of children across generations and genders also enables us to better understand work-family responsibilities as potential sources of stress for physicians. For example, preschool children typically place significantly greater child care demands on their parents compared to older school-aged children (Press et al., 2006, Craig, 2007, Wallace and Young, 2008). When comparing these family situations across the two generations, we found that more of the GXs have younger children currently living at home compared to the BBs, whose children living at home tend to be teenagers. When comparing female and male physicians, most are married, especially the men. More of the women than the men have children currently living at home and of the women with children, more are likely to have preschool aged children. This likely reflects the fact that many of the female physicians are younger on average than their male colleagues, as discussed in the section above on demographic shifts.

We asked the physicians in our study to report how often they find their work demands interfere with their family life. About 20% of the physicians reported that this occurs almost every day or every day and there was no difference by gender or generation. The percentage of physicians who report this is relatively low, likely because physicians try to protect their family life as much as they can. Other areas of their life are more likely to suffer first, such as time for oneself, exercise and sleep. This has been reported in other studies where, particularly for mothers, their ability to work and care for their children was "financed" by reductions in personal care time, including sleeping, and in passive leisure, such as watching television sometimes at the expense of the mother's own health and well-being (Hill and Stafford, 1980, Duxbury and Higgins, 2001, Zukewich, 2003). The following quote is from a male surgeon describing how he tries to juggle his regular work hours and family life:

> *Well, I come to work usually between 7 and 7:30 and I go home…by 5:30 to 6, or one of us has to be home because we have childcare issues, so, it's usually 10 to 11 hour days for 5 days a week…and then when the kids go to bed, that's when I sit down and do my paper work so between 10 and midnight I do paper work.* (Wallace and Lemaire, 2008)

In summary, the key points are that more GX physicians have younger children living at home than BBs. More female physicians have younger children living at home than male physicians.

Does Responsibility for Household Tasks Vary According to Generation and Gender?

As indicated above in the background literature, male and female physicians spend different amounts of time in their paid work and unpaid home activities. Results from our study add to this literature. We asked participants in our study to report who is usually responsible for most of the household tasks in their home. Fifty percent of the female physicians reported that they usually or always do most of the household tasks compared to 4% of the male physicians. There were no generational differences in the distribution of household tasks between male and female physicians. These results, in conjunction with those reported above from the CMA, strongly suggest that despite advancements in the workplace that are moving toward greater gender equality, and despite a new generation entering the workforce, women's family roles have not changed significantly over recent decades and women continue to assume the majority of household and family responsibilities. This "stalled revolution" (Hoschchild, 1989) has been reported in general population studies across all western nations, where men continue to be expected to fulfill the male breadwinner role while their involvement in household work has not changed significantly, and women, regardless of their increased involvement in paid work or whether they are professionals or not, continue to be primarily responsible for the household and family (Baxter, 2002). As discussed previously in this section, this added home workload may contribute to female physicians' perceptions of greater workplace workload and burnout. The following thoughts from a physician who responded to the survey illustrates these concepts:

> *Very difficult as a female physician working full time to balance having 2 young children (3 yrs and 1 yrs) at home. Still expected to do majority of housework and childcare when we get home. Hard to leave work to get kids from daycare if they are sick (when men leave work for child-care reasons it's seen as a wonderful, great and caring thing for them to do, when a woman leaves work it is not looked upon as well).* (Wallace and Lemaire, 2009)

In summary, the key point is that female physicians report significantly greater household responsibilities than male physicians and this does not differ by generation.

Do Physicians' Spouse's Employment Status Vary According to Generation and Gender?

Work family issues are also influenced by the support that physicians may receive from their spouse, another dynamic that will be discussed in greater depth when we address physicians' coping strategies. The employment status of a physician's spouse will likely impact on their ability to provide support.

When comparing physicians' spouse's employment status, there are notable differences by gender and generation. Male and female physicians differ dramatically in terms of their spouses' employment situation. Most female physicians (88%) report that their husbands are employed compared to just over half (62%) of the male physicians. In addition, most of the female physicians' employed husbands (83%) work full-time compared to less than half (39%) of the male physicians' employed wives. Although about three quarters of the spouses of both generations of physicians are employed, more of the GXs (71%) have spouses who work full time compared to the BBs (56%). The following quote is from a female physician who highlights the importance of her husband's support for her and qualifies his employment status:

> *I do well because I have a phenomenal spouse who is not a professional. I watch my colleagues with less supportive spouses struggle with the stress.* (Wallace and Lemaire, 2008)

This next physician identifies the support he receives from his wife who works part time.

> [She], *is very supportive in terms of helping get other things done that need to be done, like looking after the kids and different things that need to be looked after, maintenance type things, home type things.* (Wallace and Lemaire, 2008)

In summary, the key points are that more GX physicians have spouses who work full time compared to BBs. Female physicians are more likely than male physicians to have spouses who are employed and more likely than male physicians to have spouses who work full time.

PHYSICIANS' COPING STRATEGIES AND SOURCES OF SUPPORT

In this section, we examine several different types and sources of coping resources that physicians may use in dealing with work-related stress at work and after leaving work. We compare their use in terms of generation and gender, the extent to which they are associated with feelings of burnout and the different types and sources of social support that physicians may receive from others.

Physicians' Coping Strategies at Work

In the first stage of our study, we interviewed physicians to ask them what coping strategies they use. The most frequently described coping strategies were then added to the mail-out survey. We could then determine how often physicians used these strategies and also which coping strategies were associated with more frequent feelings of burnout.

The aggregate results for all physicians in our study have been recently published (Lemaire and Wallace, 2010). The article describes how most of the physicians reported that they often cope with stress while they are at work by concentrating on what to do next. Many also indicated that they regularly make a plan of action, use humor to lighten the situation (refer also to Chapter 4), or keep the stress to themselves. Fewer physicians reported that they often talk with their colleagues, go on as if nothing has happened or take a time-out to cope with stress while they are at work. Not all of the coping strategies were associated with lower levels of burnout. Keeping it to themselves, concentrating on what to do next and going on as if nothing has happened were related to *higher* levels of burnout. These three strategies appear to reflect denial and avoidance responses that do not involve actually dealing with the source of stress in a constructive manner and overall were used more frequently (refer also to Chapter 8). It is possible that these strategies reflect professional norms, and although potentially harmful to the individual physician, may improve the physician's ability to continue to accomplish critical work tasks despite extremely stressful situations in the workplace. The coping strategies that were associated with lower levels of burnout include: taking a time out (which doctors rarely do), using humor, talking to colleagues, and making a plan of action and working through it, which tend to reflect more active problem solving strategies.

We also analyzed the study responses of how often physicians use these coping strategies according to the physicians' generation or gender (unpublished data). First, when comparing male and female physicians, women are more likely to talk things over with colleagues (38% vs. 24%, respectively) often or most of the time in coping with work-related stress. In contrast, men are more likely than women to concentrate on what to do next (82% vs. 74%, respectively), go on as if nothing has happened (32% vs. 23%, respectively), and keep it to themselves (49% vs. 33%, respectively) (strategies related to higher levels of burnout) and use humor to lighten the situation (50% vs. 39%, respectively) (refer also to Chapter 4). With respect to generational variation, there was no difference between the GXs or the BBs in how often they used the coping strategies that were associated with higher levels of burnout (i.e. keeping it to themselves, concentrating on what to do next and going on as if nothing has happened).

We then explored the coping strategies that were associated with lower levels of burnout (taking a time-out, using humor and talking to colleagues, and making a plan of action and working through it) according to generational variation. For example, we found that talking to colleagues was used more often by GXs (37%) than by BBs (29%). However, because we know that women are also more likely to use this as a coping strategy, we further analyzed the data by gender. We found that BB men (25%) were just as likely as GX men (29%) to use this coping strategy, yet GX women (46%) were more likely to use this strategy than BB women (35%). These data suggest that the generational effect is indeed entangled with the gender effect. In a similar example, BBs (50%) were more likely than GXs (39%) to use humor as a coping strategy. Again, further analysis demonstrated that, GX men (51%) were just as likely as BB men (50%) to use humor, and the generational variation seemed to come from the women, where female physician GXs (28%) were less likely than their BBs counterparts (50%) to use humor. The following comments added to the survey are from a female physician who indicates how humor is an important coping strategy in her workplace:

> *I am lucky. I work in a setting where the physicians are very mindful of work-life balance. We use humor extensively in our clinic to deal with a very high stress environment.* (Wallace and Lemaire, 2009)

This physician who responded to our survey explains how she uses a time-out as a coping strategy:

> *It was mandatory during my psychiatric training that all residents get out of the clinic and take the full hour for lunch—a pattern that I have followed, and expanded upon, ever since. For decades now I have been taking 2 hours off at noon to exercise, do errands, enjoy the sun, etc.* (Wallace and Lemaire, 2009)

In summary, the key points are that female physicians are more likely to use coping strategies associated with lower burnout, such as talking things over with colleagues, compared to male physicians. Male physicians are more likely to use coping strategies associated with higher burnout, such as keeping stress to oneself, compared to female physicians. There were no generational differences in how often physicians use harmful coping strategies at work. It is somewhat difficult to disentangle the effect of generation and gender when exploring how often physicians use effective coping strategies at work.

Physicians' Coping Strategies Outside of Work

In our recently published study of aggregate data for all physicians, we identified the coping strategies physicians use outside of work for dealing with the stresses of their work, how often they use these strategies and which ones were associated with lower levels of burnout, regardless of gender and generation (Lemaire and Wallace, 2010). The two most popular strategies physicians use involve their families, where they regularly spend time with their family and/or talk to their spouse after having a difficult day at work. Many frequently find time to exercise and others leave work at work or make quiet time for themselves outside of work. All of these coping strategies are associated with lower burnout. It appears that the break from work, whether it is in quiet time, exercise, spending time with one's family or spouse or simply leaving work at work, are beneficial in reducing physicians' feelings of work-related stress.

When comparing male and female physicians, we found differences when considering two of the coping strategies used outside of work. More of the women report they regularly spend time with their family or talk to their spouse after a stressful day at work compared to about half of the men. The following comments added to the survey illustrate how a physician recognizes the beneficial effect of self-care time outside of work:

> It really does help to take Wednesdays off to go golfing (or whatever). (Wallace and Lemaire, 2009)

When comparing these coping strategies used outside of work across the two generations of physicians, we note some interesting findings. For example, BBs are more likely than GXs to report using exercise or setting aside some quiet time for themselves. This finding holds true even when we explore each generation by gender. Men GXs and women GXs both use these coping strategies less than men BBs and women BBs. This may be due to the increased time available for BBs to engage in these activities, given that their children are grown, they have more spousal support, and time away from work is more their own. We must also consider that this is not only a cohort effect due to the attitudinal differences between generations, but that it could also be an effect due to aging. That is, once the Gen Xers enter the life stage that the BBs are currently in (i.e., in their 50s), we may see that two generations hold share similar attitudes when they are at the same age in their lives. Again, these arguments are difficult to resolve given the entanglement between the two related variables of age and generation.

In summary, the key points are that BB physicians are more likely than GXs to use exercise or to set aside some quiet time for themselves, and female physicians are more likely than male physicians to spend time with their family or talk with their spouse after a stressful work day. See Table 13.1 that lists the most important findings.

Types and Sources of Physicians' Support

Physicians' support arises from two main sources: their colleagues and their spouses. In addition, there are three key types of support—emotional, informational and

TABLE 13.1 Learning Points

- There are more women and a new generation of physicians entering the practice of medicine
- There are more physicians retiring from medicine and most are men
- Physicians from different genders and generations may enter different specialties that are more lifestyle/ family friendly
- The generations and genders face distinctive career and family challenges
- These challenges may translate into both different and similar stressors and coping strategies
- Recognizing the diverse challenges facing physicians, we need to develop more flexible work arrangements
- We need to make the practice of medicine more family friendly, as family issues impact both female physicians and the younger generation of male and female doctors
- Further research is needed to identify ongoing stressors and effective coping strategies, in particular as they relate to generation and gender
- Despite generational and gender differences, physicians share positive attitudes toward their profession and the patients they care for

instrumental. Emotional support refers to the concern, interest, empathy or understanding that individuals may share with one another that helps them cope with their work stress (King et al., 1995). Informational support refers to the suggestions, solutions, ideas or advice that individuals may share to help one another in responding to work-related stress (Wills, 1985). Instrumental support refers to colleagues working together and helping each other out, or spouses taking on more of the household responsibilities, to help the physician cope with a stressful day at work (King et al., 1995). Based on our statistical analyses, all three forms of collegial support (emotional, informational and instrumental) appear effective in reducing physicians' feelings of burnout. Emotional support and informational support from one's spouse are also effective in this regard.

Using interview data from the earlier qualitative part of our study, we explored the gender variations in the source and types of support and found that male and female physicians tend to rely on different people for support in coping with the stresses of practicing medicine (Wallace and Lemaire, 2008). From our interview data, we found that men are more reliant on their spouses, whereas the majority of women rely on colleagues and friends in and outside of work, which is consistent with the literature reported above. From the survey data, on a scale from 1 (low) to 5 (high) support, we found that female physicians report receiving more emotional (mean = 3.5) and informational support (mean = 3.5) (e.g., advice on difficult patient care issues) from their colleagues compared to male physicians (mean = 3.3, mean = 3.3, respectively). In contrast, male physicians, more than female physicians, report receiving more emotional (means = 3.9 vs. 3.8, respectively) and instrumental support (means = 3.5 vs. 3.1, respectively) (e.g., help with housework and childcare) from their spouses. When comparing the two generations, GX physicians report more coworker support across all three types than BBs. GX physicians also report more spousal emotional (means = 3.9 vs. 3.8, respectively) and instrumental support (means = 3.4 vs. 3.2, respectively) than BBs. These comments added to the survey by a female physician explain how talking to others with whom she works offers her support:

> *Though I work alone in my office practice, I frequently consult in other locations. I have friends who are other physicians (including psychiatrists) who are supportive. I work with many other health-related professionals (e.g., psychologists; social workers; teachers; youth workers) and find my relationships with them to be positive and supportive as well. I feel very appreciated by them.* (Wallace and Lemaire, 2009)

This next physician, who has been married for 27 years, identifies his wife as an important source of support:

> *Probably my wife. Yah, she knows me better than anybody else. The* [office staff] *who work for me have a pretty good idea but I mean my wife knows me like the back of her hand.* (Wallace and Lemaire, 2008)

In summary, the key points are that female physicians receive more support from colleagues and friends in and outside of work than male physicians. Male physicians receive more support from their spouse than female physicians. GX physicians report more coworker support and more emotional and instrumental spousal support than BBs.

PHYSICIANS' ATTITUDES TOWARD MEDICINE

Throughout this chapter, we have outlined many similarities and differences between physicians of both generations and genders, as they relate to workplace stressors, such as work and on-call hours, perceived workload, burnout, work-family issues, coping strategies and sources of support. As noted above, it is often assumed that when younger physicians or female physicians have more family responsibilities, they may be less committed to their patients or to their careers. In our study, despite the many gender and generational differences in work stress, family situations and coping strategies, physicians from both generations and genders were equally satisfied in their jobs. Also, regardless of gender or generation, about three quarters of physicians would choose to be a physician if they were to start over again, which is interpreted as an indicator of their career commitment. Almost all of the physicians found working with patients is very rewarding. It is also interesting to note that despite the gender and generational differences in their family situations and activities in and out of work, over half of the physicians studied felt they generally have a pretty balanced life. This also does not differ by gender or generation.

The following comments sent in addition to the survey illustrate some examples of physicians' attitudes toward medicine.

Even though I am fairly new to practice (about 14 months), I feel my general satisfaction with work and lifestyle is because I put my family first and don't work full-time. (Wallace and Lemaire, 2009)

I consider it a great privilege to practice medicine. The best part is understanding the interactions/effects of physiology, environment, psychology and personalities. Fascinating! (Wallace and Lemaire, 2009)

I enjoy seeing patients and talking to patients and their families and sorting out problems for people on a fairly regular day-to-day basis. That's what I get my kicks out of. So I guess that's the part that satisfies me the most is being able to do things for people and hopefully at the end of the day improve their life somehow. (Wallace and Lemaire, 2008)

In summary, the key point is that there were no generational or gender differences in reports of job satisfaction, commitment to medicine, patient care attitudes or work life balance.

LEARNING POINTS AND LOOKING TO THE FUTURE

We have reviewed the literature and presented emerging research findings that examine stress and coping for physicians with particular attention to generation and gender. Several learning points bear consideration both as new knowledge and for future reflection, as we address the challenges the physicians of today and in the future face in their personal and professional lives.

There are more women and a new generation of physicians entering and practicing medicine. The generations and genders face very distinctive career and family challenges, which may translate into both different or similar stressors and coping strategies. Given these generational and gender shifts, we need to consider more flexible strategies for physicians to carry out their work and to deliver health care. While still prioritizing excellence in patient care, we must recognize the diverse and changing needs and responsibilities of the physician work force in order to sustain the health and wellness of physicians, their families, and health care systems. We need to make the practice of medicine more family friendly for physicians, as both women and the younger generation of physicians juggle their work and family lives and as older physicians begin to wind down their careers. For example, the introduction of more flexibility in work hours and scheduling, and more opportunities for job sharing and part-time positions, would be welcomed by physicians throughout the continuum of life and career stages.

We need to emphasize physician wellness as a positive and necessary contributor to the effective delivery of health care, given that care provided by burned out physicians may be suboptimal. Through ongoing research, we need to further identify and evaluate work place stressors and work life issues contributing to stress, as well as the coping strategies physicians use in response, as they pertain to physicians of both genders and generations. Lastly, despite the many generational and gender differences in workplace stress and coping strategies, physicians generally share positive attitudes toward their profession and the patients they care for, as well as the importance of their family life. These shared professional and family values continue to form the basis for collegial support amongst physicians and quality patient care.

REFERENCES

Abramson, S., Stein, J., Schaufele, M., Frates, E. & Rogan, S. 2000. Personal exercise habits and counseling practices of primary care physicians: a national survey. *Clin J Sport Med, 10*, 40–48.

Arnetz, B. B. 2001. Psychosocial challenges facing physicians of today. *Soc Sci Med, 52*, 203–213.

Baldisseri, M. R. 2007. Impaired healthcare professional. *Crit Care Med, 35*, S106–S116.

Baxter, 2002. Baxter, J. (2000). The joys and justice of housework. Sociology, 34, 609-631.

Barnett, R. C., Brennan, R. T. & Gareis, K. C. 1999. A Closer Look at the Measurement of Burnout. *Journal of Applied Biobehavioral Research, 4*, 65–78.

Brotherton, S. E., Rockey, P. H. & Etzel, S. I. 2005. US graduate medical education, 2004–2005: trends in primary care specialties. *JAMA, 294*, 1075–1082.

Borges, N., Manuel, S.R., Elam, C.L & Jones, B.J. 2006. Comparing millennial and generation X medical students at one medical school. *Academic Medicine, 81*, 571–576.

Buddeberg-Fischer, B., Stamm, M., Buddeberg, C., Bauer, G., Hammig, O., Knecht, M. & Klaghofer, R. 2010. The impact of gender and parenthood on physicians' careers- professional and personal situation seven years after graduation. *BMC Health Services Research, 10*, 1–10.

Burton, K. R. & Wong, I. K. 2004a. A force to contend with: The gender gap closes in Canadian medical schools. *CMAJ, 170*, 1385–1386.

Burton, K. R. & Wong, I. K. 2004b. The gender gap in Canadian health care. *CMAJ, 171*, 1154–1154.

Campbell, D. A., Jr., Sonnad, S. S., Eckhauser, F. E., Campbell, K. K. & Greenfield, L. J. 2001. Burnout among American surgeons. *Surgery, 130*, 696–702; discussion 702–705.

Campolieti, M., Hyatt, D. & Kralj, B. 2007. Determinants of Stress in Medical Practice: Evidence from Ontario Physicians. *Relations Industrielles/Industrial Relations, 62*, 226–257.

Canadian Institute For Health Information 2007. *Supply, Distribution and Migration of Canadian Physicians.* Ottawa, Ontario: Canadian Institute for Health Information (CIHI).

Caplan, R. D., Cobb, S. & French, J. R., Jr. 1975. Relationships of cessation of smoking with job stress, personality, and social support. *J Appl Psychol, 60*, 211–219.

Carr, P. L., Ash, A. S., Friedman, R. H., Scaramucci, A., Barnett, R. C., Szalacha, L., Palepu, A. & Moskowitz, M. A. 1998. Relation of family responsibilities and gender to the productivity and career satisfaction of medical faculty. *Ann Intern Med, 129*, 532–538.

Carter, T. 2001. a New Breed. *ABA Journal, 87*, 36.

Chan, B. T. 2002. From perceived surplus to perceived shortage: what happened to Canada's physician workforce in the 1990s? Ottawa, Ontario: Canadian Institutes for Health Information.

Craig, L. 2007. How Employed Mothers in Australia Find Time for Both Market Work and Childcare. *Journal of Family and Economic Issues, 28,* 69–87.

Dorsey, E. R., Jarjoura, D. & Rutecki, G. W. 2003. Influence of controllable lifestyle on recent trends in specialty choice by US medical students. *JAMA, 290,* 1173–1178.

Dumelow, C., Littlejohns, P. & Griffiths, S. 2000. Relation between a career and family life for English hospital consultants: qualitative, semistructured interview study. *BMJ, 320,* 1437–1440.

Dunn, L. B., Moutier, C., Green Hammond, K. A., Lehrmann, J. & Roberts, L. W. 2008. Personal health care of residents: preferences for care outside of the training institution. *Acad Psychiatry, 32,* 20–30.

Dunstone, D. C. & Reames, H. R., JR. 2001. Physician satisfaction revisited. *Soc Sci Med, 52,* 825–837.

Duxbury, L. & Higgins, C. 2001. Work-Life Balance in the New Millennium: Where Are We? Where Do We Need to Go? Ottawa: Canadian Policy Research Networks.

Fairchild, D. G., Mcloughlin, K. S., Gharib, S., Horsky, J., Portnow, M., Richter, J., Gagliano, N. & Bates, D. W. 2001. Productivity, quality, and patient satisfaction: comparison of part-time and full-time primary care physicians. *J Gen Intern Med, 16,* 663–667.

Fay, W. B. 1993. Understanding "Generation X." *Mark Res, 5,* 2.

Firth-Cozens, J. 2001. Interventions to improve physicians' well-being and patient care. *Soc Sci Med, 52,* 215–222.

Flaherty, J. & Richman, J. 1989. Gender differences in the perception and utilization of social support: theoretical perspectives and an empirical test. *Soc Sci Med, 28,* 1221–1228.

Fong, R. O. 2002. Retaining Generation X'ers in a Baby Boomer Firm. *Capital University Law Review, 29,* 911–921.

Frank, E., Mcmurray, J. E., Linzer, M. & Elon, L. 1999. Career satisfaction of US women physicians: results from the Women Physicians' Health Study. Society of General Internal Medicine Career Satisfaction Study Group. *Arch Intern Med, 159,* 1417–1426.

Fritz, N. E. & Lantos, J. D. 1991. Pediatrician's practice choices: differences between part-time and full-time practice. *Pediatrics, 88,* 764–769.

Fuhrer, R. & Stansfeld, S. A. 2002. How gender affects patterns of social relations and their impact on health: a comparison of one or multiple sources of support from "close persons." *Soc Sci Med, 54,* 811–825.

Galinsky, E., Kim, Stacy, S. & Bond, J. T. 2001. Feeling overworked: When work becomes too much. *Families and Work Institute,* 1–14.

Gjerberg, E. 2001. Medical women—toward full integration? An analysis of the specialty choices made by two cohorts of Norwegian doctors. *Soc Sci Med, 52,* 331–343.

Grant, L., Simpson, L. A., Xue Lan, R. & Holly, P.-G. 1990. Gender, parenthood, and Work Hours of Physicians. *Journal of Marriage & Family, 52,* 39–49.

Grayson, M.S., Newton, D.A., Patrick, P.A. & Smith, L. 2011. Impact of AOA status and perceived lifestyle on career choices of medical school graduates. *J Gen Intern Med, 26,* 1434–1440.

Gross, E. B. 1997. Gender differences in physician stress: why the discrepant findings? *Women Health, 26,* 1–14.

Gursoy, D., Maier T.A. & Chi, C.G. 2008. Generational differences: An examination of work values and generational gaps in the hospitality workforce. *International Journal of Hospitality Management, 27,* 448–458.

Hafferty, F. W. & Light, D. W. 1995. Professional dynamics and the changing nature of medical work. *J Health Soc Behav,* Spec No, 132–153.

Heiliger, P. J. & Hingstman, L. 2000. Career preferences and the work-family balance in medicine: gender differences among medical specialists. *Soc Sci Med, 50,* 1235–1246.

Hill, C. R. & Stafford, F. P. 1980. Parental Care of Children: Time Diary Estimates of Quantity, Predictability, and Variety. *The Journal of Human Resources, 15,* 219–239.

Hochschild, A. 1989. *The Second Shift: Working Parents and the revolution at Home.* New York, Viking Penguin Inc.

Izraeli, D. N. 1994. Money Matters: Spousal incomes and family/work relations among physician couples in Israel. *Sociological Quarterly, 35,* 69–84.

Janning, M. 2006. Put Yourself in My Work Shoes. *Journal of Family Issues, 27*, 85–109.

Jovic, E., Wallace, J. E. & Lemaire, J. 2006. The generation and gender shifts in medicine: an exploratory survey of internal medicine physicians. *BMC Health Serv Res, 6*, 55.

Jurkiewicz, C. L. 2000. Generation X and the public employee. *Public Personnel Management, 29*, 55–74.

Katz, J., Monnier, J., Libet, J., Shaw, D. & Beach, S. R. 2000. Individual and crossover effects of stress on adjustment in medical student marriages. *J Marital Fam Ther, 26*, 341–351.

Keene, J. R. & Reynolds, J. R. 2005. The Job Costs of Family Demands. *Journal of Family Issues, 26*, 275–299.

Keizer, M. 1997. Gender and career in medicine. *Neth J of Soc Sci, 33*, 94–112.

Kennedy, M. M. 2003. Managing different generations requires new skills, insightful leadership. *Physician Exec, 29*, 20–23.

Kessler, R. C. & Mcleod, J. D. 1984. Sex Differences in Vulnerability to Undesirable Life Events. *American Sociological Review, 49*, 620–631.

King, L. A., Mattimore, L. K., King, D. W. & Adams, G. A. 1995. Family Support Inventory for Workers: A New Measure of Perceived Social Support from Family Members. *Journal of Organizational Behavior, 16*, 235–258.

Kletke, P. R., Marder, W. D. & Silberger, A. B. 1990. The growing proportion of female physicians: implications for US physician supply. *Am J Public Health, 80*, 300–304.

Larson, D. L. 2003. Bridging the generation X gap in plastic surgery training: part 2. A proposed solution— identifying a "best practice" in a plastic surgery training program. *Plast Reconstr Surg, 112*, 1662–1665.

Lemaire, J. B. & Wallace, J. E. 2010. Not all coping strategies are created equal: a mixed methods study exploring physicians' self reported coping strategies. *BMC Health Serv Res, 10*, 208.

Levinson, W. & Lurie, N. 2004. When most doctors are women: what lies ahead? *Ann Intern Med, 141*, 471–474.

Linn, L. S., Brook, R. H., Clark, V. A., Davies, A. R., Fink, A. & Kosecoff, J. 1985. Physician and patient satisfaction as factors related to the organization of internal medicine group practices. *Med Care, 23*, 1171–1178.

Linzer, M., Gerrity, M., Douglas, J. A., Mcmurray, J. E., Williams, E. S. & Konrad, T. R. 2002. Physician stress: results from the physician worklife study. Presented in preliminary format at the AMA International Conference on Physician Health, Victoria BC, Canada, May 1998, and in final form at the AMCOGG symposium on mental. *Stress & Health: Journal of the International Society for the Investigation of Stress, 18*, 37–42.

Marks, S. R. & Macdermid, S. M. 1996. Multiple Roles and the Self: A Theory of Role Balance. *Journal of Marriage & Family, 58*, 417–432.

Martin, S. 2003. Family matters. *CMAJ, 168*, 1174.

Mckenzie Leiper, J. 2006. *Bar Codes: Women in the Legal Profession.*, Vancouver, B.C., University of British Columbia Press.

Mcmurray, J. E., Cohen, M., Angus, G., Harding, J., Gavel, P., Horvath, J., Paice, E., Schmittdiel, J. & Grumbach, K. 2002. Women in medicine: a four-nation comparison. *J Am Med Womens Assoc, 57*, 185–190.

O'neil, E. 2002. Shaping America's health care professions: how the health sector will respond to "generation X." *West J Med, 176*, 139–141.

Okun, M. A. & Keith, V. M. 1998. Effects of positive and negative social exchanges with various sources on depressive symptoms in younger and older adults. *J Gerontol B Psychol Sci Soc Sci, 53*, P4–P20.

Olkinuora, M., Asp, S., Juntunen, J., Kauttu, K., Strid, L. & Äärimaa, M. 1990. Stress symptoms, burnout and suicidal thoughts in Finnish physicians. *Social Psychiatry and Psychiatric Epidemiology, 25*, 81–86.

Ontario Medical Association, H. R. C. O. 2002. Position paper on physician workforce policy and planning. Toronto, Ontario: Ontario Medical Association.

Panagopoulou, E., Montgomery, A. & Benos, A. 2006. Burnout in internal medicine physicians: Differences between residents and specialists. *Eur J Intern Med, 17*, 195–200.

Peeters, M. C. W. & Le Blanc, P. M. 2001. Toward a match between job demands and sources of social support: A study among oncology care providers. *European Journal of Work and Organizational Psychology, 10*, 53–72.

Press, J., Fagan, J. & Bernd, E. 2006. Child Care, Work, and Depressive Symptoms Among Low-Income Mothers. *Journal of Family Issues, 27*, 609–632.

Phelan, S. 2010. Generational issues in the ob-gyn workplace: "Marcus Welby, MD" versus "Scrubs." *Obstetrics & Gynecology, 116*, 568–569.

Reilly, J. M. & Ring, J. M. 2007. Physician, heal thyself: tools for resident well-being. *Med Educ, 41*, 522–523.

Robinson, G. E. 2003. Stresses on women physicians: Consequences and coping techniques. *Depression & Anxiety (1091–4269), 17*, 180–189.

Ross, C. E. & Mirowsky, J. 1989. Explaining the social patterns of depression: control and problem solving—or support and talking? *J Health Soc Behav, 30*, 206–219.

Ryan-Wenger, N. A., Sharrer, V. W. & Campbell, K. K. 2005. Changes in children's stressors over the past 30 years. *Pediatr Nurs, 31*, 282–288, 291.

Santos, S. R., Carroll, C. A., Cox, K. S., Teasley, S. L., Simon, S. D., Bainbridge, L., Cunningham, M. & Ott, L. 2003. Baby boomer nurses bearing the burden of care: A four-site study of stress, strain, and coping for inpatient registered nurses. *J Nurs Adm, 33*, 243–250.

Sargent, M. C., Sotile, W., Sotile, M. O., Rubash, H. & Barrack, R. L. 2004. Stress and coping among orthopaedic surgery residents and faculty. *J Bone Joint Surg Am, 86-A*, 1579–1586.

Sarma, S., Thind, A. & Chu, M. 2011. Do new cohorts of family physicians work less compared to their older predecessors? The evidence from Canada. *Social Science & Medicine, 72*, 2049–4058.

Schwartz, R. W., Haley, J. V., Williams, C., Jarecky, R. K., Strodel, W. E., Young, B. & Griffen, W. O., Jr. 1990. The controllable lifestyle factor and students' attitudes about specialty selection. *Acad Med, 65*, 207–210.

Scott, I., Gowans, M. C., Wright, B. & Brenneis, F. 2007. Why medical students switch careers: changing course during the preclinical years of medical school. *Can Fam Physician, 53*, 95, 95:e 1–5, 94.

Shanafelt, T. D., Novotny, P., Johnson, M. E., Zhao, X., Steensma, D. P., Lacy, M. Q., Rubin, J. & Sloan, J. 2005. The well-being and personal wellness promotion strategies of medical oncologists in the North Central Cancer Treatment Group. *Oncology, 68*, 23–32.

Smith, C., Boulger, J. & Beattie, K. 2002. Exploring the dual-physician marriage. *Minn Med, 85*, 39–43.

Sobecks, N. W., Justice, A. C., Hinze, S., Chirayath, H. T., Lasek, R. J., Chren, M. M., Aucott, J., Juknialis, B., Fortinsky, R., Youngner, S. & Landefeld, C. S. 1999. When doctors marry doctors: a survey exploring the professional and family lives of young physicians. *Ann Intern Med, 130*, 312–319.

Sotile, W. & Sotile, M. 2001. Medical couples: the most stressed (and surprised) segment of married people. *Iowa Med, 91*, 16–19.

Swanson, V. & Power, K. G. 1999. Stress, satisfaction and role conflict in dual-doctor partnerships. *Community, Work & Family, 2*, 67–88.

Swanson, V., Power, K. G. & Simpson, R. J. 1998. Occupational stress and family life: A comparison of male and female doctors. *Journal of Occupational & Organizational Psychology, 71*, 237–260.

Shrestha, D. & Joyce, C.M. 2011. Aspects of work-life balance of Australian general practitioners: Determinants and possible consequences. *Australian Journal of Primary Health, 17*, 40–47.

Tattersall, A. J., Bennett, P. & Pugh, S. 1999. Stress and coping in hospital doctors. *Stress Medicine, 15*, 109–113.

Tesch, B. J., Wood, H. M., Helwig, A. L. & Nattinger, A. B. 1995. Promotion of women physicians in academic medicine. Glass ceiling or sticky floor? *JAMA, 273*, 1022–1025.

Thoits, P. A. 1995. Stress, coping, and social support processes: where are we? What next? *J Health Soc Behav*, Spec No, 53–79.

Twenge, J. 2010. A review of the empirical evidence on generational differences in work attitudes. *J Bus Psychol, 25*, 201–210.

Uhlenberg, P. & Cooney, T. M. 1990. Male and female physicians: family and career comparisons. *Soc Sci Med, 30*, 373–378.

Umberson, D., Chen, M. D., House, J. S., Hopkins, K. & Slaten, E. 1996. The Effect of Social Relationships on Psychological Well-Being: Are Men and Women Really so Different? *American Sociological Review, 61*, 837–857.

Umehara, K., Ohya, Y., Kawakami, N., Tsutsumi, A. & Fujimura, M. 2007. Association of work-related factors with psychosocial job stressors and psychosomatic symptoms among Japanese pediatricians. *J Occup Health*, 49, 467–481.

Visser, M. R., Smets, E. M., Oort, F. J. & De Haes, H. C. 2003. Stress, satisfaction and burnout among Dutch medical specialists. *CMAJ*, 168, 271–275.

Wallace, J. E. 2006. Work commitment in the legal profession: a study of Baby Boomers and Generation Xers. *Int J Legal Prof*, 13, 137–151.

Wallace, J. E. & Lemaire, J. 2007. On physician well being-you'll get by with a little help from your friends. *Soc Sci Med*, 64, 2565–2577.

Wallace, J. E. & Lemaire, J. B. 2008. Determinants of Physician Well-Being: Stage One Report. Prepared for the Alberta Heritage Foundation for Medical Research and the former Calgary Health Region, now Alberta Health Services (AHS).

Wallace, J. E. & Lemaire, J. B. 2009. Determinants of physician well-being: results from the physician survey (stage two report). Report prepared for the Alberta Heritage Foundation for Medical Research and Alberta Health Services (AHS).

Wallace, J. E. & Young, M. C. 2008. Parenthood and productivity: A study of demands, resources and family-friendly firms. *Journal of Vocational Behavior*, 72, 110–122.

Weiner, E. L., Swain, G. R., Wolf, B. & Gottlieb, M. 2001. A qualitative study of physicians' own wellness-promotion practices. *West J Med*, 174, 19–23.

Weinstein, L. & Wolfe, H.M. 2007. The downward spiral of physician satisfaction. An attempt to avert a crisis within the medical profession. *Obstetrics & Gynecology*, 109, 1181–1183.

Weisman, C. S., Teitelbaum, M. A., Nathanson, C. A., Chase, G. A., King, T. M. & Levine, D. M. 1986. Sex differences in the practice patterns of recently trained obstetrician-gynecologists. *Obstet Gynecol*, 67, 776–782.

Wills, T. 1985. Supportive functions of interpersonal relationships. *In:* Cohen, S. & Syme, L. (eds.) *Social Support and Health*. New York: Academic Press.

Wright, B., Scott, I., Woloschuk, W., Brenneis, F. & Bradley, J. 2004. Career choice of new medical students at three Canadian universities: family medicine versus specialty medicine. *CMAJ*, 170, 1920–1924.

Zukewich, N. 2003. Unpaid informal caregiving. *Canadian Social Trends*, . (Autumn/cat.no. 11-008): 14–18.

/// 14 /// TREATMENT AND PREVENTION WORK

Center for Practitioner Renewal

DAVID KUHL, DOUGLAS CAVE, HILARY PEARSON, AND PAUL WHITEHEAD

SCENARIO

A 78-year-old woman with a long standing history of cancer lies in her hospital bed still groggy from the general anesthetic she received for the surgical removal of a mass in her groin. In the distance (the doorway of her room), she hears her doctor's voice, "Oh by the way we were wrong, it is cancer. I have made an appointment for the oncologist in a few days." His voice sounds particularly cold and distant, and after those few words, the doctor walks away. No discussion, no touch, no empathy. The woman is left with her many unanswered questions, her concerns about how her family will receive this message, her thoughts of "if only ... " and her rage at how she has just been told that what she had been led to believe was benign is cancer. A decade later she recounted that day as though it had occurred only days earlier: "The way in which the doctor spoke with me was more painful than the disease itself." In that instance, the doctor added to the patient's suffering by the way in which he spoke to her. His interaction with her might be regarded as iatrogenic suffering, that is, the healer (namely the physician) is the source of the suffering experienced by the patient.[1]

CONTEXT

How is it that people who have chosen a profession that works to reverse disease processes, eliminate pain, and alleviate suffering actually contribute to the suffering of their patients? For the most part it is done unintentionally and may be unknown to the physician. In the case of iatrogenic suffering, one might consider the question, who suffers? Is it only the patient and the patient's family, or might it also be the health care provider? What are the features that contribute to the suffering of health care providers? Those are the questions that contributed to the creation of the Center for Practitioner Renewal.

Health care is about curing and healing, art and science, mind and heart, skills and knowledge, technology and compassion, life and death, living and dying. It is often based on a business model of efficiency, while the work we do is about relationship—relationship with self, other, and Other. Too often relationship is sacrificed to action, task and efficiency.

Consider the larger present day health care context. Mental and emotional health problems in the workplace result in astronomical social and economic costs. Researchers agree that the majority of workers are struggling in the face of constant and unrelenting change and that there is a large cost associated with this in terms of increasing disability rates and decreasing productivity for workers and companies.[2] According to the World Health Organization (WHO), by the year 2020 depression among workers in industrialized countries is expected to reach epochal levels.[3]

In Canada, current estimates of absenteeism and lost productivity due to mental health-related disability costs are $33–$45 million annually.[3,4] In addition to lost productivity, impoverished mental health and well-being detrimentally affect the personal and family lives of those who are ill, the workplace climate, and society at large.

Health care is recognized as an environment in which it is very easy to become and remain ill because of the constant exposure to other people's suffering, the heavy physical and emotional demands of the work, and the reluctance to disclose personal distress.[5]

Social isolation is a significant determinant of mental health problems, and in the medical culture personal difficulties are often denied or go unnoticed until they reach a critical point because of the stigma that surrounds mental health issues and seeking help for those issues.[5,6–10] There is evidence that the current health care environment has exacerbated what was already a critical situation and placed the sustainability of health care practitioners and their families at even greater risk.[11,12] This has resulted in increasing numbers of health care professionals who are unable or unwilling to continue practicing because of the overwhelming stress experienced in their work, as well as decreasing patient satisfaction and growing numbers of people without ready access to the health services they need.[3]

In health care, research studies related to stress and burnout have largely focused on the experiences of physicians and registered nurses and much remains to be understood about the experience of other (allied) health care providers.[13]

Among nurses, researchers report astonishing levels of burnout, illness, and injury.[14-16] Staff shortages, increased workloads, restructuring, lack of perceived support, intercollegial frictions, and exposure to verbal or physical abuse and bullying have been associated with disturbing levels of job dissatisfaction and a rate of absenteeism and work loss due to illness, injury, burnout, or disability among Canadian nurses almost double that of the general labor force.[13,17]

In 2002, the Canadian Labor and Business Center estimated that over the course of a year, 16 million nursing hours (the equivalent of 9,000 full time positions) are lost to injury and illness.[13] As a reference point, Canada's population is just over 33 million; the population of the United States is nearly 304 million. In terms of population, the number of people in Canada is closer to that of California whose population is nearly 38 million.

If all things were equal, the comparative numbers regarding nursing hours lost to injury and illness in the United States may be 10 times that of the Canadian numbers. All things remaining equal, this could mean there are 160 million nursing hours (the equivalent of 90,000 FTEs) lost to injury and illness annually in the United States.

In Canada, as elsewhere, there is evidence of a significant decline in physician morale and levels of burnout that are markedly higher than those in the general population.[18,19] Almost half of the respondents (46%) to the Canadian Medical Association's 2003 Physician Resource Questionnaire reported that they were experiencing an advanced stage of burnout.[5] Changes in the medical climate have left many physicians experiencing a sense of increased demands, decreased personal control over their work, and reduced social support—a combination of factors that is a recognized recipe for burnout.[12]

In several studies, burnout among physicians has been linked to lost productivity, depression and substance misuse, significantly higher rates of suicide compared to the general population, distress in physicians' family lives, suboptimal medical care, and increased patient suffering.

Recent initiatives to support physician well-being and employee assistance and other wellness programs are intended to aid workers. Attention has been drawn to the urgent need to develop effective workplace interventions to reduce isolation, transform the stigma attached to disclosing mental health difficulties, and enhance the prevention and early detection of problems.[20,21]

Researchers describe the tendency to rely on remedial, individual-focused strategies for reducing work related stress.[10,13] They also underline the critical contribution of organizational culture in moving toward primary prevention models, the need for a continuum of integrated prevention and health promotion strategies, and the importance of grounding research in theoretical models that can more adequately capture the complex interplay of psychosocial risk factors, facilitate the development of contextually effective interventions, and improve knowledge translation.

BUILDING TOOLS FOR RENEWAL

Currently, Providence Health Care (PHC) is one of the largest Catholic health care organization in Canada. PHC operates six facilities—three hospitals and three residential care facilities that provide care for 350,000 (1422 beds) patients and residents per year. As part of PHC, the Center for Practitioner Renewal was conceived in order to help sustain health care providers in the workplace. That included approximately 6000 nursing, allied health, and managerial staff, as well as 1000 physicians associated with Providence Health Care. The physicians and staff at PHC work in all areas of health care, including some of the most advanced medical programs in the country, with some of the most disadvantaged populations of the downtown core of one of Canada's largest cities and the multicultural diversity that characterizes Vancouver and Canada.

The health care providers that the CPR seeks to support experience all of the intensity and demand that has been noted elsewhere in health care generally. As part of one of the largest tertiary health care facilities in the province, they have been keenly aware of how budgetary constraints and financial restructuring have eroded the resources available to them in recent years. It was in this context that the need to support health care providers was recognized by both senior leadership at PHC and a small number of front line providers who were in a position to create the Center for Practitioner Renewal.

The Center for Practitioner Renewal (CPR) is dedicated to understanding the psychological, emotional, and spiritual needs of health care providers as they care for patients and residents. In defining our work, we ask three questions:

1. How do we sustain health care providers in the workplace?
2. What is the effect of being in the presence of suffering?
3. What would be reparative and healing or restore resilience for health care providers?

Experiencing an illness or receiving care in a hospital is more than a physical event. It is a human, social, and spiritual process for the patient as well as for the health care provider. The essence of the work that is done by health care providers is based on relationship(s)— relationship with oneself, with colleagues, with patients and their families, and perhaps even with one's sense of the spiritual or divine.

Our initial understanding of the work of the Center was informed by the growing body of literature on burnout among physicians and nurses. We also took into account that other researchers were identifying additional constructs such as compassion fatigue/secondary traumatic stress and moral distress,[9] which we hoped could help in developing a more refined understanding of the stress experienced by health care providers. While maintaining an open and exploratory approach, we differentiated between these constructs in order to guide our interventions and support.

Burnout has been identified as having to do with the nature of external demands versus the resources to meet those demands, while the other theoretical stress constructs have to do with the internal experience of working closely with suffering patients. Maslach and Leiter identify six work-related areas where a mismatch between personal expectations and the realities of the job could lead to burnout: workload, control, reward, community, fairness, and values. At the CPR we understood that our ability to address some of these realities was limited, and that our ability to provide support would be undermined if we took on the role, for example, of advocating for improved working conditions or became involved in labor relations concerns. However, we saw that we could work with individuals and groups to improve their sense of control and increase their experience of community, thus empowering them to address their workplace situation more effectively.

On the other hand, at the CPR we expected the constructs of vicarious trauma,[22] compassion fatigue/secondary traumatic stress, and moral distress to be particularly salient for health care providers. These constructs look at the impact of caring for the suffering of others, which delineates an area of stress for health care providers that is quite independent of the situational or systemic factors in the workplace, although clearly complicated by them.

We have learned in the past years that health care providers experience a considerable degree of estrangement—from self, others, and Other. Of the parent/child relationship Carl Jung stated that the greatest burden a child must bear is the unlived life of the parent. In health care it might be said that the greatest burden patients must bear are the unrecognized/unresolved psychological and spiritual issues of the health care provider. In that context it is important for health care providers to ask some difficult questions of themselves: What brought me to health care? What are some of the unresolved issues in my life that come with me from my family of origin, from my past relationships, and from my current life situation? Do I have a need to be liked? What type of relationships give me meaning? What did/do I expect of myself and others in the health care workplace?

Physicians tell us they don't have time to speak with other physicians any more—doctor's lounges have been closed because of the need for space or the need for equality (other disciplines don't have discipline specified lounges); doctors are expected to see more patients in less time; systemic changes happen without physicians being consulted. The result can easily be a sense of estrangement from the workplace.

Exposure to suffering of others, especially in an environment that does not encourage "healing connections," may result in a sense of estrangement from a Higher Power, a loving God or Goddess, a sense of goodness in the world. This certainly seems to be a feature of the workplace and characterizes those who experience vicarious trauma: a darkening of one's worldview, spirituality, and relationships.[22]

There are many features that are a challenge to well-being in health care: economic restraint and restructuring, rapidly developing technologies, increased access to information (and misinformation), increased patient complexity and an aging population, shortage of practitioners and multigenerational issues, decreased numbers of beds, and a more critical and litigious social climate. Professional barriers to well-being include heavy physical and emotional demands coupled with consistent exposure to suffering; a culture of stoicism, self-sufficiency and silence; stigma about mental health issues and help seeking; perfectionism and compulsiveness that are sanctioned and reinforced by work pressures and societal expectations; reluctance to disclose personal or a peer's distress; lack of sufficient and easily accessible resources. Personal barriers to self-care include internalized stigma, feeling over burdened and lacking peer support; denial, minimization, or trivialization; prior experience of being "shamed and blamed"; unwillingness to become a patient and/or challenges in being treated as a patient; fear of loss of license and livelihood; fear of possible diagnosis; concerns about family/friends/colleagues not accepting or negatively judging them.

Essentially the work of the CPR focuses on 2 broad domains. We provide individual therapy and group therapeutic interventions. The Individual therapy follows a traditional psychotherapeutic model. As doctoral-level trained therapists, we are informed by a range of therapeutic approaches that are appropriate for the chief complaint/concern of the health care provider.

Group therapeutic interventions include process-oriented group therapy, team interventions, resolution of unfinished business between and among employees and medical staff, and a variety of psycho-educational workshops related to promoting well being and effective interpersonal skills. Group counseling models suggest that creating a climate maximally conducive to effective interpersonal interactions, support and learning requires paying attention to group members' basic needs. To that end, the groups we conduct are informed by two related approaches to group process. Schutz proposed that group members have three basic needs: the need for inclusion; the need for control;

and the need for intimacy/trust. Pursuant to definitions given by Schutz and for ease of remembering, we renamed the needs as SIT:

Safety clarity about the structure, ground rules, the facilitator's responsibilities, and degree of personal control/safety

Inclusion a sense of belonging, feeling accepted by other group members and the facilitator, and experiencing the group climate as supportive

Trust a deepening of mutual trust and sense of we-ness/community among group members

Following a comprehensive investigation of many different approaches to group psycho-therapy, Yalom[23,24] delineated eleven factors that can contribute to therapeutic change, while noting that these factors are interdependent and do not function in isolation:

1. Installation of Hope (hope that situations can be different and better)
2. Universality (commonalities with others)
3. Group Cohesiveness (a sense of we-ness)
4. Imparting Information (psycho-education, sharing knowledge/resources)
5. Altruism (support, reassurance, normalization)
6. The Corrective Recapitulation of the Primary Family Group (early family conflicts are relived and revised correctively)
7. Development of Socializing Techniques (basic social skills)
8. Imitative Behavior (of leaders and other group members)
9. Interpersonal Learning (learning from other's experiences, working through trans-ference, and having a corrective emotional experience)
10. Catharsis (a release of stored or pent-up feelings)
11. Existential Factors (issues of meaning, purpose, life and death)

Yalom noted that group cohesiveness is more than a potent therapeutic force in its own right and is often a necessary precondition for the other factors to function optimally. It is therefore vital that group leaders be actively engaged in creating and maintaining a supportive group climate, are cognizant of general stages of group development, and are skilled in helping the group reestablish safety should misunderstandings and ruptures occur.

Each CPR group intervention is tailored to meet the unique needs of the "client" and bounded by explicitly stated and constantly revisited group agreements. The acronym

CENTRE (Canadian spelling) represents the type of agreements that can be valuable in establishing a foundation of safety:

Confidentiality (with standard limits)
Equal airtime
Non-judgmental listening
Timeliness
Right to pass
Engaged

FEATURES OF OUR WORK

Self-Care of the Team

As a part of our commitment to the work of supporting health care providers we are also committed to supporting the cohesion and healthy functioning of our own team. Even, or perhaps especially, when the demand for our services is high, we consider our weekly team meetings to be an important part of our own resilience and a model of balancing the tasks at hand with a commitment to the self-awareness of each team member and mutual support among the team. One of our first avenues of intervention with a poorly functioning team is to encourage a similar commitment to regular staff meetings when there is time to attend to both the business at hand and some level of individual "check-in."

Team Agreements

As teams or groups come together, most teams will implicitly agree about how they will be together. Implicit team agreements potentiate the risk of disagreements within the team. Conversely when team agreements are explicitly defined, the risk for challenges is more easily managed. As with any group process, when the guidelines of how the group will work together are understood and accepted by each member, the process of working together is easier.

1. Leadership. Each team must have a leader. Being the physician on the team is not reason enough to be the leader. The position would best come with a job description and role definitions. The leader would determine with the team how decisions would be made, explaining his or her relationship to the organization with regard to decision making processes and responsibilities. The leader would hold a vision for the team and also have management skills such that the vision can be translated into action.

2. Job Descriptions. Each person on the team must have a job description that is usually the contract that has been signed by that individual.
   - My contract says...
   - The most important part of the job is...
   - The least important part of the job is...

3. Role Definitions. Who does what, how, when, and where are features of role definitions. In health care, many features of the work we do within a particular discipline are shared by team members who represent different disciplines. Poorly defined roles, unspoken assumptions, and unexpressed expectations usually result in tension and conflict. Unexpressed expectations that contribute to conflict often stem from poorly defined roles.
   - I will know I'm performing my role when...
   - I will know I'm not performing my role when...
   - Decisions are made by...
   - Disagreements will be resolved by...

4. How to be together at work. How are we going to be together in the workplace? How will we make decisions? How will we express emotions that might cause awkwardness between us?
   - What I bring is...
   - What I am able to give to others and to the team is...
   - What I would value from others on the team is...

5. Enhanced Communication Skills. (See Communication and Interpersonal Skills Training, below) Health care providers have strong communication skills pertaining to their discipline. Giving one another difficult information, evaluation or feedback is not part of our training. For that reason many of us avoid difficult conversations— until such a time when we blurt something out, simply to get it off our backs.
   - How I would like to receive feedback is...
   - How I can give feedback is...

6. Core Values. Each team identifies their own values. This could include values such as
   - Confidentiality
     - Respect each other's right to privacy when a colleague asks us to keep personal information they have shared with us confidential.
   - Inclusion
     - Commit to keeping colleagues (especially new team members) appraised of information that is important to their work and to our work together as an effective team
     - Commit to welcoming new people who join the team

- Nonjudgmental climate: No blaming or shaming
  - Challenge ideas, not each other, and strive to use "I" statements rather than "You did..."
  - To decrease the likelihood of engendering defensiveness, avoid generalizations such as "always" and "never" and questions that begin with "Why" did you...
  - Assume responsibility for our own actions
  - Check out assumptions
- Interpersonal respect
  - Avoid gossip and scapegoating
  - In a nonemergency situation, when you need to interrupt a colleague check out the timing with them (i.e. ask for permission to interrupt or establish a time when both parties are free to talk)
- Commitment to resolve interpersonal difficulties and misunderstandings
  - Commit to deal with difficult issues in a timely way
  - If you think you may have inadvertently offended a colleague, check it out with them
  - When difficulties arise with a colleague, address the issue(s) one-on-one with that person and recognize that it may take more than one meeting/discussion to resolve the difficulties
  - If the issue/conflict cannot be resolved between you, then seek out leadership assistance
  - Recognize that providing clear, concrete facts about a challenging situation will allow your team leader to assist you more effectively in finding resolution
- Express expectations
  - Hopes
  - Wants
  - Desires
- What I value the most is...
7. Expectations. Team members frequently have expectations of themselves and of each other. Often these are unexpressed and may therefore lead to unmet expectations and misunderstandings. Questions for team members to answer and share with other team members are
  - What you can expect from me is...
  - What I hope from you is...
  - What I desire for us is...

8. Conflict Resolution (external help if needed). We prefer to refer to a process of forgiveness and reconciliation. Begin with difficult conversations, outlined in the next section (Communication and Interpersonal Skills Training)
   - Guidelines
   - Permission
   - I give you permission to...
   - I would like permission from you to...
   - Boundaries
   - What I cannot tolerate is...
9. Authenticity
   - You will know I'm being authentic when you see me...
10. Frequency and Format of checking in with team and reviewing/renegotiating agreements

COMMUNICATION AND INTERPERSONAL SKILLS TRAINING

Experiential group training in communication skills is offered to employees and medical staff and incorporated into the behavioral medicine modules for family practice residents and international medical graduates at PHC.

Skills are taught by the members of the CPR ream in an experiential, participatory manner rather than being "talked about" as is the case of many commujnication skills courses. The model is based on a program known as Excellence in Cultural Experiential Learning and Leadership (ExcelL) which is the product of a collaborative effort between researchers from Canada and Australia.[25] ExcelL is a skills-based group training program that is grounded in human learning theory, promotes augmentation and empowerment (as opposed to assimilation or replacement), and recognizes potential psychosocial barriers across cultures. The program emphasizes that leaders are required to pay close attention to establishing a supportive learning environment and addressing group dynamics. They actively demonstrate the skills and provide micro-skills coaching and constructive feedback as participants role rehearse each skill. Generic skills are broken down into four stages of interaction: Approach, Bridge, Comment, Develop/Closure (ABCD). The ABCD template provides a step-by-step description of what would generally be considered an effective way to communicate in a given situation. Learners can use the basic road map to focus their practice and simultaneously experiment with how to incorporate their own indvidiual style, learn from observing other group members' practice, and expand their range of interpersonal flexibility.

The CPR team effectively adapted the ABCD model to optimize the communication skills competencies, interpersonal flexibility, and inter-collegial learning that are essential in the health care workplace.[26] We have applied the template to a range of key health care competencies applicable to defined situations. Topics include discussing code status, giving life-altering news, the challenging doctor-patient interaction, refusing unreasonable requests, and having difficult conversations (among health care providers and between health care providers and patients/patients families).

While retaining the ABCD (Approach, Bridge, Contact, Develop) format (which health care providers appreciate because of its similarity to existing medical algorithms), we have added a more explicit focus on the first Approach stage of the model. We have renamed this stage Attend to emphasize the importance of mindfulness as we engage in potentially complex conversations—being mindfully self-aware and intentionally mindful of the social context and what other people may be experiencing. The basic template would follow the format below:

Attend

SELF: What am I experiencing? What am I aware of (e.g. nervousness, dread, fatigue, irritation, hope)?

OTHER: What do I imagine/sense the other person experiencing?

What is going on in the present context (i.e. noise, business, tension, quiet)?

Bridge

Introduce the topic.

Check if the timing is appropriate for discussion or whether an alternate time has to be established.

Remain aware of relationship issues (e.g. sensing your own or other's defensiveness, anxiety, withdrawal etc.).

Comment

Give your message.

Ask for what you need or hope for.

Be open to listening actively to the other person.

Check for mutual understanding (clarification, paraphrasing etc.).

Develop Contract/Relationship

Thank the other person for taking time to listen.

Acknowledge impact on the other person.

Establish time line/follow-up/immediate plans.

Close the conversation.

GROUP-BASED LIFE REVIEW

Individually and collectively, storytelling is fundamental to human experience. We are born into and live among stories. Our familial, community, and cultural stories shape our perspectives on the world and, in turn, we each create and share stories to help us make sense of our unique life experiences and deepen bonds of connection and belonging. The positive impact of biographical learning is well documented and physician-authors such as Rita Charon have drawn attention to the importance of narrative medicine as a way to foster effective medical practice and bridge the divides that separate physicians from patients, from themselves, from colleagues and from society.

In the fast-paced world of doctoring it may feel impractical or self-indulgent to consider dedicating time to reflect on and articulate our own life stories. However, pausing to take stock of who and how we are in the world allows our complex story to evolve more consciously; it provides space to tap into our ordinary wisdom and an opportunity to face the future with greater self-understanding, equanimity, and resilience.

Guided Autobiography[27] is an adult education model that has been shown to have naturally therapeutic benefits among a variety of populations. It uses a small group format (usually 5–7 people) and a structured process of reflecting and writing on preselected life themes followed by sharing parts of these personal reflections in the confidentiality of the group. Birren and Deutchman summarized the benefits from 22 life review studies. Among them were increased role clarity, self-esteem and self-understanding; an increased sense of resolution about past resentments, regrets and negative feelings; recognition of past adaptive strategies and their relevance to current needs or difficulties; development of supportive relationships with other group members; greater sense of meaning and purpose in life.

Pearson[28] researched the viability of a group-based professional development life review program for family doctors as a way to promote well-being, collegiality, and sustainability. Some of the themes included in her research were branching points, family of origin, death and dying, work experience as a physician, and meaning, value, and purpose. The feedback was overwhelmingly positive and the participants strongly recommended that opportunities for this type of personal-professional development be expanded. Currently the CPR has offered several (interdisciplinary and intradisciplinary) Professional Development Life Review pilot programs for PHC employees and physicians. The programs are grounded in group counseling theory and practice to facilitate the creation of a climate of safety, and the scheduling of each program varies to address the needs of group members. Inevitably scheduling six to eight sessions (three to four hours long, depending on the size of the group) can be challenging. We have been fortunate that senior leadership have endorsed the value of this professional development opportunity, and we continue to explore how we can maintain the integrity of the process while flexibly responding to the exigencies of life in health care.

TOOLS FOR WORKING WITH INDIVIDUALS

FIFEing Yourself: A Self-Reflective Tool

Originating from the Patient-Centered Care Model, the Feelings, Ideas, Function, Expectations (FIFE) tool is a technique originally designed for physicians to assess patients' Feelings (What are your feelings, especially your fears, about the disease?), Ideas (How do you explain or understand what is going on with regard to the disease?), Function (How does the illness impact you on a daily basis?), and Expectation (What do you expect/hope from your physician and the disease?) of patients' illness.[29] Believing that all relationships are reciprical, FIFE has been innovated as a self-reflective tool. Four broad questions have been adapted for physicians to assess their own affect, cognition, behavior, and meaning-making of a relationship or experience. Each domain has a broad question for reflection. In the questions, "patient" may be replaced by any relevant noun (i.e. colleague, self, etc.).

1. What am I feeling about my patient? (affect)
2. What is my impression (judgment) about myself regarding my patient? (cognition)
3. What are the effects of this patient on my functioning? (behavior)
4. What expectations do I have of myself? (meaning-making)

Time Lines

The following exercise can be done on your own, with a friend, or in a group. Consider a time line. On a sheet of unlined paper, draw a six-inch horizontal line. On the left side, write the word "Birth," on the right the word "Death":

Birth ——————————————————————— *Death*

Think of this line as representing your lifetime. Write your birth date under the word birth. Consider your own history of illness/well-being, your family history, the longevity of your parents and/or grandparents. Place an X on the line to indicate where you believe you are at present. That is, if you believe that you have lived half of your life, place the X midway between Birth and Death. If you believe that you have lived two-thirds of your life, place the X two-thirds along the line. After placing the X on the line, write your name below it. Once you have written your name below the X, take note of your feelings. Do you have a sense of relief? Of anxiety? Of fear? A realization that much of your life has passed?

Next think of five significant events, internal processes, relationships, or experiences in your life: examples may be meeting your spouse or partner, the birth of a child, the death of a friend, an exciting vacation, a failure, a good financial investment, graduation from university, an illness, a period of depression, a realization that you had an addiction, a divorce, the birth of a grandchild, a car accident. Number the events 1 through 5 and place the numbers on the line between your birth and the X.

- What emotions do you feel about each of those events?
- What about the emotion you feel about your life as a whole?
- Are you satisfied with the life you have lived?
- Do you wish that some things had been different?
- Is there something missing in your life that affected who you are today?
- Are there features in your life that you wish were not present?
- Are there events that ought to have been placed on the line but because of the pain they caused you omitted them?
- How might your life have been different if any or all of these features had not been part of your life?

Focus on the line between the X and Death.

- How might you best embrace life in the time that remains?
- If you didn't have to live up to the expectations of anyone else, how would you live, who would you be?
- Are there features of the past that are absent that you wish would be present and therefore you would like to work toward incorporating them into your future?
- Are there things you would like to do? Places you would like to visit? People you would like to spend more time with? Conversations you would like to have? Events you would like to attend—the baptism of a grandchild, the graduation of your eldest child, a birthday, a bar mitzvah, a wedding, an anniversary?

Choose five events, relationships of importance, or experiences you anticipate or choose to create. Number the events beginning with the number 6 and place those numbers on the line between the X and Death.

- How do you feel about each of those events, the people involved in them, and your life as a whole?
- How would you feel if those events didn't happen?
- What do you need to do in order to make them happen?

Birth ————————————————— X ————————————— Death

1	6
2	7
3	8
4	9
5	10

There are several other time lines that are pertinent to the exercise. Other time lines address features of mortality, belonging, significant relationships, estrangement in relationships, leaving a legacy, understanding oneself in the context of the family of origin, and spirituality.

MINDFULNESS/MEDITATION

Another feature that can contribute to the well-being of health care providers is that of mindfulness and meditation. In their book, *From Age-ing to Sage-ing,* Schachter-Shalomi and Miller speak of various contemplative practices: "To a Hindu, for example, meditation might refer to mantra chanting, to a Christian of the contemplative tradition, it might mean concentrating on the sacred heart of Jesus, to a Jew, it might mean chanting the prayer "Shema Yisrael" ("Hear, O Israel") and entering into the stillness pointed to by these sacred words, to a Buddhist meditation might refer to breath control and the impartial observation of thoughts, and to others it might mean quieting the mind and receiving guidance from the Higher Self."[30] (p. 126)

There are many forms of meditation. Many communities offer courses on the various forms of meditation. The following are some resources for consideration.

RESOURCES

Chodron, Pema. *The Places That Scare You: A Guide to Fearlessness in Difficult Times.* Boston: Shambhala Publications Inc., 2002

Goldstein, Joseph and Kornfield, Jack. *Seeking the Heart of Wisdom.* Boston: Shambhala Publications, Inc., 1987

Kabat-Zinn, Jon,. *Full Catastrophe Living: Using the Wisdom of Your Body and Mind to Face Stress, Pain and Illness.* _city? Delta, 1991

Kabat-Zinn, Jon. *Wherever You Go There You Are: Mindfulness Meditation in Every Day Life. [city?]* Hyperion, 1994, 2005

Keating, Thomas. *Open Mind, Open Heart, The Contemplative Dimension of the Gospel.* New York: The Continuum Publishing Company, 1992

Schachter-Shalomi, Zalman, and Miller, Ronald S. *From Age-ing to Sage-ing, A Profound Vision of Growing Older.* New York: Warner Books, 1995 pp. 124–134

REFERENCES

1. Kuhl, D. Exploring the lived experience of having a terminal illness. Journal of Palliative Care, 2011, 27(1), 43–52.

2. Curren, D. (2001, February 15). Canada's output keeps pace with US: StatsCan study on productivity growth. Financial Post, p. C7.

3. Dewa, C. S., Lesage, A., Goering, P., & Caveen, M. (2004). Nature and prevalence of mental illness in the workplace [Electronic Version]. HealthcarePapers, 5(2). Retrieved March 21, 2008 from http://www.longwoods.com

4. Disability management forum: Tackling depression and mental health. (2005). Benefits Canada, 29(8), 1 (Special Supplement).12.

5. Myers, M. (2003). Editorial: Getting better at being well. In M. Myers, T. Watkins & G. Microys (Eds.), *CMA guide to physician health and well-being: Facts, advice and resources for Canadian doctors* (pp. 3–4). Ottawa, Ontario, Canada: Canadian Medical Association.

6. Sullivan, P. (2004b). *MD's own health finally attracting medicine's interest.* Ottawa, Ontario, Canada: Canadian Medical Association.

7. Sullivan, P. (2004a). *Huge wave of MD retirements nearing: Survey.* Ottawa, Ontario, Canada: Canadian Medical Association.

8. Gunderson, L. (2001). Physician burnout. Annals of Internal Medicine, 135(2), 154–158.; Myers, M. (2003). Editorial: Getting better at being well. In M. Myers, T. Watkins & G. Microys (Eds.), CMA guide to physician health and well-being: Facts, advice and resources for Canadian doctors (pp. 3–4). Ottawa, Ontario, Canada: Canadian Medical Association.

9. Pfifferling, J., & Gilley, K. (2000). Overcoming compassion fatigue. *Family Practice Management,* 7(4).

10. Vezina, M., Bourbonnais, R., Brisson, C., & Trudel, L. (2004). Workplace prevention and promotion strategies. *HealthcarePapers,* 5(2). Retrieved March 21, 2008 from http://www.longwoods.com.

11. Firth-Cozens, J., & Payne, R. L. (Eds.). (1999). Stress management in health professionals: Psychological and organizational causes and interventions. New York: Wiley.

12. Sotile, W. M., & Sotile, M. O. (2002). *The resilient physician. Effective emotional management for doctors and their medical organizations.* Chicago, IL: American Medical.

13. Advisory Committee on Health and Human Resources. (2002). Our health, our future: Creating quality workplaces for Canadian nurses. Final report of the Canadian Nursing Advisory Committee. Retrieved June 5, 2006, from http://www.hc-sc.gc.ca.

14. Stanton, M. W., & Rutherford, M. K. (2004). Hospital nurse staffing and quality of care. *Agency for Healthcare Research and Quality: Research in Action Issue 14,* 1–9.

15. Storch, J., Hartrick Doan, G., Rodney, P., Starzomski, R., & Varcoe, C. (2006). Re: *Goal 4. To enhance all jurisdictions' capacity to build and maintain a sustainable workforce in healthy safe work environments.* Vancouver, British Columbia, Canada: Nursing Ethics Research Group: University of Victoria and University of British Columbia Schools of Nursing report for: Federal/Provincial/Territorial Advisory Committee on Health Delivery and Human Resources (ACHDHR): A framework for collaborative Pan-Canadian health Human Resources Planning (September 2005).

16. Varcoe, C., & Rodney, P. (2006). *Constrained agency: The social structure of nurses' work.* Manuscript in preparation.

17. Bourbonnais, R., & Mondor, M. (2001). Job strain and sickness absence among nurses in the province of Quebec. *American Journal of Industrial Medicine, 39*(2), 194–202.

18. Shanafet, T. D., Sloan, J. A., & Haberman, T. M. (2003). The well-being of physicians. *The American Journal of Medicine, 114,* 513–519.;

19. Sullivan, P., & Buske, L. (1998). Results from CMA's huge 1998 physician survey point to a dispirited profession. *Canadian Medical Association Journal, 159*(5), 525–528.

20. Myers, M. (2004, June 21–23). *Vicarious trauma in medicine* Paper presented at the Exploratory Workshop: Vicarious Trauma in the Workplace Conference, Vancouver, British Columbia, Canada.;

21. Remen, R. N. (2001). Recapturing the soul of medicine: Physicians need to reclaim meaning in their working lives. *The Western Journal of Medicine, 174*(1), 1–4.

22. Pearlman, L. A., & Saakvitne, K. W. (1995). Treating therapists with vicarious traumatization and secondary traumatic stress disorders. In C. R. Figley (Ed.), *Compassion fatigue: Coping with secondary traumatic stress disorder in those who treat the traumatized* (pp. 150–177). Levittown, PA: Brunner/Mazel.

23. Yalom, I. D. (1985). *The theory and practice of group psychotherapy.* New York: Basic Books.

24. Yalom, I. D. (1998). *The Yalom reader: Selections from the work of a master therapist and storyteller.* New York: Basic Books.

25. Mak, A.S., Westwood, M. J., Barker, M. C., & Ishiyama, F. I. (1998). Developing sociocultural competencies for success: The EXCELL programme. *Journal International Education, 9,* 33–38.

26. Westwood, D., Pearson, H. (2000). *Sociocultural competencies: Communication skills for career and employment success,* Log No 1535. Victoria: Centre for Curriculm Transfer and Technology.

27. Birren, J. E., & Deutchman, D. E. (1991). *Guiding Augobiography groups for older adults exploring the fabric of life.* Baltimore: The Johns Hopkins University Press.

28. Pearson, H. M. (2005). *Exploring group-based life review with family physicians: constructing narratives of experience and meaning.* Unpublished doctoral dissertation, University of British Columbia, Vancouver.

29. Stewart, M., Brown, J.B., Weston, W.W., McWhinney, I.R., McWilliam, C.L., Freeman, T.R., (2003). *Patient-centered medicine: transforming the clinical method.* 2nd ed. Oxford: Radcliffe Medical Press.

30. Schachter-Shalomi, Zalman, and Miller, Ronald S. *From Age-ing to Sage-ing, A Profound Vision of Growing Older.* New York: Warner Books, 1995, p. 126.

/// 15 /// PROMOTING RESILIENCE AND POSTTRAUMATIC GROWTH IN PHYSICIANS

JANE SHAKESPEARE-FINCH

Across the lifespan, traumatic experiences are common; more people experience such events than not. Within the context of being a medical professional, trauma may result from a direct experience (e.g., in a person's personal life) but may also occur vicariously. For example, a medical professional may be traumatized during the course of their employ as they come to the aid of a trauma survivor. Although there can be long-term negative sequale for trauma survivors (e.g., PTSD, depression), the majority of people who experience trauma, vicariously or otherwise, are resilient to long-term effects, and some people grow or develop beyond their pre-event level of functioning. Therefore, in addition to interest in antecedents and correlates of pathology, research examining the predictors and correlates of resilience and growth has gained notable attention. This chapter discusses the fundamental assumptions of the salutogenic theory. Salutogenisis refers to the study of the origins of health and to that end has a goal to determine factors involved in promoting and maintaining health. The chapter then goes on to describe posttraumatic growth, a term used to denote positive posttrauma changes, as well as resilience, including discussion of the similarities and differences between these two constructs. The chapter then identifies ways of promoting growth and resilience in medical professionals. It concludes with discussion of ways in which individuals can enhance their potential for growth and also of ways in which the organization they work for can best facilitate and promote resilience and growth in its employees.

In the mental health world, resilience has been a buzz word of the 2000s. Whereas research in mental health has traditionally been dominated by a pathological paradigm in which the primary focus seeks to diagnose psychological disorders and alleviate the symptoms and suffering that may be experienced, the last decade saw a plethora of literature dedicated to exploring and building resilience (e.g., Bonanno, 2004; 2009; Cohn, Hodson, & Crane, 2010; Mancini & Bonanno, 2006; Masten, 2001). Cathy Ridson and Sue Baptiste also offer a discussion of stress and resilience within the context of medical training curricula in Chapter 5 of this book. Within the social sciences trauma literature, there has also been a steady increase in researchers seeking to understand biopsychosocial factors involved with positive posttrauma changes. Such changes have been termed posttraumatic growth (Tedeschi & Calhoun, 1995). Rather than focus on pathology, the posttraumatic growth research and practice focal point is in identifying variables associated with positive posttrauma transformation, processes of change, and ways in which to promote posttrauma adaptation. Importantly, a focus on growth does not discount the continued distress that may accompany perceptions of positive change, the development of a new narrative about one's life, or an enhanced sense of wisdom.

Although still in its infancy, research has begun to emerge that examines posttraumatic growth and resilience within a work context of relatively high exposure to potentially traumatizing events. For example, resilience and growth have been examined in nurses, (McAllister & Lowe, 2011), police officers (e.g., Shochet et al., 2011), paramedics (Shakespeare-Finch, Smith, Gow, Embelton & Baird, 2003; Shakespeare-Finch, Gow, & Smith, 2005), psychotherapists (Shiri, Wexler, Alkalay, Meiner, & Kreitler, 2008), and physicians (Kearney, Weininger, Vachon, Harrison, & Mount, 2009). Peter Huggard, Beth Hudnall Stamm, and Laurie Anne Pearlman in Chapter 7 highlight the potential for vicarious posttraumatic growth in physicians within a broader discussion of compassion satisfaction.

In general such research has provided evidence that particular work roles can also afford the potential for significant growth from negotiating extremely difficult experiences in the context of employment, in addition to the challenges experienced in a person's nonwork life.

Medical professionals are subject to numerous challenges in the course of their roles, many of which are discussed in other chapters in this book. For example, Chapter in this volume highlights ethical and moral dilemmas that can stem from incongruences between physicians' motivations and the constraints of flawed systems acting to produce a crisis of meaning and subsequent burnout. The potential for encounters with situations that can elicit a traumatic response is also elevated in medical professionals when compared to the general population. When working in an environment that has the potential to expose workers to a large variety of stress and trauma, it is important to focus on the things that can be implemented to assist people in successfully negotiating the sometimes extreme emotional and cognitive challenges.

This chapter first discusses the nature of trauma as it may be experienced within the emergency and/or medical/health context. In keeping with the salutogenic theory underpinning this chapter, the terms *health* and *medical* are used interchangeably when referring to work roles. In this way, it should become clear that the traditional biomedical paradigm of health is subsumed by a salutogenic paradigm (Antonovsky, 1979). The chapter then explores the research that adopts a salutogenic approach to understanding and promoting mental health rather than solely exploring mental ill-health. Following a discussion of what salutogenic theory is, the chapter explains the model of posttraumatic growth (PTG; Tedeschi & Calhoun, 1995). It argues that adopting a salutogenic approach to understanding mental health within a context of potential trauma, or the constant threat of traumatization, offers a more useful approach to promoting mental health. The chapter also discusses resilience insomuch as it is suggested that resilience is not only the default state of a human following extreme challenges, but that it can also be a step beyond growth, as well as a precursor to it. The chapter ends with a section that outlines practical ways that can promote personal growth in physicians, nurses, paramedics, and other health care providers and the positive changes that can come from the very challenges that may have been perceived initially as traumatic, with all that a traumatic experience entails.

TRAUMA WITHIN THE CONTEXT OF BEING A MEDICAL PROFESSIONAL

Being a health care professional, such as a doctor, nurse, or paramedic, can at times be mundane and at others be extremely challenging. Long nights on shift with little happening can drag out, but there are also times when apparent chaos reigns—times filled with an assortment of challenges. Such challenges may include a lack of specific equipment, overcrowded departments, interpersonal difficulties with colleagues, superiors, patients, family members, or peers, fatigue, loss of life, gruesome scenes, and the myriad challenges associated with shift-work. There are also occasions in which a medical professional's coping strategies may be overwhelmed by experiences that are perceived to be traumatic. For a long time it was touted that people who enter medical professions, and other roles in which exposure to highly arousing events are inherent (e.g., emergency services personnel more broadly), are more stoic than the general population and that they are in some way immune to the psychological challenges that are faced within the context of their work-role (Miller, 1995). As of course this is not the case, there is a body of research that has examined ways in which medical professionals' mental health may be compromised.

In an example of such research, Mealer, Shelton, Berg, Rothbaum, and Moss (2007) found an increased prevalence of posttraumatic stress disorder (PTSD) in a sample of critical care nurses, and Regehr, Goldberg, and Hughes (2002) reported an extremely high prevalence of PTSD symptoms in Canadian ambulance personnel. High levels of psychological distress and emotional exhaustion in nurses have also been found, relative to general population data (Bourbonnais, Comeau, & Vezina, 1999), in addition to a negative relationship between job strain and functional health status (Cheng, Kawachi, Coakley, Schwartz & Colditz, 2000). In an interesting study that used a biological measurement of stress in medical personnel, Sluiter, van der Beek, and Frings-Dresen (2003) found that cortisol levels were higher during and after dealing with clinically challenging (i.e., life threatening) cases. Their results refuted the habituation hypothesis in which it is suggested that personnel in professions that expose them to medical emergencies ought to become accustomed to arousal and hence cortisol levels should not fluctuate as a function of case complexity.

However, these findings of elevated levels of stress and trauma responses in medical personnel is not always the case. For example, Lubin and colleagues found very low levels of PTSD and acute stress disorder (ASD) in doctors and medics who had faced horrific experiences during their time with the Israeli Defense Forces. Only 1 of 141 medics was reported to have PTSD in this group, a point the authors focus on to remind us that the nature of the event is not as important in predicting psychopathology as the subjective attitude of the person experiencing the event. It may be that the participants in this research sought to provide a good impression of their mental health, but it may also be that they were adequately prepared for the role they were to face and that adequate supports were available to personnel in dealing with instances they found initially overwhelming.

Within a health care role a personnel may experience trauma as a direct result of their own experience. For example, surviving a threat to their own life. However, emergency and medical personnel may also be vicariously traumatized. Vicarious trauma is the experience of trauma as a function of attending to someone else in crisis. It may be that hearing about the suffering of others can be difficult, particularly for those who get the opportunity to bond with patients. Vicarious trauma tends to occur when the attending health professional connects the person to the context of his or her life. For example, attending to the severe injuries of a child and feeling sure that the injuries were at the hand of the child's care-giver, or connecting the patient with something or someone in the worker's own life. Regardless of the mechanism for traumatization, the symptoms of distress seen as a result of vicarious trauma mimic those symptoms found in people who are direct trauma survivors.

The studies that focus on the potential to develop pathology, prevalence rates of pathology, correlates and predictors of PTSD and other difficulties, and how to relieve symptoms are based in a pathogenic approach to research and human understanding. While no doubt a worthy endeavor, such research tends to be to the exclusion of the many potential human responses and outcomes of experiencing highly charged and traumatic experiences. Long-term suffering as a consequence of experiencing extremely confronting situations impacts a minority of the population, although the majority of people, let alone medical professionals, are subject to such experiences more often than not (Creamer, Burgess, & McFarlane, 2001; Kessler, Sonnega, Bromet, Hughes, & Nelson, 1995). Antonovsky (1979) and others (e.g., Bonanno, 2009; Calhoun & Tedeschi, 2006) suggest a more useful approach to the promotion of mental health is in considering people on a continuum of health. This alternative to a pathogenic approach includes examining what is involved in the more common outcomes of resilience and growth as a more fruitful ways of assisting people to adapt to and manage life's onslaught.

THE FUNDAMENTAL ASSUMPTIONS OF THE SALUTOGENIC THEORY

It was through conducting research examining functionality between women who had survived the Holocaust and many other traumatic experiences in the years that followed (e.g., living in displaced person's camps, illegally migrating), and women who had not, that medical sociologist and anthropologist, Aaron Antonovsky (1979), first became enthused to embark on a career dedicated to understanding salutogenesis. Rather than using a pathological theoretical underpinning in research, the salutogenic theory quite literally seeks to understand the origins of health. Whereas quantities of illness, disease, and disability are the focus of pathology (i.e., origins of pathology), *salutogenesis* is defined as "origins of health" and therefore quantities and qualities of health are measured. Antonovsky's focus was on the question "Whence the strength?" (p. 7). This is a question of why some people manage to stay healthy and others not; and it recognizes the innate strength of people. The question is not only addresses those who have experienced stressful and traumatic experiences, but also every person, on the premise that "the human condition is stressful" (p. 9). Antonovsky marvels at how any of us manage to stay healthy in a world where we are constantly bombarded with potential stressors, for example, from pollutants to natural disasters, disease, and war.

The simplicity of a continuum, the linearity with which hypotheses are tested, is seductive as researchers aim to discover the answer to why people lie where they do on a health/disease dimension. Yet human wellness is complex. It is multivariate across potentially infinite combinations of continua. If we are to promote mental health, identifying ways in which people manage life's inevitable tensions, fostering and promoting avenues to successful adaptation, focusing on flexibility of mind and on making sense of the world is surely more productive for all than leaving biopsychosocial research only to the realm of pathogenesis. So what may people who are resistant to stress and trauma have in common?

The cluster of variables that reflect resistance to stress have been termed in a number of ways and are difficult to define given the multiple factors that comprise the proposed resistance characteristics. A "sense of coherence" is Antonovsy's term (1979), and although not the same, it is related to Kobasa's concept of "hardiness" (1979), and Bonanno's explanation of "resilience" (2009). Such concepts aim to define the dispositional characteristics of a person, their cognitions, self-concept, and coping orientations, that predispose their potential to be able to withstand the myriad stressors life may present to them. Of course an individual resides within social and relational contexts that also form part of the sense of coherence that Antonovsky explains.

Within the medical professional context, there are a variety of stressors and a potential for psychopathology as described, but there is also the potential for personal development beyond pre-event levels of functioning, as a result of negotiating the fallout from experiencing extremely challenging and/or traumatic times. Posttraumatic growth (PTG) is a construct situated in the theoretical basis of salutogenesis. The model is anchored in personal pre-trauma but it has a particular focus on cognitions including the strength of understanding the meaning of personal narratives in promoting mental health. For more discussion of a narrative approach to promoting mental health, please also refer to Chapters 3 and 4 of this book. The PTG model is more concerned with process and outcome following life crisis than exploring individual difference variables pretrauma. Given the small amount of variance in posttrauma wellness attributed to individual difference variables such as personality (e.g., Shakespeare-Finch et al., 2005; Tedeschi & Calhoun, 1996), it makes sense that process variables, and the context within which they take place (e.g., cognitions, social supports, disclosure, cultural context), be the current focus of growth research.

AN INTRODUCTION TO POSTTRAUMATIC GROWTH

Posttraumatic growth is a term coined by Richard Tedeschi and Lawrence Calhoun (1995; 1996). It refers to positive changes that may occur for some people as a result of negotiating the struggle a person engages in when coming to terms with life following an experience of trauma. Growth appears to occur in three broad areas: Changes in a person's philosophy of life, in relationships with others, and in self-perceptions such as those of personal strength (Tedeschi & Calhoun, 1995). The posttraumatic growth (PTG) model depicts the experience of trauma as one that devastates pre-event schemas, challenges core beliefs about the world and one's position in the world, and can act as a catalyst for significant positive changes in addition to ongoing distress and the development of wisdom and a new life narrative (Calhoun, Cann, & Tedeschi, 2010). Therefore, inherent in the model is a variety of posttrauma outcomes and processes; a landscape for sometimes seemingly divergent avenues and outcomes. This primarily cognitive model of growth highlights the pivotal roles of rumination, disclosure and its consequences, support and other sociocultural variables. Calhoun et al. (2010) position their model within a salutogenic theoretical orientation (Antonovsky, 1979) that, as discussed, sees a person on a continuum of health rather than on a dimension characterized (and measured) as the absence or presence of illness. Such a paradigm shift has many clinical implications which are discussed in the final section of this chapter.

In order to be able to quantify PTG, the Posttraumatic Growth Inventory (PTGI) was designed to measure positive post-trauma changes (Tedeschi & Calhoun, 1996). Following the development of scale items based on qualitative research and years working as clinicians, Principle Components Analysis supported a five factor solution to the PTGI. Measured changes are in (1) personal strength, (2) renewed appreciation of life, (3) changes on life's priorities, (4) relationships with others, and (5) religious and spiritual domains. Although there are some cultural differences in PTGI solutions (e.g., Weiss & Berger, 2010), the five-factor structure has also been replicated outside of the United States (e.g., Morris, Shakespeare-Finch, Rieck, & Newbery, 2005).

PTG research has been conducted primarily with direct trauma survivors, but slowly research is emerging that examines positive posttrauma changes as a result of vicarious trauma experienced through the course of a person's work-role. Early results indicate that the prevalence of PTG is a far more common outcome than the presence of pathology in such populations (e.g., Shakespeare-Finch et al., 2003; Shiri et al., 2008), which is consistent with symptoms of pathology as a result of direct or vicarious trauma. Shiri and colleagues (2008) examined both positive and negative posttrauma outcomes in a sample of physicians, nurses and psychotherapists (N = 138). All of the hospital workers in this study reported some levels of posttraumatic growth, again consistent with findings in a large sample of paramedics (Shakespeare-Finch et al., 2003).

One finding that has been consistent in PTG research is that this form of transformation is not seen to the same extent in the absence of perceiving an experience to be significantly traumatic. The perception of the severity of an event is more strongly related to the potential for the experience to provide an opportunity for change (Morris et al., 2005). Taubman-Ben-Ari and Weintroub (2008) examined growth and meaning in a group of physicians ($n = 58$) and a group of nurses ($n = 66$) who worked on various pediatric wards. Nurses experienced higher levels of growth than the physicians in this study but consistent with Shiri and colleagues (2008), they found that growth was also related to higher levels of vicarious traumatization. In other words, an event must be perceived as traumatic in order for the experience to afford higher levels of growth (Shiri et al., 2008). Therefore it may be that the nurses in this research had perceived their experiences of trauma to be more prevalent or more severe than the physicians sampled.

The findings that confirm the coexistence of positive and negative posttrauma outcomes are convincing (e.g., Calhoun & Tedeschi, 2006; Maercker, & Zoellner, 2004; Shakespeare-Finch et al., 2003) but the nature of the relationship is not. For example, a relationship between higher levels of symptoms of pathology and higher scores the PTGI has been found. A curvilinear relationship has also been detected between PTGI scores and PTSD symptoms in physicians, nurses and psychotherapists (Shiri et al., 2008) and some research reports no relationship between these constructs (Ho, Kwong-Lo, Mak, & Wong, 2005). However, on closer examination of the data, there are sometimes differences in the relationships between subscales of the PTGI and factors associated with PTSD and anxiety, rather than total inventory scores (e.g., Shakespeare-Finch & de Dassel, 2009). It may be that the nature of the event differentiates between PTSD symptoms and perceptions of growth. For example, survivors of childhood sexual assault have been found to report higher levels of growth in the personal strength domain when compared to bereaved persons who report significantly higher levels of changes in relationships and appreciation of life (Shakespeare-Finch & Armstrong, 2010). Essentially this research demonstrates that the experience of trauma is not uncommon but that the journey for an individual is unique. For some growth will occur and exist with ongoing distress, for others the balance will tip in a particular direction. What is clear is that one thing is not true for all but that trauma can provide a catalyst for profound change.

A model presented by Ickovics and Park (1998) simplifies the relationship between trauma and posttrauma functioning, arguably to the point of error. It depicts a flat-line of functioning which is interrupted by a life crisis. The model shows all people experiencing such events as drastically dropping in their level of functioning but in time, returning to a level of functioning, be that continued impairment or suffering, resilience (depicted as a rebound to the original line), or to a position of growth in which the model depicts superseding previous levels of functioning. Research, however, attests that this is not necessarily the case such as the examples provided above where symptoms of PTSD and PTG have been found to coexist in some people. In the Shakespeare-Finch and de Dassel research (2009) that was conducted with survivors of serious sexual assault, moderate levels of growth were reported by all of the participants, yet 95% of the sample also recorded clinical levels of PTSD symptoms. This result is consistent with the PTG model (e.g., Calhoun et al., 2010) and may indicate something unique about adult survivors of childhood sexual assault (e.g., elevated levels of hyperarousal are in fact normal in this population), or simply highlight the relationship between severity of an event and growth. Before we go on to discuss ways in which positive posttrauma outcomes can be promoted, the following section provides a brief discussion about resilience and more importantly, the ways in which growth and resilience are similar, yet different.

PTG AND RESILIENCE: WHAT ARE THEY AND DOES ONE PRECEDE THE OTHER?

Posttraumatic growth and resilience share some common characteristics (e.g., both aim to understand and promote adaptation), but are not the same. Whereas PTG is about personal development beyond pre-trauma status, resilience can be conceptualized as the capacity to rebound from challenges. Originally a term used in the hard sciences (e.g., physics, biology) to describe the rebound of physical structures such as bridges or a plant's ability to return to an equivalent level of functioning to that before a major disruption, resilience tends to be portrayed in the social sciences as the capacity to bounce back from stress and/or trauma (e.g., Bonanno, 2004; 2009). A limitation in the current literature on resilience is that in the vast majority of cases research has operationalized resilience as an absence of pathology (e.g., Levine, Laufer, Stein, Hamama-Raz, & Solomon, 2009). This is problematic for a number of reasons, not the least of which is that the approach assumes resilience, pathology and growth are somehow situated on a linear continuum. As seen with the relationship or lack thereof between growth and pathology, the linear conceptualization is problematic. Further, the instances that precipitate resilience and PTG are different.

Some writers suggest that posttraumatic growth is a step beyond resilience and others that resilience may be a usual response to stress, whereas PTG is related to trauma. But is it? It may be that resilience is inherent in the individual (e.g., Kobasa, 1979), dispositional and learned (e.g., a sense of coherence; Antonovsky, 1979), or that resilience is a step beyond growth (e.g., Westphal & Bonanno, 2007). Resilience being a step beyond growth supposes that successfully negotiating trauma can increase the proficiency with which coping strategies and resources are used when the person is confronted by a subsequent crisis. The individual does not actually experience the dramatic decrease in functioning as depicted in the Ickovics and Park model (1998) mentioned above. In other words, the successful negotiation of an extremely challenging event can increase a person's capacity to cope or refine their resources in order to more readily perceive that the demands of a situation do not outweigh the resources and strategies they have to cope with demands. An anecdotal example of this notion of resilience following growth comes from a local general practitioner who has her surgery in the center of a large-scale natural disaster zone in which there were multiple fatalities. In this disaster massive flooding impactedBrisbane, Australia and nearby areas with devastating consequences (van den Honert, & McAneney, 2011). Three months on this GP commented that a number of people had needed support but that she was surprised at some of the patients she would have expected to be "vulnerable" to the impact of these fatal waters. One person, who has significant physical stressors and had lost a child two years earlier, did very well psychologically following this flood in which she lost her home and all her worldly possessions. According to the doctor, the patient had not actually experienced the sharp decrease in functioning that is associated with experiencing an event as traumatic, and hypothesized that the response was due to the negotiation of her previous trauma. In other words, she displayed resilience when faced with this natural disaster.

PROMOTING PERSONAL GROWTH IN PHYSICIANS, NURSES, AND THEIR FAMILIES

This section provides a review of strategies and resources that can promote growth and resilience. Such an endeavor is applicable for all people but most especially, for people within work contexts that are often charged by highly emotional situations, clinical challenges, and personally confronting experiences associated with assisting others in various states of distress. Different adaptive strategies and resources may be employed depending on the circumstance. Many coping factors have been highlighted elsewhere in this text (e.g., humor, social support), so some of the following suggestions relate to tapping into individual factors and others relate more to the organizational context and culture.

Individual experience and response. In the main health workers self-select for their vocation and therefore, at least initially, hold a belief that they will be able to deal with the demands of the particular role. Yet there are likely to be experiences in such work roles that are sudden in onset and may be chaotic and overwhelming, and of course there are also quieter experiences that can have a significant impact on a person's mental health. For example, some physicians may struggle to come to terms with the loss of a patient they have been treating for some time or with the process of caring for patients at the end of their lives (Kearney, Weininger, Vachon, Harrison, & Mount, 2009). Kearney and colleagues suggest reflective practices are beneficial in promoting wellness in physicians. Through self-awareness and self-care, doctors are more likely to ward off the potential for vicarious traumatization and compassion fatigue. Positive posttrauma changes in the Taubman-Ben-Ari and Weintroub (2008) samples were associated with higher levels of self-esteem regarding their professional selves. A sense of professional self-esteem can be developed through the reflective practices discussed by Kearney et al. (2009), by physicians' revisiting their personal framework regarding grief in order to reflect and refine their knowledge of themselves (Moon, 2011); through examination of personal life narrative (Calhoun & Tedeschi, 2006); and through a strengths-based focus to prevention and intervention.

Bannink (2008), Calhoun & Tedeschi (1999), and Tedeschi and Kilmer (2005), among others, have provided some useful insights into the practical ways in which posttraumatic growth and resilience can be encouraged when working with traumatized clients. These strategies can be used by the health care professional in assisting traumatized patients, family and peers but also promote self-care through processes such as personal reflection. An example of the positive aspects of self-reflection comes from an intensive care paramedic who was part of a group deployed to Banda Ache following the Boxing Day Indian ocean tsunami. Not long after returning from his deployment to the devastated area, he said that he had assisted an injured homeless person when off duty because he had a different sense of the person's needs after his experiences. He said that he "now value[d] that person differently, not for what he isn't, but for what he is" (Shakespeare-Finch & Scully, 2008, p. 97). Part of this new view was associated with the paramedic's sense of meaningfulness in relation to the mass loss he had seen that developed into a renewed appreciation for his own life and of those in it. He was more acutely aware of the disparities between those who have and those who have much less. This finding suggested that meaning in a context of extreme challenge can be translated into growth through processes of deliberate rumination (Calhoun & Tedeschi, 2006), which may also be aptly called self-reflection. Importantly, in this instance the reflection occurred within the intrapersonal and interpersonal aspects of this man's life. Whereas elevated levels of intrusive or negative rumination following crisis have been perceived as predictive of maladjustment, higher levels of rumination about a traumatic event, soon after the event and deliberate rumination more recently, has been found in other research to positively correlate with PTG (Calhoun, Cann, Tedeschi, & McMillan, 2000).

Bannink (2008) provides a number of practical ways to assist people in moving through crisis using a solution focused approach to therapy. Although a detailed discussion of solution focused therapy is beyond the scope of this chapter, some of the key elements found to be useful include looking for success stories in a person's past; in your own past. By focusing on resilience, competence, coping resources and strategies, new positive neural networks are created and can replace the older negative connections (p 218). Dwelling on problems increases cortisol levels, which is related to increases in anxiety and depression (Bannink, 2008). Bannink (2008) and Calhoun and Tedeschi (1999) also promote the use of discourse as important, for example, viewing yourself and others you may be assisting to see themselves as survivors rather than victims. Strength-based interventions may be aimed at individuals who identify with difficulties or as a training component, especially relevant to people entering professions where there is likelihood of high trauma exposure (Calderon-Abbo, Kronenberg, Many, & Osofsky, 2008; Shochet et al., 2011). Calderon-Abbo et al. (2008) examined the impact of direct and indirect exposure to trauma in health care workers within the context of disaster. They concur that incorporation of self-care strategies in disaster management both in a proactive way and as part of a reactive intervention program is productive.

Organizational attributes in promoting resilience and growth. Incorporating the best practice for organizations in supporting psychological well-being is easier to idealize than achieve, let alone achieve within a dynamic health care context. Because of the unique needs of any organization, standards of employee support programs are just as varied as their composition. Some organizations' staff employees have a relatively low risk to their psychological well-being and others have inherently higher risk, as already discussed. Within the emergency, military, and health contexts, debriefing became the primary (and reactive) intervention that was adopted around the world throughout the 1980s and 1990s. Despite being intended for emergency service personnel and not developed in response to scientific scrutiny of options for support, this intervention was adopted across the community as a stand-alone posttrauma group intervention. Perhaps the lack of original rigor in developing the program is why the practice was widely discontinued when research caught up with the potential for negative effect in practice (e.g., Cochrane review, 2001).

There are also some organizational factors that have received research support in recent years in terms of their ability to promote well-being. For example, well thought out and carefully constructed psycho-education and support programs, constantly being open to scrutiny and development, can produce extremely high satisfaction levels in medical personnel (e.g., Shakespeare-Finch & Scully, 2004; Scully, 2011). In stark contrast to providing a comprehensive employee assistance program, Regehr and her colleagues (2002) report that, in a paramedical organization that does not have a comprehensive program of psycho-education and support, personnel report extremely high (i.e., 40%) levels of stress associated with dissatisfaction with services that are not available. As organizational stressors are reported to be accountable for more factors relating to pathological posttrauma outcomes in a work context than individual difference variables (e.g., Gist & Woodall, 2000), it is important for organizations to take note of protective factors that are supported by research. For example, a lack of consultation due to poor workplace communication, coupled with a perception that the organization is unsupportive, are significant risk factors for difficulties in adjusting to extreme stress and trauma at work (Shakespeare-Finch, 2007). Positive outcomes for an employee promote positive outcomes for their patients, families, colleagues, and ultimately, the broader community. Particularly in highly charged work contexts, it is important for people to feel that they are valued and recognized for doing their job well. It is important that such endorsements are forthcoming from both peers and those who have immediate influence. Superiors and peers can remind each other formally and informally that trauma can be seen as a learning experience—a valuable opportunity for personal and social growth.

Just as in individual experiences of posttraumatic growth, growth, change, and development in organizations can be spurred on by challenges and by failures. When medical professionals are part of organizations that have been challenged by or have not performed well in a given situation, an opportunity is available for organizational change as well as individual change. There are various principles that should be followed to support individuals when searching for ways for the organization to function better. Dunning (2003) and Paton (2006) describe some of the principles that organizations should follow to promote growth in both the individuals and the organization. They point out that it is important to respect the ways individuals use their own frames of reference and mental models to understand the events that might have challenged them and the organization, and encourage the telling of stories about these experiences with colleagues. Monrouxe and Sweeney (Chapter 3) and Rees and Monrouxe (Chapter 4) also highlight the importance of peers in promoting mental health. Recognition should be given to those who have responded to difficult circumstances, and their stories and various points of view can be utilized and combined to practice future response. Medical professionals who are highly trained should be allowed to use creative and innovative methods, while the organization provides a framework to ensure important policies and laws are met. Highly meaningful outcomes may occur through exercising professional skills, which is rarely possible in routine contexts (Shakespeare-Finch, 2007). Managers who stay connected to the reality of the work in the field and what is happening to their workers can do a better job of providing organizational support that encourages growth and builds resilience. It is important that all the medical professionals understand the shared intentions and goals of the organization and how to work toward these goals even under the most adverse conditions. A shared primary motivation among those doing this kind of work is the desire to help people through what are often the most difficult times of their lives. Sometimes those in the health care arena can benefit from reflecting on that.

In summary, health carers are in a unique work position that can sometimes challenge their psychological foundations. Caring for people in the last days, hours, or minutes of their lives, being exposed to sometimes gruesome sights, seeing children in pain and families grieving can take an emotional toll. However, with a sense of capacity to deal with the challenges inherent in these work roles, strategies and resources to draw on when needed, and a culture of caring from an organizational perspective, a health care professional is afforded a unique opportunity for significant growth as a result of adjusting to the cognitive and emotional challenges associated with the same incidents that are, at first, overwhelming. Indeed, growth and resilience to such challenges characterizes the human response; responses that in the long term are far from being an exception.

ACKNOWLEDGMENTS

I would like to thank my colleagues, Professors Richard Tedeschi and Lawrence Calhoun, for their review and comment on this chapter and for their on-going support and friendship.

REFERENCES

Ablett, J. R., & Jones, R. S. P. (2007). Resilience and well-being in palliative care staff: A qualitative study of hospice nurses' experience of work. *Psycho-Oncology 16*, 733–740.

Almedom, A. (2005). Resilience, hardiness, sense of coherence, and posttraumatic growth: All paths leading to "light at the end of the tunnel"? *Journal of Loss and Trauma, 10*, 253–265. doi: 10.1080/15325020590928216.

American Psychiatric Association (2000). *Diagnostic and Statistical Manual of Mental Disorders (4thed—TR)*. Washington DC: American Psychiatric Association.

Antonovsky, A. (1979). *Health, Stress, and coping*. San Francisco: Jossey-Bass.

Bannink, F. (2008). Posttraumatic success: solution-focused brief therapy. *Brief Treatment and Crisis Intervention, 8*, 215–225. doi: 10.1093/brief-treatment/mhn013.

Bonanno, G. (2004). Loss, trauma, and human resilience: Have we underestimated the human capacity to thrive after extremely aversive events? *American Psychologist, 59*, 20–28.

Bonanno, G. (2009). *The other side of sadness: What the new science of bereavement tells us about life after loss*. New York: Basic books.

Bourbonnais, R., Comeau, M., & Vezina, M. (1999). Job strain and evolution of mental health among nurses. *Journal of Occupational Health Psychology, 4*, 95–107.

Calderon-Abbo, J., Kronenberg, M., Many. M., & Osofsky, H. (2008). Fostering Health care providers' post-traumatic growth in disaster areas: Proposed additional core competencies in trauma-impact management. *American Journal of Medical Sciences, 336*, 208–214. doi: 10.1097/MAJ.0b013e318180f5db.

Calhoun, L. G., &Tedeschi, R. G. (2006). The foundations of posttraumatic growth: An expanded framework. In L.G. Calhoun & R.G. Tedeschi (Eds.), *Handbook of Posttraumatic Growth: Research and Practice* (pp. 3–23). New Jersey: Lawrence Erlbaum.

Calhoun, L. G., & Tedeschi, R. G. (1999). *Facilitating posttraumatic growth: A clinicians guide*. New Jersey: Lawrence Erlbaum.

Calhoun, L. G., Cann, A., &Tedeschi, R. G. (2010). The posttraumatic growth model. In Z. Weiss & R. Berger (Eds.), *Posttraumatic growth and culturally competent practice: Lessons learned from around the globe* (pp. 1–14). Hoboken, New Jersey: John Wiley & Sons, Inc.

Calhoun, L. G., Cann, A., Tedeschi, R. G., & McMillan, J. (2000). A correlational test of the relationship between posttraumatic growth, religion, and cognitive processing. *Journal of Traumatic Stress, 13*, 521–527.

Cheng, Y, Kawachi, I., Coakley, E., Schwartz, J., & Colditz, G. (2000). Association between psychosocial work characteristics and health functioning in American women: Prospective study. *British Medical Journal, 320*, 1432–1436.

Cohn, A., Hodson, S., & Crane, M. (2010). Resilience training in the Australian Defence Force. *InPsych*, *32*, 16–17.

Creamer, M., Burgess, P., & McFarlane, A. C. (2001). Post-traumatic stress disorder: Findings from the Australian National Survey of mental health and well-being. *Psychological Medicine*, *31*, 1237–1247.

Dunning, C. (2003). Sense of coherence in managing trauma workers. In D. Paton, J.M. Violanti, & L.M. Smith (Eds.) *Promoting capabilities to manage posttraumatic stress: Perspectives on resilience* (pp. 119–135). Springfield, IL: Charles C. Thomas.

Figley, C. (Ed.). (1995). *Compassion Fatigue: Coping with secondary traumatic stress disorder in those who treat the traumatised*. New York: Brunner/Mazel.

Gist, R., & Woodall, J. (2000). There are no simple solutions to complex problems. In J. M. Violanti, D. Paton, & C. Dunning (Eds.), *Posttraumatic stress intervention: Challenges, issues, and perspectives* (pp. 81–95). Springfield, IL: Charles C Thomas.

Ho, S. M. Y., Kwong-Lo, R. S. Y., Mak, C., & Wong, J. S. (2005). Fear of Severe Acute Respiratory Syndrome (SARS) among health care workers. *Journal of Consulting and Clinical Psychology*, *73*, 344–349.

Ickovics, J., & Park, C. (1998). Paradigm shift: Why a focus on health is important. *Journal of Social Issues*, *54*, 237–244.

Janoff-Bulman, R. (2006). Schema-change perspectives on Posttraumatic Growth. In L. G. Calhoun & R. G. Tedeschi (Eds.), *Handbook of posttraumatic growth: Research and practice* (pp. 81–99). Mahwah, New Jersey: Lawrence Erlbaum Associates, Inc.

Kearney, M., Weininger, R., Vachon, M., Harrison, R., & Mount, B. (2009). Self-care of physicians caring for patients at the end of life. *The Journal of the American Medical Association*, *301*, 1155–1164. doi: 10.10001/jama.2009.352.

Kessler, R., Sonnega, A., Bromet, E., Hughes, M. & Nelson, C. (1995). Posttraumatic stress disorder in the National Comorbidity Survey. *Archives of General Psychiatry*, *52*, 1048–1060.

Kobasa, S. C. (1979). Stressful life events, personality and health: An inquiry into hardiness. *Journal of Personality and Social Psychology*, *37*, 1–11.

Levine, S., Laufer, A., Stein, E., Hamama-Raz, Y., & Solomon, Z. (2009). Examining the relationship between resilience and posttraumatic growth. *Journal of Traumatic Stress*, *22*, 282–286. doi: 10.1002/jts.20409.

Linley, P. A., & Joseph, S. (2004). Positive change following trauma and adversity: A review. *Journal of Traumatic Stress*, *17*, 11–21.doi: 10.1023/B:JOTS.00000.14671.28856.7e

Maercker, A., & Zoellner, T. (2004). The Janus face of self-perceived growth: Toward a two-component model of posttraumatic growth. *Psychological Inquiry*, *15*, 41–48.

Mancini, A., & Bonanno, G. (2006). Resilience in the face of potential trauma: Clinical practices and illustrations. *Journal of Clinical Psychology*, *62*, 971–985. doi: 10.1002/jclp.20283

Masten, A., (2001). Ordinary magic: Resilience processes in development. *American Psychologist*, *56*, 227–238. doi: 10.1037/0003-066X.56.3.227

McAllister, M., & Lowe, J. (Eds) (2011). *The resilient nurse*. New York: Springer.

Mealer, M., Shelton, A., Berg, B., Rothbaum, B., & Moss, M. (2007). Increased prevalence of Post-traumatic Stress Disorder symptoms in critical care nurses. *American Journal of Respiratory and Critical Care Medicine*, *175*, 693–697.

Miller, L. (1995). Tough guys: Psychotherapeutic strategies with law enforcement and emergency service personnel. *Psychotherapy*, *32*, 592–600.

Moon, P. (advanced online viewing, 2011). Untaming grief? Palliative care physicians. *American Journal of Hospice and Palliative Care*. doi: 10.1177/1049909111406705.

Morris, B. A., Shakespeare-Finch, J., Rieck, M., & Newbery, J. (2005). Multidimensional nature of posttraumatic growth in an Australian population. *Journal of Traumatic Stress Studies*, *18*, 575–585.

Paton, D. (2006). Posttraumatic growth in disaster and emergency work. In L. G. Calhoun & R. G. Tedeschi (Eds.), *Handbook of posttraumatic growth: Research and practice* (pp. 225–247). Mahwah, New Jersey: Lawrence Erlbaum Associates, Inc.

Regehr, C., Goldberg, G., & Hughes, J. (2002). Exposure to human tragedy, empathy, and trauma in ambulance paramedics. *Journal of Orthopsychiatry*, *72*, 505–513.

Scully, P. J. (2011). Taking care of staff: A comprehensive model of support for paramedics. *Traumatology*, *17*(4): 35–42, doi:10.1177/1534765611430129

Shochet, I. M., Shakespeare-Finch, J., Young, R., Brough, P., Craig, C., & Roos. C., Wurfl, A., & Hodge, R. (2011). The development of the Promoting Resilience Officers (PRO) program. *Traumatology, 17*(4), 43–51. doi:10.1177/1534765611429080

Shakespeare-Finch, J. (2007). Building resilience in emergency service personnel through organisational structures. *Proceedings of the 42nd Australian Psychological Society,* 362–365.

Shakespeare-Finch, J., & Armstrong, D. (2010). Trauma type and post-trauma outcomes: Differences between survivors of motor vehicle accidents, sexual assault and bereavement. *Journal of Loss and Trauma, 15,* 69–82.

Shakespeare-Finch, J., & Barrington, A. (advanced online view, July, 2012). Behavioural changes add validity to the construct of posttraumatic growth. *Journal of Traumatic Stress.* DOI: 10.1002/jts.21730.

Shakespeare-Finch, J., & De Dassel, T. (2009). A mixed methods analysis of posttraumatic growth as a function of childhood sexual abuse. *Journal of Child Sexual Abuse, 18,* 326–332. *Journal of Loss and Trauma, 15,* 69–82.

Shakespeare-Finch, J., & Enders, T. (2008). Corroborating evidence of posttraumatic growth. *Journal of Traumatic Stress, 21*(4), 421–424.doi: 10.1002/jts20347

Shakespeare-Finch, J. E., Gow, K, M., & Smith, S. G. (2005). Personality, coping and posttraumatic growth in emergency ambulance personnel. *Traumatology 11,* 325–334.

Shakespeare-Finch, J., & Morris, B. (2010). Posttraumatic growth in Australian populations. In Z. Weiss & R. Berger (Eds.), *Posttraumatic growth and culturally competent practice: Lessons learned from around the globe* (pp. 157–172). Hoboken, New Jersey: John Wiley & Sons, Inc.

Shakespeare-Finch, J., & Scully, P. (2004). A Multi-method Evaluation of an Emergency Service Employee Assistance Program. *Employee Assistance Quarterly, 19*(4), 71–91.

Shakespeare-Finch, J. & Scully, P. J. (2008). Ways in which paramedics cope with, and respond to, natural large-scale disasters. In K. Gow & D. Paton (Eds.). *The phoenix of natural disasters: Community resilience.* New York: Nova Science publishers.

Shakespeare-Finch, J., Smith, S.G., Gow, K. M., Embelton, G., & Baird, L. (2003). The prevalence of posttraumatic growth in emergency ambulance personnel. *Traumatology, 9,* 58–70.

Shiri, S., Wexler, I., Alkalay, Y., Meiner, Z., & Kreitler, S. (2008). Positive psychological impact of treating victims of politically motivated violence among hospital-based health care providers. *Psychotherapy and Psychosomatics, 77,* 315–318. doi: 10.1159/000142524.

Sluiter, J., van der Beek, A., & Frings-Dresen, M. (2003). Medical staff in emergency situations: severity of patient status predicts stress hormone reactivity and recovery. *Occupational & Environmental Medicine, 60,* 373–375. doi:10.1136/oem.60.5.373.

Taubman-Ben-Ari, O., & Weintroub, A. (2008). Meaning in life and personal growth among pediatric physicians and nurses. *Death Studies, 32,* 621–645. doi: 10.1080/07481180802215627.

Tedeschi, R. G., & Calhoun, L. G. (1995).*Trauma and transformation: Growing in the aftermath of suffering.* Thousand Oaks, California: Sage Publications Ltd.

Tedeschi, R. G., & Calhoun, L. G. (1996). The Posttraumatic Growth Inventory: Measuring the positive legacy of trauma. *Journal of Traumatic Stress, 9,* 455–472.

Tedeschi, R. G., & Kilmer, R. (2005). Assessing strengths, resilience, and growth to guide clinical interventions. *Professional Psychology: Research and Practice, 36,* 230–237. doi: 10.1037/0735–7028.36.3.230.van den Honert, C., & McAneney, J. (2011). The 2011 Brisbane Floods: Causes, Impacts and Implications. *Water, 34,* 1149–1173. doi:10.3390/w3041149.

Weiss, T., & Berger, R. (Eds). (2010). *Transformation in context: Posttraumatic growth across cultures.* Wiley: New York.

Wessley, S., Rose, S., & Bisson, J. (2000). Brief psychological interventions ("debriefing") for trauma-related symptoms and the prevention of posttraumatic stress disorder [Cochrane review]. In: *The Cochrane Library;* Issue 3, 2000. Oxford.

Westphal, M., & Bonanno, G. (2007). Posttraumatic growth and resilience to trauma: Different sides of the same coin or different coins? *Applied Psychology, 56,* 417–427. doi: 10.1111/j.1464-0597.2007.00298.

/// 16 /// ETHICAL DECISIONS

Stress and Distress in Medicine

JEFFERY SPIKE AND NATHAN CARLIN

Medicine as a profession possesses unique conditions to create stress on a daily basis. There is probably no profession that takes so many years of training yet results in a practice with so much regulation. It is not surprising that doctors might expect that after 7–10 years of training they will be considered sufficiently expert to wield a large degree of professional autonomy, and so are often surprised to find so many people limiting or disputing their right to make decisions based on their perceived expertise.

Each of these common situations can create restrictions on professional judgment and become potential sources of physician stress: lawyers trolling for plaintiffs, Health Maintenance Organizations (HMOs) limiting payments on the basis of performance, state licensing rules requiring Continuing Medical Education (CME) courses, patients asking "too many" questions when only 15 minutes have been scheduled, patients seeking excuses to give to their boss for absences from work, or to an airline for changes in travel plans, or to Social Security and Occupational Safety and Health Administration (OSHA) for work related injuries, upset family members who want to restrict what a patient knows or force certain things on them (such as moving to a nursing home or removing their driver's license), patients who don't take their medications or accept good medical advice such as controlling their weight, stopping smoking, or cutting back on drinking, insurance companies with reimbursements below cost, pregnant women who demand medically unnecessary c-sections and other pregnant women who refuse medically indicated c-sections, and drug companies who mine prescribing data. And that is only a tiny representation of the problems doctors face daily. It is not surprising that a number of physicians end up with drug and alcohol problems, even without the additional factor of unusually easy access to these drugs, which their profession also enables. Many American physicians see themselves by and large as an overworked and underappreciated lot; and the fact that the public sees them as relatively rich and powerful only adds to the sense of isolation or dissonance that some physicians feel.

Furthermore, the stakes are high, both ethically and legally: patients' lives are in the balance, and mistakes can be fatal. It can be hard for physicians to know if they want more responsibility or less. It can feel as though they get too much of the blame when something goes wrong and too little of the credit when something goes well.

One way to understand the source of physician stress is that doctors (especially in the United States) are the victims of a terrible health care system (if it can even be called a system), one in which professional judgment has been severely limited in importance. The power and the money are in the hands of the insurance companies and the pharmaceutical companies, and to a lesser extent in the hands of lawyers and the government, leaving doctors practically indentured servants. In countries with better systems such as Canada, Japan, Israel, and most European countries, doctors can practice with more autonomy, leading to greater satisfaction, even if the pay is a little lower.

Anyone who understands the concept of a profession should have some sympathy for the doctor's plight. At some point it becomes apparent to most people that getting more money is not enough to make up for the loss of other things one cherishes.

Another way to understand this stress is to focus on the loss of seeing medicine as a service profession. In this view physicians have historically been seen as altruistic and wise, rather than as rich and powerful. Mid-career doctors wrote sincere application essays to medical school earlier in their lives to get into the medical profession because they professed these values, and there is no reason to cynically discount the sincerity of those essays. Many doctors are unhappy with their profession not because of reimbursement issues, but because of the injury (even if it sometimes self-inflicted) to their self-image as helpers or healers—a loss of respect from their patients, but also a loss of self-respect. When they complain, they feel guilty for complaining—doubling their sense of dissatisfaction. We believe the concept of moral distress is the most fruitful way to understand the psychological discomfort many physicians feel when they feel thwarted in their actions to do something that they believe is the ethical thing to do.

In a pair of recent editorials in the *New England Journal of Medicine* and the *Journal of the American Medical Association,* national physician leaders have remarked on these dual sources of physician dissatisfaction. In "Money and the Changing Culture of Medicine," Hartzband and Groopman discuss how "social" or "communal" relationships in medicine have been displaced by "market" or "exchange" interactions in which one naturally asks "what's in it for me." Ultimately there will be less satisfaction when the doctor's role is seen in this way, as there is no final goal; greed can always demand higher reimbursement, especially when it is meant to compensate for an unhappy life.

In "The Ethical Foundation of American Medicine: In Search of Social Justice," Kirch (the President of the American Association of Medical Colleges) and Vernon focus squarely on ethical causes of dissatisfaction and conclude that the body of research that describes inequalities in US health care support the conclusion that the US health system does not meet the criteria for being just. Many people are uninsured, many have insurance that doesn't cover what the patients need, or have such high deductible expenses built into them that patients can't afford treatment. Physicians who entered the field hoping to help people might naturally feel submerged and suffocated by becoming a part of such an unjust system.

PHYSICIAN STRESS AND BURNOUT AS SYMPTOMS OF ETHICAL VIOLENCE

In "Faculty Health and the Crisis of Meaning," Thomas Cole and Nathan Carlin (2009) used Theodor Adorno's (2000) concept of "ethical violence" to understand the various stresses that faculty, particularly physicians and scientists, face in academic health science centers. While their chapter focused on faculty health, their insights are also applicable to physicians practicing in hospitals or other health care settings. Indeed, Cole and Carlin (2009) have subsequently taken up the broader topic of physician suffering beyond academic health science centers in a reflective piece in *The Lancet*.

What did Adorno mean by "ethical violence"? Cole and Carlin note that when Adorno used the term he used it in the context of political history. Adorno argued that ethical rules and maxims must be reasonably achievable. When they are impossible or near to impossible to fulfill, such rules and maxims inflict a kind of violence on the person or group trying to uphold them. A simple example of this might be when a powerful majority upholds a universal ethical principle—such as, for example, do not steal—over a powerless minority who needs to steal to eat (an example in the medical context might be asking a group of, say, eight medical students to perform pelvic exams on an unconscious patient—the medical students might sense something wrong about this scenario but would also feel pressures about their grade—see Chapter 4 in this volume on the professional lapses of medical students). In any case, Adorno argues that ethical norms must be able to be appropriated "in a living way," that is, in a way that is possible to live out.

Cole and Carlin apply this insight to the suffering of physicians. They note that most physicians are good people who all try to do the "right thing." However, when the daily stresses of the lives of physicians reduce their vocation to a job, and when that job cannot be completed in a meaningful and moral way because there is another patient to see, another article to read, more paperwork to fill out, the result is ethical violence, the symptoms of which include guilt, shame, disillusionment, frustration, disease, and burnout (cf. Edelwich, & Brodsky 1980; Bruce, et al., 2005; Chapman, 1997; Chopra, et al., 2004). The busy-ness and business of medicine, in other words, often obscure the reasons doctors pursued medicine in the first place (cf. Selder & Paustian, 1989). And this, we suggest, is the meaning of burnout: that is, burnout is a crisis of meaning.

HOW TO PRESERVE OR RESTORE MEANING AND ETHICAL IDEALISM

We offer a number of suggestions that one might try in order to help a physician who feels disillusioned with his or her practice, and we suggest these with the hope that they will inspire readers to try to find their own solutions.

One way to begin is to ask what first attracted you to the job, what inspired you to be a physician, and when was the last time the job seemed to achieve those goals you once had. Try to regain some of that appreciation for the job. For example, if you chose to go into medicine rather than a career in science because you wanted to talk to people and help them with their problems, rather than work in a lab, then what things in your job could you adjust to give you more time with patients or to do other things in medicine that you enjoy?

You might consider trying to renegotiate your contract so that you spend a little more time with each patient. Or you could insist on having an open slot in mid-morning and one mid-afternoon so you can run overtime if necessary without slowing up too many people on the appointment schedule after that one. Each time a patient waits 45 minutes for you, you may be unintentionally sending a message (or they may be accidentally getting a message) that you think you are more important than they are, and that may in turn make each of those interactions less pleasant for both of you.

Also, chronic illnesses are the fastest growing and most time-consuming diagnoses. Finding a more efficient and effective way to deal with patients with chronic illness can revitalize a practice quickly. Some of the ideas that have been tried by some physicians include having evening hours one night a week, and/or having group appointments (which can combine patient education and a support group). Adding a person to run the support groups can also add a new dimension to your practice, giving you new perspectives on treatment modalities beyond your own.

For other practitioners, especially those in rural areas, the use of more telephone, videophone, and email patient encounters might lend variety to your practice.

Most important, remember that the practice of medicine can be a calling, can provide rewards more important than reimbursement, and should be something that brings fulfillment. If the system or culture of medicine seems to make that impossible, then it may be better to fight the system. For example, if you feel pressured to rush through appointments, and find yourself pressuring patients in turn, you may fall into the trap of only listening to patients for 14 seconds when you ask them what brought them in to the appointment (and dreading it if they have more than one answer). Remember that most patients, if given a chance to talk, still only talk for less than 30 seconds. In return for your patience, you may find some of the joy returning to the job. Listening to patients' stories not only improves their satisfaction, but has the potential to improve your satisfaction as well (Beckman 1984, Tallman 2007).

Lastly, for those practicing in a system such as that in the United States, where over 40 million people are uninsured and many more have insurance that demands unfair resources from you in order to get reimbursed, consider taking drastic action. Here are some options: first, speak out about the uninsured with as much passion as others speak about the "malpractice crisis" or "tort reform." You will always seem more altruistic if your concerns center around the injustice done to others than that done to yourself. Second, act decisively. Do something about it. For example, volunteer one half day a week or one half day a month at a free clinic, women's shelter, or homeless shelter. This will make you a wonderful role model for your profession, and will probably do more for your self-esteem than any boost in income. And then use the other half of that day to relax and exercise either your mind or your body. Go to a movie, attend an art opening, or do something else that will take your mind off of your job for a few hours.

USING HUMOR TO PROMOTE RESILIENCE

In this chapter, we have been concerned with the matter of promoting physician stress resilience, particularly when facing difficult ethical decisions. One strategy that we have recommended involves time management, and we offer practical advice such as renegotiating contracts to allow one day off a week, or, if that is not possible, just one day off a month. We also suggest doing things that not just are relaxing, such as fishing or meditating, but we also suggested doing things that bring back the good feeling of being a doctor, such as volunteering in a homeless shelter or woman's shelter. These activities, we believe, can help physicians regain the sense of their vocation.

We would also like to recommend another strategy to promote resilience: cultivating a humorous outlook on life. There is a good deal of writing and research on humor and medicine (see, e.g., Bennett, 2003; Wender, 1996; Martin, 2002; Berger, Coulehan, & Belling, 2004; Yoles & Clair, 1995; Billig, 2005). But we focus here on the counsel of Sigmund Freud, a physician whose life was filled with stress and interpersonal conflict, especially with his colleagues (see, e.g., Homans, 1989).

One way that Freud (1927) suggested saving mental energy was cultivating a humorous outlook in one's life, and we believe that Freud's insights might be applied to situations in the everyday lives of physicians today—with a great payoff. Cultivating a humorous attitude is one strategy, in addition to the previous strategies that we have mentioned, that promotes physician resilience, perhaps especially when the previous strategies have failed or have had limited success. Sometimes one just has to laugh at the things that happen in life, when confronted with events that are unexpected or unwanted. Indeed, the way in which affect can influence how one sees an event, coloring it so as to seem either funny or sad, is one of the most important determinants of resilience.

SIGMUND FREUD ON HUMOR

As many people know, one way that Freud conceived of the human psyche was by dividing it into an ego, an id, and a superego (cf. Freud, 1923). As many people also know, Freud also thought that the superego functions as our conscience. The superego is the psychic internalization of right and wrong, which human beings acquire through culture, primarily one's parents. And so the superego also produces guilt and punishes the ego when we have done something wrong. What many people do not know is that Freud (1927) also attributed the function of humor to the superego as well. Why? The superego, as noted, serves a kind of parental function, putting guilt on the ego when we have done something wrong. But the superego, also like a parent, wants to protect the ego from painful situations that might crush the ego.

Freud (1905) assumed that we run on a limited amount of mental energy. He also assumed that some emotions cost us more than others. Feeling ashamed or depressed, for example, might cost us more than feeling joyful. And to make his point, Freud (1927) told a joke about a man on his way to his own execution. Now it happened to be Monday, and as the man approached the gallows, he said to a couple of people in the crowd, "Well, this is a good start of the week!" Now the man could have expressed rage, horror, or whatever. But instead, the man displayed a humorous attitude, demonstrating that humor has a liberating element, even in—*especially* in—painful situations. Freud suggests that humor "spares oneself the affects to which the situation would naturally give rise and dismisses the possibility of such expressions of emotion with a jest" (p. 162). What, then, is humor? Freud is suggesting that it is an attitude or a point of view. Sometimes this attitude can be expressed in the form of jokes. But it can also be expressed in laughing at oneself or at a stressful situation—it is taking life less seriously.

Humor, Freud suggests, is not resigned but rebellious: "The grandeur in [humor] lies in the triumph of narcissism, the victorious assertion of the ego's invulnerability. The ego refuses to be distressed by the provocations of reality, to let itself be compelled to suffer" (p. 162). Freud also notes that the humorous attitude, which he related to the superego, is not likely to cause one to burst into laughter, as when one hears a joke (which Freud felt is related to the unconscious). And Freud also notes that not everyone is capable of the humorous attitude: "It is a rare and precious gift, and many people are even without the capacity to enjoy humorous pleasure that is presented to them" (p. 166).

Whether Freud was right about his structural model of the mind—id, ego, and superego—is beside the point for our purposes here. What we are endorsing is Freud's *economic* model of the mind, which seems plausible—that is, human beings run on a limited amount of psychic energy (cf. Freud, 1905), and that some situations cost us energy while others might recharge us. The logic of Freud's writings on humor, when applied to medicine, suggests that part of being or becoming a resilient physician is learning how to make the best use of one's mental resources, and cultivating a humorous outlook on life is one way to do so, thus letting go of things that are beyond one's control. However, we should also keep in mind Freud's counsel that humor is "a rare and precious gift." Freud does not say that one cannot cultivate a sense of humor, so, if one does not happen to have a sense of humor, this should not dissuade one from trying to cultivate one.

RECENT RESEARCH ON HUMOR AND HEALTH

While common sense suggests that humor is good for one's health, that having a sense of humor would help to relieve stress or, as Freud puts it, save psychic energy, the empirical research on the health benefits are mixed, and many questions remain unanswered (cf. Benett & Lengacher, 2006). And the methodologies of most studies of humor have been found to be inadequate (Martin, 2002). Donald Capps (2008) has also recently reviewed the literature on humor and health, and he concludes, "if a cheerful heart is a good medicine, it's a medicine that works like a placebo—it probably doesn't have any physiological benefits, but it does seem to have psychological benefits" (p. 3). Capps notes three such psychological benefits—namely, a humorous outlook may help to (1) reduce life-stress, (2) alleviate milder forms of depression, and (3) reduce anxiety.

A CLINICAL EXAMPLE OF A HUMOROUS OUTLOOK OF A MEDICAL STUDENT

We now turn to a clinical example of a medical student who exemplifies a humorous outlook on life. We could also give an example from the life of a physician, but since there is less writing about the experiences of medical students as compared with the writing about the experiences of physicians—there are countless memoirs written by doctors, whereas the same cannot be said about medical students—we have decided to focus on the experience of a medical student. This student (we will call him Max) wrote about his experience during his third-year rotation in OB/GYN, and he has given us permission to tell his story.

Max begins his entry by writing, "Today I feel like I am fresh out of an episode of the TV show *Scrubs*." He continues,

"Let me set the stage. Fridays are clinic days for the gyn surgery team. Each student is randomly assigned to a resident in order to help see patients. The residents are all different in how they interact with patients and students, as well as in what they expect from students. Today I had the opportunity to work with two different residents, Dr. O. and Dr. B."

Max notes that he spent the morning with Dr. O., who "knows how to laugh with her patients and how to make them laugh, but she doesn't ignore the occasional patient that needs time to cry."

Max also describes an interaction that he had with a woman who was about 60 or so: "She had multiple tattoos," Max notes, and "was missing teeth and had been a smoker for 30+ years." She was here today to have a polyp on her cervix removed. Dr. O. assigned Max to the task. Max writes:

"There I sat, shy little me, on a stool in between this woman's legs staring eye to eye with her cervix. In one hand I wielded an incredibly long pair of medical 'pliers' with the ends shaped like a donut (in order to grab onto things) and in the other hand a Q-tip that made me look like I went through a shrinking machine—it's literally a foot and a half long with a tip the size of a marshmallow. My job was to grab onto this pea-sized polyp and 'with a flick of the wrist' pull that sucker off. I am not one to resist a challenge, so in I went: grab, twist-twist, pluck, done! No more polyp (at least that's the short and sweet version of the story)."

Max adds: "Possibly the best part is that at the end of it all our patient offered a sincere thanks to me for helping with her care."

In the afternoon, Max switched to working with Dr. B. "Dr. B," Max notes, "is much more serious than Dr. O." This very contrast—the contrast between Dr. O. and Dr. B.—is what makes for much of the humor in what is about to follow.

Max and Dr. B. were seeing a patient who was undergoing diagnostic cystometry, meaning that they were evaluating different functional qualities of her bladder, such as "how much it held, how much urine made her feel like she needed to go to the bathroom, and if she had any 'leak' with a full bladder." Max writes,

"It is not difficult to envisage that this can be an embarrassing procedure—imagine having to sit with your rear end nearly hanging off the edge of the table while you don't have any pants on (just a sheet draped over your knees) with three separate people staring at the tube that is sticking out of your bladder. Now that we have that established, stop imagining that you are the half-dressed woman on the table and begin to imagine that you are the medical student in the room having the various causes of urinary incontinence explained to you while staring at said tube. You are seated in the chair at the foot of the bed a few arm's lengths from this woman's weak urethra in a cramped room in which you are the sole male.

Max was seated where he was on Dr. B.'s orders, in order to, as she put it, "facilitate the learning process." And Max reports that he did in fact learn a lot from this process. Indeed, he believes that he is much more likely to get test questions correct on issues related to this whole procedure.

As noted, they were basically trying to find out why the woman was having problems with her bladder. Was it due to weak muscles, or was it due to spasms of the bladder muscles? Or could it have been something else? They needed these answers because each situation would require a different type of treatment. Max described the discernment process in this way:

"Once the bladder has been filled with sterile water to the point that our patient says she feels the urge to urinate, we remove the catheter from her bladder and evaluate whether a stress component of incontinence is present. This is where I come in. Our all-knowing Chief Resident Dr. B placed me in what she anticipated would be an innocuous location and allowed me to watch the stress test."

Max then continues with his narrative. He notes that Dr. B. instructs him to sit eye level with the woman's vagina and to get close, not to be shy. He was to part the labia so that he could observe the external urethral orifice, because "[t]his small hole will give us the answer that we are looking for, it will tell us what the root of this woman's problem is." Dr. B. then instructed the patient to give a hearty cough. And cough she did. Max writes, "Before I relate the outcome of this 'cough,' please gather an image in your mind. Think of Old Faithful or the fountains in front of the Belagio or sitting near the tank of Shamu at Sea World." Max humorously continues,

"There I was, at arms length from this lady's perineum when that fateful cough was summoned. We discovered that our patient had a significant component of stress incontinence. With her cough she "leaked" (with extreme force) all ~250ml of sterile water that we had injected into her bladder. As though she were sitting on a fire hose this woman forcefully soaked my white coat, tie, button down shirt and slacks (missing my face) with fluid from her bladder."

Dr. B. then said to Max: "I certainly didn't expect that to happen. Why don't you go change?" Max ends his entry by writing, "Now I understand that reality truly can be stranger than fiction."

What we would like to point out here is that Max likely experienced various kinds of emotions: embarrassment about his location in the examining room, confusion over what exactly he was supposed to do and to learn, or frustration with Dr. B.'s serious attitude (in comparison with Dr. O.'s more light-hearted spirit). Max could have been angry about having water sprayed all over him, or this, too, could have embarrassed him. He could have experienced anxiety, asking himself, could there be anything harmful to me in these fluids? There are all sorts of emotions that Max could have experienced. But the fact that he took a humorous outlook suggests to us that Max, in the future, will, we believe, prove to become a resilient physician, capable of handling the many stresses he will face.

The contrast between Dr. O. and Dr. B. is also important. Dr. O. likes to laugh and have a good time with patients, even though she also knows when to be serious with her patients. Dr. B., however, is not portrayed by Max in this way. She is called his "all-knowing Chief Resident," a phrase that is used sarcastically by Max, especially when he reports her words later in his entry: "I certainly didn't expect that to happen." Max's point here does not seem to be that Dr. O. would have laughed when the woman sprayed Max—and we are not suggesting that this is what Dr. B. should have done. His point, rather, seems to be that Dr. O.'s humor makes her more enjoyable to be around, maybe because her humor makes her come across as a little more humble, in contrast to all-knowing Dr. B. But if, after the spraying incident, the patient would have laughed, then we can imagine that Dr. O. and Max would have laughed as well, and Max could have responded: "I've found the leak!"

This journal entry, then, is about more than Max's experience as a medical student. It is also about the role of humor in the lives of physicians. Perhaps at one point or another every physician feels as though she is on her way to the gallows. We do not doubt the severity or intensity of the stress that physicians face, especially when it comes to making difficult ethical decisions. But when physicians find themselves at the end of their rope, so to speak, they do have some choice in how they look at their situation. And perhaps a humorous outlook, such as the outlook of Dr. O., will make all the difference. Realizing one is not omnipotent, and not taking oneself too seriously, can be the first step in appreciating the world around you, and being able to "look on the bright side of life."

DOCTOR JOKES AS A MEANS OF CULTIVATING A HUMOROUS OUTLOOK

We believe that one way one can cultivate a humorous outlook is by reading jokes that are relevant to one's life and work. Jokes, Freud (1905) pointed out, have a certain logic to them, like dreams. By reading jokes, the logic becomes clearer to us and, we believe, the development of this logic can aid us in seeing humor in situations that are presented to us, enabling us, as Freud (1927) put it, to refuse "to be distressed by the provocations of reality." So in this context, this means reading doctor jokes.

As we were looking around for doctor jokes, we came across a website that is dedicated to the topic: doctorjokes.net. On this website, individuals can contribute their own jokes. Like Max's journal entry, these jokes demonstrate that although the hospital is filled with pain and suffering, it is also filled with various types of humor. We will outline some in the form of jokes.

It should be no surprise that many doctor jokes focus on humorous aspects of the human body. Dr. Susan Steinberg from Manitoba, Canada submitted the following joke:

"One day I had to be the bearer of bad news when I told a wife that her husband had died of a massive myocardial infarct. Not more than five minutes later, I heard her reporting to the rest of the family that he had died of a 'massive internal fart.'"

This, it seems, could very well have been an actual occurrence. What seems especially humorous about this scenario is that, if the man's wife really did take the nurse to be saying that her husband died from a massive internal fart, it did not occur to the woman to question the nurse about this, which perhaps suggests that she was used to massive external farts by her husband. We can imagine that Dr. Susan Steinberg faces many deaths and that she has to be the bearer of bad news on a regular basis. And we know from reading the memoirs of physicians that being the bearer of bad news often causes doctors to question their self-worth, because death is, as it were, the enemy (cf. Grim, 2000, pp. 24–25). Being able to see the humor in painful situations can help protect one's sense of self-worth.

Another joke that we found comes from Dr. Steven Swanson in Corvallis, Oregon. He submitted the following joke:

"While acquainting myself with a new elderly patient, I asked, 'How long have you been bedridden?' After a look of complete confusion she answered... 'Why, not for about twenty years—when my husband was alive.'"

This joke seems like it really could have happened as well. The patient's confusion over the meaning of "bedridden" is humorous. But the fact that she says she has not been "bedridden" for twenty years also adds to the humor. After all, perhaps she *had* been "bedridden" but felt that that was none of the doctor's business. How does a humorous outlook contribute to physician resilience here? Another area of significant stress that physicians face involves communication issues with patients. Often the way to proceed is uncertain (cf. Cole & Carlin, forthcoming; Grouse, 1997). In this joke, the patient was obviously confused as to what the doctor was asking, and we assume that the doctor, at least for a brief moment, would have been confused by the patient's response.

Jokes and, more generally, humor allow us to see how certain things can be both poignant and funny. One can find humor in everyday events, in television and movies and in cartoons, novels, and short stories. The people who write such works can make their audience get more out of life, energizing us for the next onslaught. In this chapter, we have chosen to emphasize the positive aspects of humor (i.e., the energy saving and stress relieving aspects of humor). We realize that humor can have negative aspects as well, such as sarcasm, which literally means "tearing of the flesh." We have done so because this essay is not about humor and medicine per se, but, rather, it is about resiliency.

CONCLUSIONS

Medicine is a combination of applied science (including both biological and behavioral sciences) and ethics. The need to constantly keep updated on the science of medicine can add to the difficulty of the job. But it is important to remember that it is the human element that really determines whether the job is fulfilling or stressful. For most physicians who find themselves burning out or disillusioned with the job, the cause is most likely the loss of the human connections that they expected when they entered the field, and the loss of their own idealism. That is not irretrievable. What is needed is the courage to identify and reinvigorate some of the illusions; the balance we seek in mid-career is not egocentric, but realizing that youthful idealism was a powerful motivator and can be recaptured by devoting energy to the pursuit of justice, while recognizing the humor of it all.

REFERENCES

Adorno, T. W. (2000). *Problems of Moral Philosophy*. Stanford, Calif: Stanford University Press.

Beckman HB, Frankel RM (1984). The effect of physician behavior on the collection of data. *Annals of Internal Medicine 101*: 692–696.

Bennett, M. P., Lengacher, C. A. (2006). Humor and laughter may influence health. I. History and background. *Evidence-based Complementary and Alternative Medicine, 3*(1), 61–63.

Bruce, S. M., Conaglen, H. M., & Conaglen, J. V. (2005). Burnout in physicians: A case for peer-support. *Internal Medicine Journal, 35*(5), 272–278.

Capps, D. (2008). *Laughter Ever After: Ministry of Good Humor*. Chalice Pr.

Chapman, D. M. (1997). Burnout in emergency medicine: what are we doing to ourselves? *Academic Emergency Medicine, 4*(4), 245–247.

Chopra, S. S., Sotile, W. M., & Sotile, M. O. (2004). Physician burnout. *JAMA, 291*(5), 633–633.

Cole, T., Carlin, N. (forthcoming). The dehumanization of medicine and the suffering of physicians. *The Lancet*.

Cole, T., & Carlin, N. (2009). Faculty health and the crisis of meaning: Humanistic diagnosis and treatment. In *Faculty Health in Academic Medicine: Physicians, Scientists, and the Pressures of Success*.

Cole, T., & Carlin, N. (2009). The suffering of physicians. *The Lancet, 374*(9699), 1414–1415.

Edelwich, J., & Brodsky, A. (1980). *Burn-out: Stages of disillusionment in the helping professions.* Human Sciences Press New York.

Freud, S. (1905). *Jokes and Their Relation to the Unconscious.*

Freud, S. (1923). *The ego and the id.*

Freud, S. (1927). Humor.

Grim, P. (2000). *Just here trying to save a few lives: tales of life and death from the ER.* Grand Central Pub.

Grouse, L. D. (1997). The lie. *Archives of Internal Medicine, 157*(18).

Hartzband, P., and Groopman, J. Money and the Changing Culture of Medicine. *NEJM,* Jan. 8, 2009,Volume *360*(2):101–103

Homans, P. (1989). *The ability to mourn: Disillusionment and the social origins of psychoanalysis.*Chicago: University of Chicago Press.

Kirch D.G. and Vernon D.J. The ethical foundation of American medicine: In search of social justice. *JAMA.* April 8, 2009. Volume *301*(14):1482–1484.

Martin, R. A. (2002). Is laughter the best medicine? Humor, laughter, and physical health. *Current Directions in Psychological Science, 11*(6), 216–220.

Selder, F. E., & Paustian, A. (1989). Burnout: Absence of vision. *Professional Burnout in Medicine and the Helping Professions, 73.*

Tallman K, Janisse T, Frankel RM, Sung SH, Krupat E, Hsu JT. Communication practices of physicians with high patient-satisfaction ratings. *The Permanente Journal,* Winter 2007, *11*:1, 19–29.

Personal Reflections

INTRODUCTION

Charles R. Figley

This final section of the book includes the editors' own reflections that attempt to summarize the major points of the book and provide a more personalized discussion, including the editors' own challenges in working in the House of Medicine.

The first chapter in this section, Chapter 17, is by Patrick Alley, a practicing medical surgeon for more than 40 years who currently practices at New Zealand's Southern Cross Hospital in North Harbour. Dr. Alley is the senior medical advisor to the Northern Clinical Training Network and a clinical associate professor of medicine at the University of Auckland. He consults for the Medical Council of New Zealand on matters of competence. He discusses the difficulties of surgery by relating to case studies. In one case study, Miriam dies unexpectedly following surgery, and in another, Jack suddenly shows up ten years after surgery as healthy, happy, and appreciative. Alley asks: "How is it then that you can remember the Miriams of this world but not the Jacks?" After 40 years of practice, Dr. Alley suggests he knows why: The Miriams of patient care are "bolts from the blue" for an important lesson in humility; despite the use of best practices and facilities and expertise, patients can still die. Both types of cases are important and always should be considered together.

Alley also talks about the importance of finding a balance in your practice: to be realistic about complication rates while taking pride in the fact that most cases go well and the outcomes are near perfect. In addition to all the other suggestions offered in this volume, Alley emphasizes the importance of forming and maintaining good collegial relationships to share the good times and the bad times. He notes that surgeons can more readily accept an objective audit of their practice by colleagues, and that such an audit is can be important to support, not just correct, the practitioner. He points out that even though complication-free medicine is a myth and an impossible dream, surgeons are expected to adapt well to complications when they occur. "Awareness of our limitations, the ability to care for ourselves and our colleagues as well as we care for our patients, and the acceptance of objective scrutiny of our practices are all requisites of sensible and reflective practice."

The challenges of physicians working in palliative care are discussed by Carol McAllum in Chapter 18. Palliative care practitioners have been shown to experience less burnout than physicians and oncologists. The word *palliative* means "to abate" or "reduce the violence of." The term *palliative care* is care that eases the symptoms. In the absence of disease-specific modifiers, a cloak of care focusing on comfort was the mainstay and is emerging into all things to do with dying. McAllum notes that the most challenging aspect of palliative care is dealing with the flood of emotions that attend a person's awareness of their mortality or their actual death. Managing the flood of emotions, as noted by Chynoweth and others in this book, is something that doctors are rarely trained to handle. This book hopes to aid in that training.

McAllum notes that patients tell her that their surgeon or oncologist said the finite phrase, "Nothing can be done." But just a simple modification matters to patients' families: "What matters now is savoring every moment." Thus she counsels other physicians and professionals, as well as patients and their families and friends, about death and dying because few of us are prepared. Her interest emerged from 16 years of general practice in rural settings, which prepared her well for a decade of work in palliative care. She talks about the first two people whose deaths she experienced, Marion and Brian, as "gifts." She also talks about Roy, a 72-year-old hospice patient who provided her latest lesson. This was a few weeks before she completed her chapter.

At the end of the chapter she notes resources available to physicians who practice palliative care. In the absence of other therapeutic interventions, practitioners of palliative care have themselves to fall back on, and this is the source of both resilience and burnout. The former can be facilitated through effective communication. The latter is complex and includes communication with self as well as others.

Terry L. Dise is both a pediatrician and medical educator at Tulane University

Health Sciences Center. In Chapter 19, focusing on pediatrics, she notes that stress management was not an issue until well into her practice, and when it became one she was not sufficiently prepared for it. In contrast to today, stress and its management were considered a "personal matter." Yet she notes that the impact of stress is easy to see: smoking, drinking, weight problems, and tense relationships with colleagues. In her role of guiding medical students it was not just about diagnosing ear infections and plotting growth points on charts, but much much more: how to thrive doing it while learning to be more focused on compassion, service, joy, love, caring, clinical detachment, and helpfulness to others. She ends her chapter with a discussion of the joy of enabling medical students to be open to caring. "Opening the heart to feel the love and fondness that we have toward our patients is a wonderful surprise, first, because it can feel so good, and second, to recognize how right it is to do so. No one tells you this in medical school."

Shailesh Kumar discusses his career as a psychiatrist in Chapter 20, Psychiatrists in Distress: When Work Becomes a Problem. Throughout his career Kumar has seen the problems of physicians placing their work ahead of family and friends and having a life, even though some saw themselves as role models. He finds that physicians often treat their patients as objects because they are tired, feel unappreciated, and no longer practice their beloved vocation with passion. Their personal lives suffer and they become bitter, unhappy people. This is a sign of burnout.

As suggested elsewhere in this volume, psychiatrists, like other physicians working in the Hippocratic tradition, place their patients first. Kumar is concerned about psychiatrists acting on emotions they do not fully understand, thus reflecting their need to rescue, not just treat patients. As a result, they experience a sense of failure when a patient's illness goes unaffected by their treatment program. They may feel powerlessness, a sense of loss, grief, and fear of becoming ill, or they make efforts to wall themselves off from patients and their families, thereby reducing their effectiveness. Kumar offers some suggestions to avoid these and other pitfalls.

Jessica Chynoweth is a family physician, graduate of the University of New Mexico Medical School and now working at the Isleta Pueblo (American Native American Tribe) family clinic in New Mexico. In Chapter 21, Medical Students and Residents, she discusses the most challenging and rewarding elements in adopting to the demands of becoming a physician. She describes the services available to students who are having trouble with the pressure and those who need extra help, especially from the teaching faculty. She found that the crunch for medical students came in the clinical years of medical school (3 and 4), a period that involves rotations in all the specialties. Each rotation is a different specialty, so the knowledge base changes frequently. Although the physical demands on medical students are enormous—often working 70 hours a week during this period, with only one day off per week—the biggest challenges are emotional regulation. Working with death and dying patients and their families is the biggest emotional challenge for which she was not prepared.

When death and dying were discussed it was solely from a medical viewpoint. "Indeed, they seem to intentionally deflect us from talking about our emotions." Repression, apparently, is the antidote to emotional pain. In addition to pressure to succeed, Chenoweth notes the long hours, studying in what little spare time you can find, so that you can be publicly quizzed the next day by your attending physician, coupled with the absence of any opportunity to process events at an emotional level. Medical school staff periodically provide lectures on finding your work versus life balance, how to eat healthy, exercise, and get lots of sleep. Then the fourth year of medical school takes on an entirely new set of expectations, such as taking the second set of medical board exams and then applying for residency, completing a "subinternship," an Intensive Care (ICU) month. Chynoweth notes that this particular month was perhaps the most difficult emotionally, seeing how families managing impending death. "The medical student," she concludes, "is placed in a situation where, no matter what you do, you know someone is going to die but yet you have to do everything in your power to be the best physician possible. This challenge is enormous, and it can take a huge toll both on one's performance at work and in school, and outside it."

In Chapter 22, Family Medicine: I Will Never Fly in a Helicopter Again, Bruce Arroll, professor and head of the Auckland University Department of General Practice in New Zealand, discusses his career as a physician in general practice. He describes an especially harrowing experience accompanying a patient on a helicopter ride to the hospital with severe wounds who suddenly stopped breathing. The lessons learned from his career are both practical and theoretical. The practical one is to train rural physicians and staff in the skills and issues of transferring sick patients. Arroll also discusses the limitations of self-criticism and the need to accept one's limitations and try to learn from mistakes, such as the use of a helicopter to transfer his patients (he never used one again). Yet he points out at the end of his chapter that every time a helicopter brings a patient to the city hospital where he now works, he gets a " welling of tears suggesting that my soul has a little scar from that night of terror."

Robin Youngson, the author of Chapter 23, Anesthesiology, created the very first anesthesiology clinic at his hospital, urging his surgical colleagues "to send me their 'worst' cases." He describes that in the case of Jessie, it was left to him to explain the "enormity of the surgical risk." She told him that her religious beliefs prevented proper medical treatment; but that she would trust Dr. Youngson's skill and God's compassion and guidance.

Youngson proposes that physicians need to acquire the right attitude, choosing humor, laughter, and compassion over self-pity with a know-it-all attitude. He notes that the patient sets the agenda, not the doctor. The doctor assumes more of the role of mentor and facilitator to augment technical skills, knowledge, caring, and compassion. Thus, the principles of humanity, interdependence, choice of an attitude, and laughter are critical to balancing skill with compassion for self and patients. "When we open our hearts to our patients, they offer us such gifts. I thought I needed to be resilient but I learned that the secret is to take off our armor, not put it on."

In the final chapter, Chapter 24, Lisa Moreno-Walton, a Tulane University emergency physician, associate professor, and medical educator, writes about her profession. Her chapter addresses three fundamental questions: Why do emergency physicians choose emergency medicine? What are the stressors? How can I see what is worst about people and still retain my faith in humanity? Dr. Moreno-Walton wryly notes that emergency physicians (EPs) are like no other for their love of action and challenge, acute care, and the life-and-death of practice of medicine in "real time." Emergency medicine provides exhilaration of those who seek and thrive in it. Yet EPs must endure an extraordinary amount of pressure to perform. Moreover, it is a challenge to work with emergency patients. She notes that it is common for her patients not to have showered in a while. They are not generally wearing their Sunday best clothes, nor are they particularly happy to be there. Her patients may be pulled from burning buildings, dragged bleeding from the scene of a domestic dispute, brought from the job site where they suddenly developed crushing chest pain, or carried off of their favorite easy chair after experiencing facial numbness and slurred speech while watching soap operas in their nightgowns. They are unprepared, angry, and frightened by their appearance in the Emergency Department (ED), and that sets the scene for both the best and the worst behaviors that human beings can exhibit. Their lives are interrupted, their bodies have failed them, they have lost control, and, as human beings are wont to do, they vent their frustrations on the people whose very presence highlights their vulnerability: the ED staff. Answering her final question of how one deals with the bad as well as the good, Moreno Walton talks about the need for perspective taking, doing so with humor and sufficient self-monitoring and the help of trusted colleagues. She suggests that EPs take only brief pauses to process their emotions. "It is often difficult to take time to feel. It hurts too much." It is difficult in part because there is so much to do anyway: the patients who have been out in the waiting room for six hours and really do want us to hurry things along and get to seeing them. And so it goes.

/// 17 /// SURGERY

PATRICK ALLEY

Miriam was a 41-year-old mother of three who had been diagnosed with ulcerative colitis in her late 20s. She had presented with worsening diarrhea and abdominal pain with the usual accompaniments of fatigue, lassitude, and mild depression. Her initial medical treatment with prednisone had been very successful, and she had managed to fulfill her roles as a manager of her household and her small business. Her three daughters had passed relatively unscathed through the hazards of teenage life and were now launched on their respective pathways in life. Her husband, a man of great talent and charm, had been her primary supporter and shared with her the challenges of not only managing her chronic illness but also the maturation of their children to successful careers.

In the several years before I met her, Miriam had begun to experience a regression and had developed more symptoms. The diagnosis was again confirmed and after all the usual checks she had been started on an escalating dose of prednisone and other immunosuppressive agents. Over that time she had half a dozen admissions for control of acute symptoms and required numerous blood transfusions, alteration to her drug regime, and management of her worsening depression. When she reached a daily total of 30 visits to the toilet for her diarrhea she was referred to me for consideration of surgery.

In 1995 the gold standard operation for this condition was a total procto-colectomy and ileostomy. It is a major procedure but in for sufferers of ulcerative colitis the benefits are enormous. The transformation three months out from their surgery was inevitably pleasing to both the patient and everyone involved with their care.

As a prelude to her surgery there were a number of family meetings punctuated by lots of diagrams and questions. Finally the date was set and she duly arrived in theater for her operation. She had asked a family friend, a senior surgeon well known to me, to come to the anesthetic room with her. I asked him to stay for the procedure if he wished. He did so, watching closely and benignly as the senior registrar, and I set about the operation. It was a very straightforward procedure and the spectator surgeon left muttering that he had never seen such a major procedure cost so little in terms of blood loss. Miriam was awake and talking soon after the procedure and already she seemed better. Two hours later I visited her in the ward and found her surrounded by flowers and family, Miriam chattering excitedly to them about the prospects of freedom from her illness and what that entailed.

Soon after midnight I was woken by a phone call from the Supervising Charge Nurse. "Just get over here, would you?" "What's the problem?" "Just get over here, please." So I did. She met me in the foyer of the hospital and gathered me in a hug. "I'm sorry," she said. "We found Miriam dead in her bed a few minutes ago—the family is on their way in." Apparently the nurses had settled Miriam for the night—all her observations were normal, she felt well and was pain free. Sometime in the intervening hour she had had some form of cardiac arrest and there was little point in attempting resuscitation when she was found cold and lifeless.

The devastation to everyone was immense. To worsen matters, the family in no way held me or the staff responsible and offered me as much if not more sympathy than I offered them. I frankly would have preferred to deal with their anger and disappointment rather than their sympathetic understanding of the situation. Her funeral was attended by nearly a thousand friends and family and the aforementioned surgeon spoke there about my surgery in praising terms—something that was of little comfort to me. Nor was the discovery three weeks later that a post-mortem analysis revealed a rare and fatal viral inflammation of her heart muscle that accounted for her untimely and unexpected demise.

There are few weeks that I do not recall Miriam's death. Occasionally I speak about it to colleagues and many of them have had similar experiences.

The point of this story is the other side of the coin of remembrance. It is this.

About a week after Miriam died, I was stopped at a roadside sandwich shop when the door of an adjacent truck opened and a huge barrel chested driver leapt out and made his way to me. His hand was out in greeting five meters before he got to me.

"You Doc Alley?" he said.

"I am" I replied.

"Bloody good to see you—you did this in 1992." Pulling up his bush singlet he displayed a multi-scarred abdomen.

"Really!" I said. "Please forgive me—I see so many people over the years and I can't always remember who is who."

"Name's Jack Fortrance, North Shore Hospital—look me up!"

So I did just that. Sure enough, he had been under my care for the nasty combined pathologies of acute cholecystitis and acute pancreatitis. The latter had required careful monitoring of his metabolic state and his gallbladder needed surgery two days after he came in. Three days later he nearly died from a massive bleed from an acute duodenal ulcer. This required further surgery. He then developed a deep vein thrombosis and a pulmonary embolus that nearly killed him, and finally he had a small bowel obstruction requiring more surgery. He survived all that and went back to his truck driving apparently none too much the worse for wear.

I had completely forgotten him but obviously he had not forgotten who I was.

How is it then that you can remember the Miriams of this world but not the Jacks? There are a number of reasons for this. The first is the expectation that you are in the business of surgery to fix surgical problems and when you do, that is entirely the norm, what is expected, and it is no big deal. Forget that one and move onto the next case. The Miriams are bolts from the blue—they serve to remind us that despite the best in technique, the best facility, and the best of your expertise, there are no matches for some pathology. The important point is to recognize that these two sorts of cases need to be considered together. Unless you can be reminded of the Jacks of this world your life is going to be dominated by the Miriams, and you will have little peace, let alone sleep. But it is sometimes a difficult task to actually effect these positive reminiscences. There is a substantial body of evidence indicating the link between our emotions and our memory, and clearly whatever a surgeon may believe about emotional control the Miriams of our lives will engender indelible memories.

There is a related phenomenon in recall of clinical cases. While the Miriams of the world are stuck irremovably into our psyche, unfavorable outcomes of less import may escape our memory. It is a sobering fact that when confronted by any measure of audit, doctors do not always do as well as they think. Therefore the dilemma is to find a balance between being realistic about our complication rates and achieving recall and taking pride in those cases in which all goes well and the outcomes are excellent.

The secret to coping with these issues is the ability to form constructive collegial relationships. The ability to share narratives of the disasters and the imperfections of clinical performance is a necessary safeguard to a situation, which if persistent, will cause harm to the practitioner. From that basis, surgeons can more readily accept the reality of objective audit of their practice and in so doing become more reflective and secure in their practice.

Nowadays there is an increasing tendency of surgeons to operate in isolation, even though they may be in large cities. Such arrangements allow the ability to specialize in an area where one's expertise can be developed to a high and potentially "complications-free" level. However, not only does that diminish the availability of collegial support when disaster strikes, but it also decreases the opportunity for an audit process that is timely, relevant to their practice, and educationally supportive.

Complication-free medicine is a myth to which the popular press aspire. In reality it is an impossible dream. However, it is a rightful expectation of the communities that we serve to have practitioners in complication-prone occupations such as surgery well equipped to manage such complications when they occur. There is a clear need for both reflective practitioners and audit systems to work in parallel so that safe practice is reasonably assured. We are powerless to change the pathology that presents to us but we are not powerless to change ourselves. Awareness of our limitations, the ability to care for ourselves and our colleagues as well as we care for our patients, and the acceptance of objective scrutiny of our practices are all requisites of sensible and reflective practice.

/// 18 /// THE GIFTS OF PALLIATIVE CARE

Sometimes Awkward, always Wholesome

CAROL MCALLUM

In the first six months of my being a doctor, two patients, Ana and Duncan, each gave me a gift. I didn't recognize they were gifts back then. Ana was in her 80s, had severe heart failure, and had just arrived on the medical ward in the early evening. It was my job to assess her and document this. Ana had not long been discharged from the same ward. She had only been at her daughter's home for just over 24 hours before this re-admission. Her daughter was exhausted. I entered Ana's space behind the curtain in the six-bedded ward. My paperwork was at hand. I knew the drill, and so did Ana. Her hand reached out to gently interrupt my introduction. She asked me to stay with her. She told me she was dying. I can't remember her exact words. She said enough to stop me from leaving her to go and get help; to get the charge nurse or my registrar; to get Ana's daughter who had just left; to get someone! I wanted to do something! I think I wanted to flee. Yet I stayed with Ana. I was full of questions for her. I could see she was tired, weak, and really just wanting to lie there. I had to choose my questions to spare her from the burden of my merely wanting to know. With our few and quiet exchanges I felt reassured that this really was her wish; that she had no outstanding matters to attend; and she wanted that her daughter not be disturbed as she too needed her rest, and she wouldn't yet have reached home anyway so she couldn't be contacted for a while. This was well before mobile telephones. I was then speechless. I was silent. I sat and watched and waited. Ana's breathing stopped. Ana died. I stayed with her a bit longer.

I then needed to make the transition back to the life beyond the curtain. Time had played its paradoxical tricks on me. Time had gone on forever and simultaneously it had stopped, or was suspended. In real time it was between twenty and thirty minutes before I emerged from behind the curtain. I recall being aware of an awkwardness that I had to break the news that Ana had died and I hadn't completed the required documentation. I was feeling more guilty about the latter than the former. In my naivety I hadn't calculated any impact beyond what was important for Ana. There was some consternation. This wasn't exactly what my registrar or the charge nurse had expected. They had some work to do to restore the proper process that this young doctor had disturbed. True to Ana's words, her daughter had just arrived back home when the registrar rang to break the news. I remember apologizing for not following due process, but I also know that a bit of me was satisfied that Ana did it her way on her terms. She died with gentleness, presence, and grace. Her gift endures.

Death and dying are best avoided at all costs. Make sure it doesn't happen, and if it's going to happen make sure it's not on your shift if you can help it. And if the worst does happen, then just make sure you haven't done anything wrong! Those were the succinct subliminal messages I learned about dying from my medical school years, if indeed I did learn anything about death and dying then. They were unwittingly reinforced for many years thereafter, despite my early experience with Ana and Duncan.

Duncan's gift is only apparent to me now as I write this. It was very well disguised. It didn't come gently as did Ana's. Duncan was a war veteran, cared for in the long-term wing of the hospital. These were the wards that young doctors only ventured into when called upon, which was none too often. It was my 24-hour shift on call. Mid morning I was asked by the nursing staff to assess Duncan, which I duly did. Duncan had indigestion. He hadn't had much indigestion in the past and it wasn't overwhelmingly distressing. He was a man of few words and uncomplaining. He asked for little, just wanted something to give him some relief. Nowadays such understatement in a man of no complaints would be sufficient enough to alert me that something was truly amiss.

My assessment included recording his blood pressure and pulse and feeling his abdomen. I remember feeling a bit at a loss about what to do. This didn't seem serious. I don't recall what follow-up plans I put in place, much less what I did at the time. I am likely to have prescribed something for indigestion. About two o'clock the following morning I was called to see Duncan, as he had collapsed. I was surprised. I hadn't expected this. I was scared. I was with Duncan in a matter of minutes. Duncan was dead when I got there. I was even more scared. What had happened was that Duncan had woken and on getting out of bed he had vomited such a large volume of blood that it was not survivable. He died within minutes.

I was worried, very worried, that I had done something wrong. I was very worried about what to write on the death certificate. I remembered that he was a man on his own, without family. By daylight I worriedly sought the counsel of my consultant. While I remember being quizzed and reassured that under the circumstances no further action was required, I feel quite sure now that I missed something then. If nothing else I underestimated Duncan's symptoms and didn't really know what I was doing, but more disturbing, I didn't ask for help. It was of little comfort then that my consultant reflected that there was most likely no other outcome for Duncan, no matter where he was, or what investigations might have been undertaken.

It's been my time in palliative care, and writing this reflection, that's brought two of Duncan's gift out of the dark. My colleagues in pediatric palliative care have embraced the term "allow natural death" for planning end of life care. This is preferred to the relatively minimalist "do not resuscitate" directives, which are particularly found in acute hospital settings. It encourages discussion about what is wanted during the last days of life, rather than what isn't. Allow Natural Death/*Te Wa Aroha* is the full title given to the end-of-life care plan at the Starship Children's Hospital in Auckland. *Te Wa Aroha* is Maori for "a time of love" or "a time of compassion" (Naylor, 2012). This is not directly applicable to Duncan's circumstances, because his death was more of a sudden nature, with little opportunity for planning. Yet I would have valued knowing about it way back then. It would have given me language.

With all the advantages of the intervening 34 years I would now talk with Duncan directly: Duncan, I'm not sure what's happening. I want to talk with my consultant. How does that sit with you? And if indeed Duncan was as reluctant about investigations or interventions as my memory attributes to him, then I would share "what if" questions. Duncan, can you tell me what's important for you and the people who matter to you? Duncan, what if this is serious, an indication of a heart attack or a bleeding stomach ulcer? These were quite likely my fears at the time, and I know I would never have asked him. I was probably hoping nothing like that was happening; hoping with fingers crossed! Even although he was a man of few words I believe it is likely he could have and would have answered questions of that nature. I know that from my subsequent encounters with people of Duncan's ilk.

Yet Duncan endowed me with other gifts. My consultant that day was the first of several senior colleagues who have at one time or another, often at short notice, listened and offered their wisdom and experience, not that they would have called it wisdom. To be propelled into that realm of continual apprenticeship was invaluable.

So in front of my very eyes, my patients were already debunking some of the subconscious learnings I had absorbed in my undergraduate years. There was more to dying than what I'd been taught. Dying happened naturally and despite doctors. It was a serious business, and not many doctors talked about it. It wasn't always comfortable for the witness. Years later I avidly read Sherwin Nuland's book *How We Die* (Nuland, 1994) and have taken from it an understanding that the body has in-built ways of leave-taking, closing down, dying. It seems to me that we experience the trauma of being born with attendant dramatic physical and physiological changes and yet for the most part it is beyond conscious recall. I muse that such transcendence might be the same at the end of our life, except for our consciousness of life's bitter-sweet nature having an impact on our anticipated experience of dying and death.

Early in my doctoring years I spent nine months in obstetrics, during which I attended a number of births. Over time I have tended many more deaths than births. The parallels are uncanny. The same cluster of feelings arises in me when I witness a child being born as when I am in the presence of a person dying. Without fail, every single time, I feel it is breathtaking. For me there is a touch of mystery. There is a sense of otherness. There is a sense of awe. The stark physical transformations embody something intangible.

As I write, it makes me wonder how much this phenomenon keeps me going. Is this the opposite of vicarious trauma? It must be vicarious something! I know the moments with those who are dying are opportunities for a smidgeon of transcendence in the course of the often chaotic, always fully overcommitted working day—unbidden and undemanding opportunities.

Just two days ago I was on the ward, working out the 24 hour dose of morphine that Alan needed to keep suppressed the pain of meningitis due to metastatic lung cancer. Wretched unremitting and increasing headache that it was, Alan retained his gracious composure. Only two weeks earlier had Alan been admitted to hospital, and not only was this the first indication of the cancer, curative treatments were not to be had. Earlier in his hospitalization I had time with Alan on his own, when he could see me. This day my time with Alan was very short. He had lost his sight, and his adult children had arrived to bear witness to the news that he chose to forego the very slender precarious benefits of chemotherapy or radiation therapy. With increasing weakness every day, Alan's outlook was short term, maybe as little as a few weeks or even days.

I might have had about seven minutes with Alan, his partner of fifteen years, and his three adult children that day. I had so many questions to ask, so much I wanted to know to fine tune the medications to suppress his symptoms of pain and nausea. There had been a proverbial "truckload" of visitors that morning, plus several doctors all doing what needed to be done. He had welcomed me to his bedside, and our hands touched lightly in introduction. Alan apologized for not being able to focus on me. He explained his eyes weren't working so well. I am always humbled by such gestures. After a few minutes Alan developed an unaccustomed and barely perceptible irritability. Apart from irritability and sleepiness being symptoms of meningitis, Alan had enough other reasons to need some peace and quiet. I withdrew and set to my work.

That involved an hour or so of scouting through the clinical records, speaking with the primary physician, the team doctors, the oncologist, the nursing staff, the physiotherapist, and the social worker; followed by compiling a workable plan. From having had no morphine a week ago, Alan now needed a modest dose and he was getting it intravenously. To be anywhere other than hospital (and I was mindful he wanted to be at home) this needed conversion to the subcutaneous route, which could be delivered continuously under the skin with the aid of a portable battery operated pump. Making this conversion, doing it accurately so that Alan neither gets too much nor too little takes all my concentration. Alan's time is short and he wants to be no more sleepy than he naturally would be, and if I overcalculate that might mean unnecessary drowsiness for a precious 24 hours or so. If I undercalculate then Alan will get more pain. I put in place a plan for either of those eventualities, which includes speaking with the nurse and medical team again.

Each patient presents some element of uncharted water for me, because of his or her uniqueness. The principles of prescribing in palliative care are now well established. We prescribe according to the patient's needs and symptoms, finding the lowest effective dose that gives relief, with the least side effects. It takes continual monitoring and frequent reviews. If there is pain, the prescription is for pain relief, analgesics. If there is nausea or vomiting, specific anti-emetics are available. For anxiety there are "anxiolytics," the most common group of medications being the benzodiazepines, which give muscle relaxation, sedation, and a sense of detachment—the same medication often used prior to surgery. Gone are the days when the blunt instrument of increasing the morphine was the panacea for all symptoms.

The prescription is but a small part of the whole, yet much emphasis is placed on it. What matters now is everything else. The prescription is to enable the everything else to happen. For Alan that was under way. The following day I was not in the hospital and there were numerous conversations involving health professionals and Alan and family as plans were forged. Going home seemed, too tenuous as Alan's symptoms were still changing. Alan and his partner took up the offer to transfer to the hospice inpatient unit for the time being. Until that day none of us health professionals knew that plans were in place for Alan to be married the following day.

It is more than enough for me to know that when my expertise was needed it was effective. I was pleased to find out that the prescription recommendations I'd made for Alan's pain and nausea "did the trick," met the need. I enjoy applying myself to the task at hand. In my early doctoring days I was none too sure about myself. I often felt alone then.

That may well have been in part due to my nature, or the essentially peripatetic life of young doctors, or a combination of both. Nowadays teamwork is essential, and I'm most fortunate that the majority of my fellow colleagues, nursing, medical, and allied health professionals alike, are collaborative and have their patients' welfare at heart. For those who aren't quite as collaborative I still have energy to work with them to get the best outcome for the patient. Sometimes in the process I detect a modicum of burnout, stress, weariness, grief, and/or cynicism that has its origins only known to that person.

I'm quite sure I was close to burnout, too, some ten years back. Subclinical burnout is the euphemism with which I adorn that period. I had two weeks' leave. At that time it was the only time I'd ever taken off from work. And for the rest, I carried on. On reflection it was a combination of working too much, doing too much, not being clear about communicating, frustrations with systems, and not being quite grounded enough. The reason I suspect burnout is because I know that now I have energy and the capacity to enjoy the highlights of my work, as well as to navigate the turmoil. Back then I focused erroneously on the frustrations of the system—the health system, an easy target.

Two years ago I was caught up in extenuating and, I hope, once-in-a-lifetime work circumstances that endured over a period of ten months. The impact on me was an almost unbearable workload. Barely a day would go by and I'd ask myself why I didn't leave. There was ample opportunity for me to work elsewhere. My ready response was that if I could get through this day, I wanted to stay where I was. The future of a truly integrated palliative care service for the region was, and still is, promising, if I could clear the hurdles of the present. Each day I found the work heavy and hard. In the midst of the organizational meltdown I had the ear of and moral support from close colleagues. This was invaluable, although I unreasonably rued that no-one could put more hours in the day. I just needed a bit more time every day! Still the magic of working in palliative care, of seeing people living so much as their lives were coming to an end, was a vital and golden thread through that dense tapestry: the vicarious gifts of palliative care. There is so much living in dying. That might be what makes it hard in a way, as living is not always easy.

I've been inspired by Makowski and Epstein's (2012) proposition that we might "lean into the dissonance of many palliative care encounters," and to this I'll take the liberty of adding the dissonance of work environments sometimes. Their paper opens with Vasily Kandinsky's Komposition 8, alongside his words: "Clashing discords, loss of equilibrium, 'principles' overthrown, unexpected drumbeats, great questionings, apparently purpose-less strivings, stress and longing [...] This is our harmony." It matches my experience of the health care setting perfectly! They cite research that experienced meditators engage more fully with another's suffering and recover themselves more quickly. They propose that being there, being present, being fully present is something that can be achieved through training. Being there is what Ana helped me to do so many years ago. Being there is the most and the least I can do when all else is done.

I've been distracted. When I started to write about my encounter with Alan, I intended to share a different story, which I will end with now. The nurse who was caring for Alan reflected back to another patient we both cared for, ever so briefly. The man was in his 20s and had suffered a catastrophic accident at work. He was an only son. In his last hours I was asked to review his management, to make sure that all that could be done was being done. The nurse recalled how I went into the young man's room, found a chair and sat with him for a time, unconscious though he was. My internal conversation as she spoke was: "That would be right. I don't think I did anything. I probably just tried to 'be there.'" She said it was so different. She hadn't seen a doctor do that before. In some way it was reassuring for her. It was a tiny gift amidst the bleakness of a young man's death and a father's overwhelming anguish. Here, some years later she gifted it back to me.

For reasons I can't truly fathom my niche is certainly palliative care. Its gifts are at times tough, disguised, long in the coming, but whatever else they are wholesome as they continually nudge and cajole me onward in the lifelong apprenticeship of understanding more about me and more about the people I live and work with.

I want to leave you with a refrain from a song sung by Leonard Cohen. It captures the reality of the weaknesses and imperfections with which I, like many others, abound. And yet it is cheekily cheerful: "There's a crack, there's a crack in everything. That's how the light gets in."

ACKNOWLEDGMENTS

I want to acknowledge my patients and their families for letting me be there, and Dr. John Gommans for his advice and timely counsel.

REFERENCES

Makoswski, S.K.E. & Epstein, R.M. (2012). Turning toward dissonance: Lessons from art, music and literature. *Journal of Pain and Symptom Management*, 43(2), 293–298.

Naylor, W. (2012). *New Zealand palliative care glossary*. Wellington. The Palliative Care Council of New Zealand, Hospice New Zealand & the Ministry of Health.

Nuland, S. (1994). *How we die*. London: Chatto & Windus.

/// 19 /// PEDIATRICS

If Only it was Just the Kids

TERRY L. DISE

I was never taught about stress management during my residency. Even afterward, as a young attending at a medical school, my senior partners didn't speak of it. I think it was a combination of not being in vogue at the time, in the late 1980s to early 1990s, to discuss such things and that handling one's inner challenges was a private matter, not to be shared. Consequently, one had to rely on oneself to manage, and not unexpected, some handled it better than others. It is easy to look around a med school and see the smoking, drinking, weight problems, and tense relationships with colleagues that are manifestations of stress.

After being an academic general pediatric physician for 16 years, I was invited to run the first and second year Foundations in Medicine course for medical students. It was at this time, since I was in a position to influence these young future doctors' minds, that I began to think more about what makes doctors (and specifically me) stressed in the practice of medicine. In my teaching of the medical students, I became more aware of the subtext of my practicing life. I realized that it was not just diagnosing ear infections and plotting growth points on charts; but watching myself, how I interacted with patients, how I felt about the children and parents I treated, and dealing with the emotions that would arise during these encounters. When I began to pay more attention to all of this and process in my head what was happening, a deeper emotional richness to my relationships with my patients arose. I have become a happier physician, which I wasn't always.

There are some areas I'd like to focus on in this chapter. These were topics that I assigned to medical students as short essays to write: clinical detachment, resilience, compassion, joy, service and helpfulness to others, love (caring), forgiveness, and patience.

I felt that if they could begin the process of reflection early in their careers, it would help them to become better doctors.

CLINICAL DETACHMENT

Doctors are taught, at one time or another, that clinical detachment is necessary to the practice of medicine. There are far too many doctors, however, that take this advice to an extreme. They become so detached that they lose the connection to their patients or never have a connection to begin with. They are cold and unemotional, seemingly brusque and uninterested. Patients are not satisfied with encounters with this type of physician. The physicians feel they are protecting themselves by staying emotionally uninvolved, but I think that harm is being done, not only to the patient, but to the doctor as well. To become unemotional when faced by patients who are suffering is to deny feelings that well up in us. Denying feelings can be stressful. I believe that the more clinically detached physicians become, the more stressed they are. It takes a lot of work to stamp down feelings, much more than acknowledging them. Most people would tell you that feeling emotions is exhausting, so it may seem intuitive that keeping emotions in is better. But what it really does is to distance the doctor from the person, so it's harder to connect with the patient and have empathy. It's uncomfortable to feel patients' pain because it can remind us of our own pain and limitations; but if you can't access the pain, you can't access the love, compassion, and joy in practice either.

RESILIENCE IN MEDICINE

We bring our personalities, prejudices, and history with us into the exam rooms of patients. It is human nature to do so. What helps us to rise above our human nature is awareness that we do this. Watching the watcher, or observing ourselves as we practice medicine, can help us realize when our own "stuff" is interfering with the care we are giving to our patients. An example of this is my own feeling about religion. I describe myself as a very spiritual person, but I do not attend organized religious services. I very much respect others' commitment to their religions, but it took me a long time in my day-to-day practice with my patients to get there. When patients of mine would say, "I'm going to pray on it" or "I will just leave it in God's hands," inwardly I would feel uncomfortable and fidgety, and I would change the topic as quickly as I could. When I was able to let this discomfort go, and appreciate this aspect of my patients' (or actually the parents of my patients) characters, I was better able to appreciate the resiliency that these parents had about dealing with their children's chronic diseases and respect them more for it. An added benefit was that my discomfort about hearing others share their religious beliefs with me stopped; in fact, when it seemed right to do so, I would recommend to patients to pray about their concerns. Doctors speak often about resilient patients who appear to rise above their illnesses somehow, who have a core of inner strength that helps them to survive an illness that another patient can't access. Why do some doctors succumb to the stress of their work while others thrive? I feel that answer lies in resiliency; finding the inner core of strength to rise above the grind, to see the freshness of every patient encounter.

COMPASSION

In my mind, compassion is in the top five in a list of important attributes of the physician. Physicians who allow themselves to feel compassion, and to express it, are much better at their craft. Because we are all humans together, patients can sense the connection of the physician to their stories. They know whether the doctor is paying attention, really investing in their words. Reading facial expressions and body language is not only the physician's domain. Patients can also read ours. Can a patient tell if the doctor is tired, cranky, or distracted by other matters? Certainly. It behooves us to remember that we are being observed by our patients too. Part of the healing of patients comes from the attentive and compassionate listening that should be done with patients by their doctors. Medical students have asked me if it's acceptable to cry with patients. They fear losing control, or not being able to function. They fear that they will be judged or criticized by fellow doctors, or perhaps even patients. These concerns come mostly from female medical students, but I suspect that it's not limited to that gender. It is seen to be a goal to stay in control, to be serious and stern and coldly clinical. My impression is that if you succeed at that goal you lose your humanity and compassion. Not every doctor feels that it's right to show such strong emotion with patients; it's a personal choice. I teach students that they each have to make the decision but assure that their ability to access their feelings doesn't get lost.

FORGIVENESS

The concept of learning to forgive patients is foreign to many doctors, I think because it simply does not occur to them that this is a valuable technique to reduce feelings of stress about previous bad outcomes. Bad outcomes can be as serious as being sued, or as commonplace as losing one's temper with a patient for being late for an appointment. Feeling angry at patients and staying angry uses up a lot of personal energy. Deciding to forgive someone, and even more challenging, to also forget the event, can be liberating. Holding grudges and resentment toward patients alters our relationship with them and saps the enjoyment of taking care of them. It doesn't do anyone any good either to stay angry; nothing is solved, there is simply a pervasive feeling of discontent. One mother in my practice helped teach me about this when I finally asked her why she missed so many appointments with me. She told me that it took three bus changes for her to get to my clinic, and so it was hard sometimes to make it on time. The feeling that swept over me after hearing that was shame; here was I feeling put upon and having my time wasted when the poor lady was doing her best to get to me. She needed my understanding, not my misplaced annoyance with her. This incident taught me to find out more about the inner lives of my patients, to understand their struggles and challenges, and to constantly remember that most people *are* doing the best that they can even if it doesn't seem so at first glance.

PATIENCE

When I teach medical students, I emphasize the importance of patience while interviewing. Physicians are very bad about interrupting patients before they finish their stories; and in our haste to get the job done, we run the risk of missing a key point in the history. There is a saying in medicine that if you listen long enough, your patient will tell you what is wrong with them. Sometimes what a patient needs more than a physical exam or lab work is for another human being to listen to them wholeheartedly, without interruption or judgment. It can be the most important treatment we offer our patients, and most doctors intuitively know this, but they are under constraints to see a patient in 15 minutes; a dictum that comes from large companies who are focused on the bottom line and not on the quality of patient care. They call patients "clients" and doctors "providers" and in my opinion the "business" of medicine is part of the deterioration of the doctor-patient relationship and a major cause of our stress in the workplace.

JOY

Is it possible to find joy, happiness, laughter, and enjoyment in practice? I firmly believe so because I live that life daily. How to incorporate these experiences is the question for many. Incorporating some of the tenets of Buddhist practice has helped me here. A key idea is learning to live in the moment, appreciating each nuance, every subtlety. Learning and practicing how to silence the incessant inner chatter. Really listening to patients without internally thinking about what you need to get from the grocery on the way home. To take calming breaths when the pace of the day becomes too much. It takes discipline and practice to excel in this endeavor, but it's well worth it. In my specialty of pediatrics, it may be easier to learn this, because children are excellent teachers. They live in the moment, hold onto their desires (at times rather loudly), and expect adults to answer every question honestly. The joyful smile of a child who finds out that no, he does *not* need a shot today can really remind an adult that it's the little things in life that are important.

When my patients are anxious about being examined or possibly needing a shot, I use humor when appropriate to lighten the mood. When parents seem overwhelmed by the responsibilities of parenthood or the current illness their child has, I try to find something to laugh about with them. Laughter is healing and releases the tension of stress. I try to laugh at myself when I can; it's not healthy to take oneself too seriously.

SERVICE AND HELPFULNESS TO OTHERS

How can we find happiness in life? Again, I turn to my Buddhist faith. It is in helping others that we find true happiness. When we put others first, we find joy and fulfillment. When we forget this and become impatient that a patient is taking too long to tell us their stories, or that it is time for our shift to be over, we have forgotten that we are there to serve. We hold detailed, hard-won knowledge that is not accessible to most people. We have been entrusted with this knowledge in order to serve. To not take the time to help our patients to understand their illnesses and concerns is selfish, and so is forgetting what we were meant to do: to serve. We are caught in the middle between what we know is right—that we should listen to our patients—and yet we are told by all kinds of people who do not understand what we do: Hurry up! See more patients! Do more paperwork! We know in our hearts that we are not staying true to what we were taught about how to interact with patients, and this is extremely stressful.

LOVE OR CARING

Opening the heart to feel the love and fondness that we have toward our patients is a wonderful surprise, first, because it can feel so good, and second, to recognize how right it is to do so. No one tells you this in medical school, probably because there is a concern about what is appropriate in the doctor-patient relationship. I am not speaking of romantic love, that is inappropriate. Even one of the editors of this book was concerned about my word choice and wanted me to rethink what I wrote about it. I think, because I am a pediatrician, I feel differently about it based on my personal experiences as a physician. How many surgeons have had a patient say to them, I love you, Doctor. I will guess, not many. I have had this experience quite a few times. It is usually a child who is three to five years old. This is an age in which usually what a child is thinking comes right out of their mouths, without any filtering. A child that age senses a feeling of fondness, and they are going to tell you that they love you, or, they may give you a hug. It was these experiences that got me thinking about it. Of course, you don't want to hurt the child's feelings by saying, "Now you know you don't really mean that, you haven't possibly known me long enough to really love me, what do you mean?" They wouldn't understand all that adult talk anyway. The point I'm trying to make is that I believe that we can develop a fondness, a sense of caring, toward patients that we've taken care of for a long time, and that we shouldn't stifle or deny those feelings either. This experience certainly is different from specialties that don't have long-term relationships with patients, such as emergency medicine doctors. Is it any wonder then that it is emergency medicine doctors that have the highest rates of burnout? People come into our clinics and offices and tell us things they would never share with other people. They cry in our offices, they tell us how guilty they feel about something they did yesterday or 30 years ago, they suffer and feel pain in front of us; yet, we aren't supposed to feel anything in return? We aren't supposed to care? We are told to shut down, tune out, and not feel. No wonder so many doctors drink, smoke, are overweight, and get divorced.

THE PARTICULARS OF PEDIATRICS

One of the questions I ask medical students when they rotate through pediatrics is, "How do you feel about parents?" The answer can be revealing! When students don't like the parent doctor interactions, they tend to shy away from doing pediatrics, even if they like interacting with the children. The pediatrician has to rely on the parents to tell him or her what is going on, but students see this as a barrier and a challenge. It can be difficult to navigate a doctor-patient relationship with one person, and here are two and sometimes three people in the room to interact with; and don't forget the grandparents either! When faced with multiple relatives in one room who all may have questions, it can get quite stressful until you turn it into a fun experience in your head. Another concept I like to discuss with medical students and residents is how to deal with patients that you dislike for whatever reason; in pediatrics, it is usually the parent, not the pediatric patient.

Related to this is if a parent says something you disagree with and they argue with you, or if they are doing something annoying, like answering their cell phone (which probably means we shouldn't answer ours either). In these situations I try the deep calming breaths, remind myself that people are doing the best that they can (me too!), try to find something I like about the person, and remember that this moment in time will pass away.

Most important though, I feel it is valuable to acknowledge that we don't always like everyone we meet, but that doesn't mean that we can't be just as good of a doctor for them as a patient or parent that we like a lot. *Every* patient deserves the best we can be.

CONCLUSION

I love being a doctor. Even after 24 years in practice, each morning as I drive to work, I look forward to seeing my patients, hearing their stories, and finding ways to help them. I hope that they feel better after they've seen me. I hope that they know I care about them, and that I want them to be happy and fulfilled. I want them to have health so that they can achieve all their dreams and reach for the stars.

I aspire to achieve each of these aspects every day at work. I am not perfect and I have bad days too. Sometimes I have things on my mind that are personal, but still, I always try to be mindful. When I am successful I feel tired yet fulfilled as I walk out to my car each evening. I also firmly believe that I am less stressed because I have found happiness in my profession.

/// 20 /// PSYCHIATRISTS IN DISTRESS

When Work becomes a Problem

SHAILESH KUMAR

Throughout my career I have seen many colleagues who placed work before their personal lives. Some of them were my role models and I aspired to be like them until I saw the damage they suffered. Tired, feeling unappreciated, and practicing their beloved vocation without passion, they treated their patients like objects. Their personal lives suffered and they ended up bitter, unhappy people. They had burned out! One of them committed suicide. His death affected me, I guess like many other colleagues who were close to him. His death also raised questions that I never had the need to ask before. I realized that psychiatrists work hard and invariably have a stressful life.

In the Hippocratic tradition, psychiatrists, like other doctors, place their patients before themselves. They respond to patients' needs and emotions with emotions of their own, which may reflect a need to rescue the patient, a sense of failure and frustration when the patient's illness progresses, feelings of powerlessness against illness and its associated losses, grief, fear of becoming ill oneself, or a desire to separate from and avoid patients to escape these feelings (Meier et al 2001). These emotions, powerful in nature, are capable of causing stress on their own right.

Unfortunately, stress is not limited to the relationships that exist between doctors and patients. Doctors are also exposed to stresses from external sources. We work in increasingly litigious and unforgiving environment, and bureaucratic requirements imposed upon us are increasing and medical knowledge is advancing rapidly with which we have to constantly keep in touch (Hughes et al 2002). As psychiatrists, we may be more vulnerable than our counterparts in other medical disciplines. This can happen for a variety of reasons. Psychiatric treatment philosophy and modalities have undergone radical transformation in recent times (Hafner 2002). We are finding ourselves working in an environment for which we were not trained, service delivery is changing from an office-based to population-based health model, we are required to fulfill administrative duties whether we like them or not and whether we have had training in them or not, and this occurs often in addition to the significant clinical commitments (Hughes et al 2002). Demand for psychiatric services is increasing exponentially, yet the number of entrants into the profession appear to be decreasing (Storer 2002). Our patients demand us to do more than just alleviate their distress from mental disorder. We are expected not only to be proficient with the advances in psychopharmacology but also know alternative treatment modalities. In other words, practicing psychiatry is almost synonymous with working in stressful conditions these days.

The impact of exposure to these stresses has been a topic of much interest in recent times. A variety of outcomes have been described in the literature, including vicarious victimization, traumatic countertransference, contact victimization, secondary traumatic syndrome, compassion fatigue, and burnout (Dutton and Rubinstein 1995; Huggard 2003). These conditions may either appear in the short or long run. An immediate effect is often described as a state of disengagement and distancing from patients, which is common to compassion fatigue. Huggard (2003) has suggested that even though disengagement and distancing is often employed as a coping mechanism by people facing burnout, it leads to a reduction in empathy. Many doctors believe that detachment from emotional engagement with patients is beneficial. Halpern (2001) has identified the main benefits of such detachment: protection against burnout, better concentration, sustained impartiality and objectivity, and better time management. Despite the benefits identified, maintaining empathy in a therapeutic relationship is beneficial and indeed may be preventative against compassion fatigue or burnout (Huggard, 2003. Halpern 2001).

Compassion fatigue is often described as the set of behaviors and emotions that result from knowledge of or exposure to a traumatizing event experienced by a significant other or from helping or wanting to help a traumatized person (Dutton and Rubinstein 1995). It is said to have a sudden onset, a consequence of doctors' exposure to their patients' experiences combined with their empathy for their patients (Benson 2005). In other words, compassion fatigue develops from doctor-patient interaction, and other factors are of little or no consequence. Doctors experiencing compassion fatigue report a feeling of being overwhelmed by work and not achieving favorable outcomes for their patients (Benson 2005). They often present with feelings of having no energy, emptiness, depleted wondering "why am I doing this?" (Wright, 2004). All of these experiences are early warning signs of adverse health outcomes; they are amenable to intervention but sadly go unrecognized. Cumulative exposure to such experiences leads to burnout.

Burnout is another condition described in the literature as a result of chronic exposure to work-related stress. It is now a term in common usage but was first coined by Freudenberger (1974) to describe the emotional exhaustion experienced by workers in the public services. Over last 30 years of research literature on burnout has accumulated, and according to an estimate over 2500 publications had appeared by 1999 (Carson et al., 1999). It is noteworthy that most of these publications have restricted the definition to human service workers, a trend that acknowledges the unique pressures of utilizing one's self as the "tool" in face-to-face work with needy, demanding, and often troubled clients.

The more popular definition of burnout is based on the work of Maslach and Jackson (1986), who used "emotional exhaustion" (tiredness, somatic symptoms, decreased emotional resources, and a feeling that one has nothing left to give to others) to mean people feeling emotionally overextended and exhausted by their work; "depersonalization" when people develop negative, cynical attitudes and impersonal feelings toward their clients and treat them as objects; and "reduced personal accomplishments" (feelings of incompetence, inefficiency, and inadequacy) to mean when people feel their work has low productivity and they are achieving little. The higher the emotional exhaustion and depersonalization score and lower the personal accomplishment score, the more a physician would be considered as suffering from burnout.

One could look at the construct of burnout as a continuum or a spectrum and conceptualize the three dimensions of burnout in the Maslach and Jackson (1986) model as three *phases*. In other words emotional exhaustion could be seen as the initial phase in which the people under stress could be simply feeling emotionally exhausted. If exposure to stress continues, it could lead to the second phase of burnout, that is, of depersonalization manifested by cynicism and devaluation of patients. At a later, third phase, people experiencing burnout may start underestimating their personal accomplishments. In this model the three dimensions are not mutually exclusive, but one leads to another. Should this model be valid one can also see similarities between emotional exhaustion (EE) and compassion fatigue (CF)—there are not only semantic similarities but also the two present similarly. In both situations doctors feel empty and devoid of empathy or the ability to give themselves to others. There are differences between the two constructs, too, which can't be ignored. While EE results from chronic exposure to workplace stress that is not only limited to the doctor-patient relationship, CF tends to develop acutely and often results from exposure to traumatic incidents.

Among doctors, psychiatrists represent a special group who may be particularly vulnerable to compassion fatigue and burnout more so than their counterparts in other disciplines (Snibbe et al 1989; Deary et al 1996). Despite their training, psychiatrists as a group are vulnerable to reacting adversely to stress due to their personality characteristics, nature of their work, and rapidly changing service delivery models (Deary et al 1996; Martin et al 1997). There is also a possibility that the risk of exposure to stress may increase among psychiatrists globally as demands on them rise due to increasing population, a progressive move to community-based treatment, increasing standards of practice, greater expectations by doctors to have time for study and relaxation, as well as diminishing numbers of entrants into psychiatry (Lazarus 1994; Pullan & Lorbergs. 2001; Draper et al 1989; Langsley & Robinowitz 1979; Kirchner & Owen 1996).

Furthermore, psychiatry has undergone significant and rapid change in a relatively short period. From their work being confined to working in asylums up to the mid 20th century, and psychiatrists themselves separated from urban culture and medicine in general, they have been exposed to the rapidly accumulating knowledge and technological progress in last few decades. Psychiatry has changed from being a custodial to a therapeutic discipline. It now requires psychiatrists to possess a variety of skills and expertise on psychological and biological fronts. Simultaneously, the expectations of society have also increased dramatically. People not only seek psychiatric help for relief from a disorder but also for manifold problems of everyday life. Professional requirements to be met by psychiatrists have also increased quantitatively and qualitatively with the change from a caring, paternalistic attitude toward the mentally ill to a therapeutic partnership. By virtue of the nature of their work, psychiatrists get personally involved with their patients—much more than other doctors. As a consequence, the stress experienced in psychiatry is immense (Hafner 2002).

With the knowledge of coping skills and strategies we are also expected to be in a better position to look after our own or our colleagues' mental health, but is that possible? We don't! In fact, just reverse is true. Among health professionals, psychiatrists are at higher risk of mental illness, burnout, and suicide (Thomsen et al 1999; Rathod et al 2000). A study reported that psychiatrists had high emotional exhaustion and depersonalization compared to primary care physicians, yet both groups scored high on personal achievement (Snibbe et al 1989). In another study, out of 55 psychiatrists who responded to a postal questionnaire (mean age 41.5 yr), 27 scored poorly on emotional exhaustion, 26 on depersonalization, and most rated favorably on professional accomplishment (Lozinskaia 2002). Psychiatrists' vulnerability to compassion fatigue and burnout can't be ignored and must be taken seriously.

ARE WE THEN DESTINED TO BE MISERABLE?

It is not all doom and gloom that we psychiatrists face in our chosen path. There is a lot that we can do that can help us continue finding enjoyment in our profession. Lifestyle factors and paying attention to one's nonprofessional life is reported to protect us from work stress (Garfinkel et al 2001). Academic work has been reported (Clark and Vaccaro 1987) to be negatively correlated with depersonalization, emotional exhaustion, and overall stress. Adding academic commitments to the busy lives of clinicians may not intuitively appear to protect against work stress. After all, teaching is yet an added responsibility and needs preparation and commitment, without any reduction in clinical workload. It has been suggested that personality traits of people with academic interests (Agius et al 1996), as well as sense of professional accomplishment from teaching (Rutter et al 2002), may offer protective effects against burnout and work stress. Such optimism needs to be cautiously balanced against the fact that intervention studies are lacking for psychiatrists' burnout. A systematic review of stress, burnout, and coping failed to find any studies that evaluated the use of stress-management interventions in psychiatrists (Fothergill et al 2004). Although well-designed interventional studies are lacking, anecdotal reports exist. For instance, Holloway et al. (2000) listed interventions focusing on the individual (such as social skills training, stress management interventions, social support, and time management) and on the organization (defining role and job characteristics, improving interpersonal relationships, encouraging decentralization in the organizational structure, and improving the physical environment of the workplace). The authors emphasized the importance of formal support through regular feedback and appraisal of psychiatrists' performance, which need to occur even in the absence of any identified problem. They concluded that management of stress and burnout among psychiatrists will need to involve partnership among psychiatrists who are prepared to accept that they are vulnerable to experiencing stress, recognize its onset early, and commit to finding work-life balance and supported by an understanding, caring, work environment.

CONCLUSIONS

Compassion fatigue is a common consequence of chronic exposure to stress. Psychiatrists may be particularly vulnerable to experiencing compassion fatigue because of internal, external, and patient-related factors. It can be seen as an early phase of burnout and therefore ameliorating compassion fatigue may have considerable preventative power, given the considerable adverse effects of burnout on the health care system, patient care, and moreover on psychiatrists' lives. Recognizing it early could help us minimize the risk of psychiatrists harming themselves and their near ones. Psychiatrists need to take responsibility for their own well-being by getting better at recognizing stress, exploring non-work-related recreational opportunities, and finding a work-life balance.

REFERENCES

Agius R.M., Blenkin H., Deary I.J. et al. Survey of perceived stress and work demands of consultant doctors. *Occup Environ Med* 1996; 53, 217–224.

Benson J (2005) Compassion fatigue and burnout: The role of Balint Groups. *Australian Family Physician.* 34: 497–498.

Carson. J and Kuipers E (1998) Stress management interventions. In *Occupational Stress: Personal and Professional Approaches* (ed. S Hardy, J Carson and B Thomas) Cheltenham: Stanley Thornes.

Carson J, Maal S, Roche S, Fagin L, De Villiers N, O'Malley P, Holloway F. Burnout in mental health nurses: Much ado about nothing? *Stress Medicine* 1999; 15: 127–134.

Clark GH, Vaccaro JV. Burnout among CMHC psychiatrists and the struggle to survive. *Hosp Commun Psychiatry* 1987; 38: 843–847.

Deary IJ, Agius RM, Sadler A. (1996) Personality and stress in consultant psychiatrists. *Int J Soc Psychiatry.* 42:112–123.

Draper R, Galbraith D, Frost B (1989) Physician recruitment in Ontario provincial psychiatric hospitals. *Canadian Journal of Psychiatry.* 34: 800–803.

Dutton MA and Rubinstein FL (1995) Working with people with PTSD: Research Implications. In *Compassion Fatigue: Coping with secondary traumatic stress disorders in those who treat the traumatised* (eds. CR Figley) NY: Brunner/Mazel, 1995.

Fothergill A, Edwards D, Burnard P. Stress, burnout, coping and stress management in psychiatrists: findings from a systematic review. *Int J Soc Psychiatry* 2004; 50: 54–65.

Freudenberger H. J. (1974) Staff burnout. *J Soc Issues* 1974; 30:159–165.

Garfinkel PE, Bagby RM, Schuller DR et al. Predictors of success and satisfaction in the practice of psychiatry: a preliminary follow-up study. *Can J Psychiatry* 2001; 46: 835–840.

Hafner H. (2002) Psychiatry as a profession (Psychiatrie als Beruf) *Nervenarzt.* 73:33–40.

Haller RM, Deluty RH (1988): Assaults on staff by psychiatric inpatients. A critical review. *British Journal of Psychiatry* 152: 174–179.

Halpern J (2001) *From detached concern to empathy: Humanizing medical practice.* Oxford: Oxford University Press.

Holloway F, Szmukler G, Carson J. Support systems. 1. Introduction. *Advances in Psychiatric Treatment* 2000;6: 226–235.

Huggard P (2003) Compassion Fatigue: How much can I give? *Medical Education.* 37: 163–164.

Hughes D; Burke D, Hickie I; Wilson A, and Tobin M (2002) Advanced training in adult psychiatry. *Australasian Psychiatry.* 10:6–11.

Kirchner JE, Owen RR (1996) Choosing a career in psychiatry. *American Journal of Psychiatry.* 153: 1372.

Langsley DL, Robinowitz CB (1979) Psychiatric manpower: An overview. *Hospital and Community Psychiatry.* 30:749–755.

Lazarus A (1994) Opportunities for psychiatrists in managed care organizations. *Hospital and Community Psychiatry.* 45: 1206–1210.

Lozinskaia, E. I. (2002) Study of stress parameters in the work of the clinical psychiatrist. *International Journal of Mental Health.* 31: 93–98.

Martin F, Poyen D, Bouderlique E, Gouvernet J, Rivet B, Disdier P, Martinez O, Scotto JC (1997) Depression and Burnout in Hospital Health Care Professionals. *Int J Occup Environ Health.* 3:204–209.

Maslach C and Jackson SE. (1986) *Maslach Burnout Inventory manual* (2nd ed) Palo Alto: Consulting Psychologist Press.

Meier, ST (1984) The construct validity of burnout. *Journal of Occupational Psychology.* 57: 211–219.

Meier DE, Back AL, Morrison RS. The inner life of physicians and care of the seriously ill. *Journal of American Medical Association* 2001; 286: 3007–3014.

Pullan SE, Lorbergs KA (2001) Recruitment and retention: a successful model in forensic psychiatric nursing. *Journal of Psychosocial Nursing.* 39: 18–25.

Rathod, S; Roy, L; Ramsay, M; Das, M; Birtwistle, J; and Kingdon, D. (2000) A survey of stress in psychiatrists working in the Wessex Region. *Psychiatric Bulletin.* 24: 133–136.

Rutter H, Herzberg J, Paice E. Stress in doctors and dentists who teach. *Med Educ* 2002; 36:543–549.

Snibbe JR, Radcliffe T, Weisberger C, Richards M, Kelly J (1989). Burnout among primary care physicians and mental health professionals in a managed health care setting. *Psychol Rep.* 65(3 Pt 1):775–780.

Snyder TG, Kumar S. Who do I serve? An experiential perspective of problems in retaining psychiatrists in New Zealand. *Australasian Psychiatry* 2004; 12: 401–403.

Storer D (2002) Recruiting and retaining psychiatrists. *Br J Psychiatry;* 180:296–297.

Thompson C. (1998) The mental state we are in: Morale and psychiatry. *Psychiatr Bull;* 22: 405–409.

Thomsen S, Soares J, Nolan P, Dallender J, & Arnetz B. Feelings of professional fulfillment and exhaustion in mental health personnel: The importance of organisational and individual factors. *Psychotherapy Psychosomatics* 1999; 68: 157–164.

Wright B (2004) Compassion fatigue: How to avoid it? (editorial) *Palliative Medicine.* 18:3–4.

MEDICAL STUDENTS AND RESIDENTS

JESSICA CHYNOWETH

I read *The House of God* by Samuel Shem after my 4th year of medical school before start-ing my intern year. For those who haven't read it, it describes the experiences of an internal medicine resident back in the 1940s at Harvard. While reading I was taken by the sheer number of "medical" dramas and comedies that have sprung from this book, in particular *Scrubs*. I also noted how many of the experiences the main character has and situations he describes occur in hospitals today on a daily basis. Medical education in a lot of ways has not really changed. You still have hierarchies that are in many ways essential to the func-tioning of the hospital. During your medical education you slowly climb from the low-est rung, that of a medical student, to the highest rung, an attending physician. There is some degree of hazing, as you move up, in the form of sometimes inhumanly long hours, although over the years, with the new duty hour regulations, this has improved.

In addition, when you are at your most exhausted, one of the residents or attending physicians will put you on the spot and quiz you on diagnoses and treatments for your own educational benefit. This is commonly referred to as "pimping." The pressure to per-form well under such circumstances are more significant during medical school in many ways. During medical school you spend a lot of time worrying how your performance is going to affect your ability to get into a "good" residency or specialty.

However, now that I am a practicing family physician thinking back on my medi-cal school years, the things that stand out for me are not the long hours and the stress I endured, but the life lessons and patients' stories that I will carry with me for the rest of my career and life. One of the most important life lessons is to be present in your life and find balance. For example, no matter how tired you are, acting like a zombie and grunting in response to a question is not an appropriate way to interact with your significant other. In addition, it is not acceptable to ignore Valentines Day just because you are having a difficult week or month. I will always be eternally grateful for my husband putting up with me for the 7 years of my medical training.

I often reflect upon the fact that as you climb the medical ladder, the amount of time that you can spend really learning about a patient decreases substantially. By learning, I don't necessarily mean book learning, although that too is valuable. I am referring more to the opportunity to really sit with patients and hear their stories. It is these interactions that I will always carry with me. The first one was appropriately during my first year of medical school. As part of our medical training we had a clinical skills class that taught us many things, including how to "interview" patients. One day we were to go into the hospital, a pretty foreign and intimidating place, and "interview" one of several patients who had been preselected for us. I felt so insecure and inadequate. It seemed a monumental task at the time. The patient chosen for me was a woman with sickle cell anemia, something that is rare in New Mexico but common many other places. I was totally tongue tied, so she just told me her story. I carry with me countless other experiences with me from my medical training, such as the schizophrenic patient on the VA psych ward who scared the wits out if me but who also tried to teach me to play chess. There have also been patent deaths, which for a long time left me crying in the bathroom. I am lucky to have a practice in which I have longer appointment times than many of my peers, but I still sometimes miss those "slow" night calls when you could just spend time in the patients' rooms, learning from them and focusing solely on true patient care.

When it all comes down to it, medical training is so much more than long hours and book knowledge. It is more than the hazing that we all go through. It is the patients and the lessons that we learn that are the most valuable.

/// 22 /// FAMILY MEDICINE

I will Never Fly in a Helicopter Again

BRUCE ARROLL

I was working in a small rural town in British Columbia in the mid-1980s. I was on call at the local hospital, which had about 25 beds, and the medical side was run by four physicians. I was called to the emergency room to see a man who had been injured in his left groin by a chainsaw. He was the person standing behind the person using the chainsaw and his job was to monitor the situation for safety. He was meant to be wearing a leather apron to prevent the injury he received from happening. The chainsaw "bucked" and jumped back and hit him in the groin severing at least his femoral artery. Blood spurted out with the expected arterial force. Unfortunately the man with the chainsaw ran for help rather than putting pressure on the wound. The injured man rapidly exsanguinated.

By the time he arrived at the emergency room he was conscious. The hospital kept packed red cells on the premises and he was given two units rapidly. There was concern that he had obviously torn his left femoral artery as he had no pulses in his leg. We felt some urgency to get him to the regional hospital. A small forestry helicopter was available. The decision was made to transfer him at about 7 P.M.—this gave us 30 minutes to get him into the helicopter and fly away. The flight rules said you had to take off in daylight but could land in the dark. We put all the resuscitation gear in the plane and loaded the patient on board. The pilot was in the front seat with me behind him and the patient was on a bed that occupied the other front and back seat. I vaguely noted as we took off that the intravenous lines had been caught under the stretcher but as the patient was conscious I was not too concerned. We rose above the 8,000 foot mountains and it rapidly became dark. To my horror the patient stopped breathing. I could not feel a pulse and assumed he had had a full cardiac arrest.

I commenced cardiopulmonary resuscitation giving mouth to mouth and cardiac massage. Every time I pushed on his chest the helicopter rocked. The pilot could only watch helplessly. All the gear I needed to intubate him was sitting, unavailable, under his stretcher bed. The thought that kept going through my mind was that we should have taken him by land in an ambulance and if we had done this we could have stopped and got him stabilized. I thought that perhaps he had started bleeding from his femoral wound as we had not had time to ensure that it would not start bleeding again.

I kept thinking of myself in the coroner's court trying to explain my decision and how I/we had made the decision that had "killed" him. As I beat up myself I could see myself being struck off the medical register for incompetence. It was such a relief to see the lights of the Royal Inland Hospital in Kamloops. The helicopter landed and the patient was transferred to the emergency department. I was physically and mentally exhausted. I sat on the floor in a corner and watched what was going on. A group of doctors took over and got to work on him. They had the occasional glance at me, sitting on the floor, but they carried on with their tasks. I assumed they had no idea what had just happened to me. He was stabilized and taken to the intensive care unit (ICU).

I had a friend who lived in Kamloops so I called him up to see if I could stay with him overnight until I could get back to my home town. In the midst of explaining what had happened I burst in to tears—he thought my wife had been killed in a car accident as I could relate so little of my story without crying. There was a general internist in the doctors' coffee room who was not expecting to have a colleague burst into tears and did not know how to comfort me. He looked uncomfortable and made no comment to me. My friend collected me and it was very cathartic to be able to talk with him and his wife about my experience.

The patient stayed in the ICU for a few days. He developed swelling of his brain, which suggested that he had at least had a respiratory arrest and his absent pulse reflected his low blood volume. He may have had a full cardiac arrest but no one will ever know. Fortunately for all concerned he survived and returned to my office a few months later to thank me. That was quite an emotional meeting to see him face to face. His mother wrote me a letter thanking me for saving her son's life.

There are a number of lessons from this. The practical one is to train rural physicians/staff in the skills and issues of transferring sick patients. Another lesson is how hard we can be on ourselves when things go wrong. Also, our general internist could use some training in how to deal with crying people (he was quite out of his depth). Had the patient died there would have been other lessons and stresses to cope with. As it was I did a locum tenens in Kamloops the following year and one of the emergency physicians complimented me on my "heroic" action. That left me feeling very healed a, far cry from the self torment of the helicopter flight. I did, however, decide I would never transfer a patient in a helicopter again and never did. I now work in a big city.

Every time a helicopter brings in a patient to the city hospital I get a welling of tears, suggesting that my soul has a little scar from that night of terror.

/// 23 /// ANESTHESIOLOGY

Personal Reflections

ROBIN YOUNGSON

INTRODUCTION

As a newly appointed anesthesiologist in a large teaching hospital, I was the master of technical expertise. But technical mastery alone, as a source of identity and self-esteem, left me vulnerable in dealing with the emotional side of medicine. I did not have the communication and relationship skills to support a patient when technical skill was not enough, especially if a patient came to harm through error. I was also not aware of the power dynamic between doctor and patient and many times failed to help my patients because I unconsciously took control. I was skilled at diverting the agenda onto technical areas of practice where I felt confident, rather than understanding the needs of the patient.

Salvation came in the guise of a wise old patient who taught me some profound lessons in compassionate practice. She taught me that caring and compassion is a two-way street, equally of benefit to the physician as well as the patient. She also taught me the power of choosing an attitude and how profoundly you can shape the world around you.

As I learned to serve my patients on their own terms, my fear and vulnerability dissipated. I replaced clinical detachment with open-hearted compassion. My practice has never been more joyful and rewarding.

MY GREATEST TEACHER

When I first met Jessie, she was 85 years young. She came to my hospital clinic in a wheelchair, looking somehow crumpled and lopsided, owing to a devastating stroke suffered many years ago. Her left side was completely paralyzed. The tissues of her face sagged in untidy folds like an unmade bed. She had only half a smile but there was mischief and light in her eyes. Despite an appalling burden of medical complaints, she still managed to live alone. I quickly began to sense an indomitable spirit.

Jessie came to my preoperative clinic because she had bowel cancer. Her surgeon was fearful of submitting her to the perils of surgery, with her advanced age and with so many complicating medical conditions.

In my hospital, I had created the very first anesthesiology clinic and I had written to all my surgical colleagues, inviting them to send me their "worst cases," those that faced life-threatening risks in contemplating surgery. I promised I would do my best to assess the level of risk and to help patients come to a decision about taking their chances with risky surgery. I took my job, and myself, very seriously.

Jessie was the most challenging patient that ever came to my clinic. It took me a long time to summarize all the information from her bulky hospital charts, to inquire into her current symptoms, and to perform a physical examination.

She was in serious trouble. Her bowel cancer was continually bleeding, causing severe anemia. She had subacute bowel obstruction. In addition to her massive stroke, Jessie had a catalogue of other serious medical problems. Heart disease headed the list and she had critical aortic stenosis, severe coronary disease, and poorly controlled heart failure. In addition, she suffered obesity, diabetes, hypertension, and renal impairment. She consumed 11 different medications. Her life hung in the balance. She reported frequent angina at rest, each bout accompanied by breathlessness.

My report to the surgeon spanned three pages. I concluded that Jessie had only a 50% chance of leaving the operating theater alive and that her prospects of ever leaving the hospital were dismal. There was little we could do to improve her condition except to correct her anemia with a blood transfusion.

With a heavy heart, I did my best to explain to Jessie the enormity of the surgical risk.

"What's the alternative?" she asked.

"If you don't have surgery, the blockage in your bowel will get worse, the bleeding will continue, and you will probably die of heart failure and bowel obstruction."

"Is there any other form of treatment for the bowel cancer?"

"No," I replied, shaking my head. "We would do our best to keep you comfortable."

"Well then, I really don't have a choice. Robin, I want you to take on my case, I want you to do my surgery. I'll take my chance. I've had a good life and if I die having surgery then it's not anyone's fault. I won't blame you."

I then began to explain to Jessie that we could reduce the risk of her surgery if we gave her a blood transfusion. In response, Jessie smiled sweetly and told me she would not accept a blood transfusion because she was a Jehovah's Witness.

She must have seen the expression of dismay on my face. In a surprising gesture, she took my hand in hers. "Robin, I put my faith in you. I know you'll do the best job you can and God will be watching over you."

I confess I felt very uncomfortable with this behavior. Clinical detachment was at threat here. Not only was she addressing me by my first name but also she was holding my hand and invoking her God to watch over me.

My next clinic patient was waiting. I told Jessie that I would write to her surgeon recommending surgery, even though the risk was very high. She thanked me for my time. As I called in the next patient, I sincerely hoped that the awful challenge of giving an anesthetic to Jessie would fall to one of my anesthesiologist colleagues.

However, fate had determined that this would be a very personal lesson for me. On the eve of surgery, I discovered to my dismay that I was the anesthesiologist allocated to the operating theatre where Jessie would have her operation. With a heavy heart I went to consult with her on the ward. I felt duty bound to explain again the dire risks she was facing and to document these concerns on the consent form.

Jessie cut me off short. "Robin, we've discussed all that already. I understand the risks I'm taking but I put my faith in you. I know you will do the best you can."

She held my hand again. This was disconcerting. She said to me, "Robin, you're looking so worried about giving my anesthetic that I think I need to cheer you up. I'm going to tell you a joke!"

Lifting her forefinger to touch her lips, she blew a lopsided and wet sounding raspberry. "What's that?" she said.

"I have no idea," I replied, shaking my head in confusion and disbelief.

"It's a fart trying to get past a g-string!" she said with a wicked twinkle in her eye.

I was now completely undone. Any semblance of the proper doctor-patient relationship had now dissolved in helpless mirth. When my tears of laughter were wiped away, I revised my estimate of her chances of survival. This was a human spirit not yet ready to depart the world. We made our farewells and to my surprise I was able to put aside my fretful worrying to sleep soundly in preparation for the next day's challenge.

Jessie had a stormy time in surgery and post-operative care. She narrowly scraped through several crises, never once complaining. I went to see her, three days after surgery, when she was back on the ward.

She held my hand again. With a twinkle in her eye, she said, "Robin, I prayed that you would survive my anesthetic, and you did!"

Those events took place many years ago. Jessie has since passed on but her spirit is ever present. She has been my greatest teacher.

Before I met Jessie, I conceived of the doctor-patient relationship as a one-way street. I was the highly trained doctor, the expert and the person with authority and control. Caring was a one-way process. I cared for patients and determined the process and the agenda. Patients didn't care for me. They were grateful, of course, they took my advice and they did what I told them. Those who didn't were "difficult patients" or "noncompliant."

But somehow, Jessie turned the tables on me. She was the one caring for me and supporting me in my difficulties. The relationship had become a two-way process.

What Jessie had recognized was my own vulnerability. She undid all of my defenses with remarkable ease but it has taken me years of reflection to recognize the source of that deep vulnerability and to heal some of my own wounds.

There's little doubt that doctors are brutalized in their training. I recall one Saturday afternoon, working as an anesthesiologist resident, in which I did my best to save three patients but instead witnessed the death in quick succession of a young mother, a baby, and a nineteen-year-old motorcyclist. In each case, after failed surgery and resuscitation, I wrote up all the notes and reported the deaths to the authorities. I was halfway through a fourteen-hour shift. There was no suggestion that I might not be in a fit state to carry on with my duties, or that I should be sent home, or receive support or counseling.

That day, I anesthetized five more patients. I first had a cup of tea and then went to see my next patient. As I asked him to sign the consent form, the internal voice in my head was saying, "Hmm, I wonder if this should be part of informed consent? Should I tell my patient that my last three patients all died?" Of course, I just kept quiet and carried on with my shift.

By any standard this is a brutally inhumane practice. It hasn't changed. Four weeks ago I witnessed one of my obstetrician colleagues undergo a traumatic event in which a healthy baby died. He carried on with a 24-hour shift and did three more Cesarean operations that night. A few hours later, in a state of exhaustion and sleep deprivation, he was performing elective surgery on a routine morning gynecology list. There was no support, no time off, and no counseling.

We are taught clinical detachment as a fundamentally important value in medical practice. It subsequently becomes a psychological defense mechanism as we attempt to avoid the emotional cost of witnessing suffering and tragic losses. We put on the cloak of the hero doctor. For myself, I can say that almost my whole sense of professional identity and self-esteem was connected with being a technical expert. As an anesthesiologist in a large teaching hospital, I was at the pinnacle of technical medicine. However, if my care failed, or my patient was harmed through error, I experienced a devastating failure of professional purpose. Moreover, I was not equipped with the communication or relationship skills to care for a patient who was harmed. I felt deeply inadequate and shunned such patients. They were cruelly abandoned at their time of greatest need. I believed that the best protection against such emotionally disturbing experiences was to have no emotional connection with my patients.

In reality, we are not able to switch off our emotions. Each of these tragedies leaves a wound in our own heart because we entered into medicine with a deep desire to provide care and compassion. These failures create an irresolvable conflict within us, which is the source of so much vulnerability and fear. We become skilled at masking the pain and strive to achieve ever-higher levels of technical competence to compensate for our feelings of inadequacy.

Jessie, though, could see through all my bravado. In truth, I was afraid of the responsibility of anesthetizing an elective patient who was likely to die on the operating table. In sensing my vulnerability, she not only offered support but also began to teach me lessons that have profoundly shaped my practice over the years. These changes have taken almost all of the fear out of my clinical practice and have led me to renewed joy and satisfaction. As my practice has deepened, I have come to believe that much that we are taught about objectivity and clinical detachment is not only wrong but also harmful. These new understandings have given me much greater resilience as a physician but also have made me much more effective and humane in my practice.

The first lesson that Jessie taught me was that caring and compassion are two-way processes; the doctor benefits from the relationship as much as the patient. There is a widespread belief among doctors that we need to limit our emotional connection with patients because all of our compassion will run out. This one-sided view of compassion is a peculiarly Western belief. In the Buddhist world, every act of compassion is seen as providing compassion equally for the giver as the receiver. That has been my recent experience; the more I bring open-hearted compassion to the care of my patients, the more love I have to give. It's a mutually sustaining practice.

In truth, when I met Jessie on the eve of her surgery, there were two people who were afraid, not just one. That we both survived the experience was owing to the mutual interdependence and support we gave each other. As my practice has deepened I have come to recognize the extraordinary privilege of being a witness to the capacity of ordinary people to deal with life's challenges. As a technical expert, I was always busy doing things to fix or to help patients. Now I appreciate that doing "nothing" is sometimes the most profound support I can offer. The quality of being I bring to the encounter may be more important than anything that I do. I have found it is helpful to be a little more humble and to judge less. In the end, we are all equal.

The second lesson from Jessie was about choosing an attitude. In the face of severe disability, constant pain, and the prospect of almost certain death over the next few days or weeks, she chose her attitude with care. She wasn't grumpy or ill-tempered. She didn't complain. She didn't dwell on her misfortune. She chose instead to show concern and compassion for me as a vulnerable human being. She gave me support, she cheered me up, and she told me a joke.

If Jessie could choose humor, laughter, and compassion in her awful circumstances, then what excuse could I have for grumpiness or self-pity? It took me some years to learn this lesson and I precisely recall the moment when this gift from Jessie finally settled into my being.

I was driving to the hospital to perform an epidural injection for pain relief in a laboring mother. It was my fourth call out of bed after a long day of dealing with a stream of emergencies. I felt exhausted, very grumpy, and sorry for myself. Quite suddenly, Jessie's remarkable example came into my mind and I felt instantly ashamed. I began to realize that filling my mind with grumpy thoughts was an idiotic waste of energy. I decided, instead, to focus on the extraordinary privilege of being invited to participate in childbirth, one of the most intimate events in our lives. It was a very deliberate process of choosing the thoughts and attitudes I would bring to the patient, replacing grumpiness with gentleness and compassion.

Over several months, an extraordinary change occurred. The quality of greeting I received in the delivery room was transformed. The midwives welcomed me warmly, anticipated my needs and assisted in getting epidural injections completed much more quickly. I noticed the rate of complications was reduced and I had fewer calls back for inadequate pain relief. After each procedure, I went home with a feeling of deep pleasure and satisfaction and I didn't care how many times I was called out of bed. Each call was a precious invitation.

At a later date I shifted my attitude toward "difficult" patients—I decided that the problem was probably a difficult doctor, not a difficult patient. I promised myself that I would try to listen better and to understand the unmet need before I rushed to judgment. The "difficult" patients seemed to melt away and I began to derive much more pleasure from my practice.

My anesthesiologist colleagues began to look at me rather oddly when I declared that, henceforth, I would try to respond to every single concern brought by my patients. What would happen, I wondered, if we assumed that no patient ever makes unreasonable demands? My colleagues' reaction arose from the universal experience of health professionals: that demand is overwhelming. Everybody knows there are just not enough beds, or doctors, or hours in the day to cope with the rising tide of health problems laid at our door. We survive only by putting up barriers to try to limit the demand.

The result of my new strategy was both unexpected and delightful. The demands from my patients grew fewer, not greater. I was puzzled until I came across a brief article by Rachel Naomi Remen, which explained the difference between fixing, helping, and serving. I knew all about "fixing" because I was a master of technical medicine. When I couldn't fix, helping seemed laudable. But I came to realize that even in the process of helping, it was I who retained the knowledge and power. I prevented patients from helping themselves. I realized that if we spend all of our time fixing and helping, then we make ourselves responsible for every single life problem presented by our patients.

It turns out that "serving" is a different quality of relationship. The hallmark of service, writes Remen, is that the people being served experience personal growth. They develop their capacity to be responsible for their own health and wellbeing, and to find their own solutions. To serve another person, you need first to understand their concerns and then to bring your knowledge, skill, and power to the service of those needs. The agenda is set by the patient, not the doctor. The doctor assumes the role of a coach, a mentor, and facilitator in addition to bringing technical skills, knowledge, caring, and compassion.

I had to learn many new skills about communication and relationships but as I did I found I could build trust and get to the heart of the matter much more quickly. In a clinic session I still see as many patients as my colleagues do. I give no more time but my patients feel that I have truly listened. It is deeply gratifying to see a patient's fear and anxiety transform into self-confidence that he or she can face the challenge. There is a deeper bond of trust. I am no longer afraid of being persecuted for complications or mistakes. My patients know that I have done my very best, that I cannot promise more, and that I care for them deeply. When things go wrong they are quick to forgive and to offer me support.

The final lesson that Jessie taught me was that laughter is the best medicine. No matter how dire the circumstances, there is a place for gentle humor or a good belly laugh. If we can learn to laugh at ourselves we open up our hearts to a deeper human connection and have the humility to learn. Laughter is a wonderful release for tension and anger. A workplace that creates fun and humor through the day is a more joyous, creative, and energizing place to work, no matter the challenges.

Chapter 16 spoke of the "ethical violence" done to physicians by the modern healthcare environment. What I learned from Jessie is how profoundly I could reshape my experience of the world by choosing my attitude, dropping my defenses, and mindfully bringing gratitude and appreciation to my daily practice. Humor too, plays its part. There's a lightness to my day that doesn't allow the arrows of misfortune to find their mark.

These simple lessons from Jessie—humanity, interdependence, choosing an attitude, and laughter—are a wonderful prescription for personal transformation and for developing open-hearted compassion. Happily, recent advances in neuroscience and positive psychology offer us a wealth of evidence that these strategies are the pathway to personal flourishing.

I still witness tragedy but my response is different. I cry with my patients and offer them a hug. The tears are the beginning of healing for both of us. I walk away with compassion in my heart, not sorrow.

When we open our hearts to our patients, they offer us such gifts. I thought I needed to be resilient but I learned that the secret is to take off our armor, not put it on.

RESOURCES

Remen, RN. In the service of life. *Noetic Sciences Review* 1996; 37:24–25.
Youngson, R. Time to Care—How to love your patients and your job. 2012. Paperback 260pp. Rebelheart Publishers, Raglan, New Zealand.

/// 24 /// EMERGENCY MEDICINE

LISA MORENO-WALTON

WHO ARE EMERGENCY PHYSICIANS?

We are happy to leave to the pediatrician the long-term monitoring and treatment of juvenile diabetes, to the cardiologist the management of congestive heart failure and adjustment of antihypertensive agents, to the neurologist the monitoring of the slow decompensation of the brain afflicted with Alzheimer's disease. Frankly, although we can understand how some of our colleagues find satisfaction in enduring relationships with their patients, we find these things boring. We would rather splint a Greenstick fracture, send our little patient on his way, and move on to the next case.

When you ask EPs why they chose their specialty, there are generally three common denominators: (1) the opportunity to use the full breadth of what was learned in medical school, (2) the excitement of never knowing what we are going to see and do and deal with on any given day when we go to work, and (3) the ability to really and truly save lives in real time.

In the House of Medicine, we all like to diagnose each other, and EPs are often accused of having two psychiatric diagnoses: attention deficit hyperactivity disorder (ADHD) and obsessive compulsive disorder (OCD). ADHD comes in very handy in a frenetically busy Emergency Department (ED) when you must be aware of everything that is going on with every patient everywhere and at every minute. And if you are an academic physician, you must be aware of what is going on with all your residents as well. We are the master multitaskers. We can be listening to a resident present a case, and taking in every detail, forming our differential diagnosis, deciding what labs and radiologic studies we will and will not order, and yet very clearly hear the conversation that is taking place to our left, just outside of our field of vision, between a patient who was already discharged and was given two days off from work and has come back in and is now trying to convince one of our medical students why he should have an entire week off.

In the ED, we are quite literally all over the place, both physically as we run from one patient to another and from one emergency to another, and mentally as we continuously run through each patient's history, physical findings, and study results putting the evidence together to reach a diagnosis and plan the next intervention. And yet we are obsessively attentive to detail. While a patient is with us, every detail of his physical exam is uppermost in our minds, every lab value is temporarily memorized even if we have 30 patients at a time, every procedure is performed perfectly, and every dressing is meticulously applied.

EPs are often described as "adrenaline junkies." We like to move quickly from case to case, we like the closure of accomplishing a rapid diagnosis, or when that is not possible, a rapid disposition on every patient. It's like a quick fix, and both the meanings are true: We fix things quickly (making the cure, the diagnosis, or the disposition) and we get our personal dose of that substance to which we are all addicted: adrenaline. You may hear ED nurses saying, "I hope it's quiet today," but an EP will never say that. At the end of a busy shift, we say, "That was a great shift!" and during a slow period, we say, "I hate when it's not busy. The time drags on and I'm so bored."

Many doctors, most doctors, save lives. The psychiatrist heals the psyche of the near suicide so that the patient returns to his family and his community and is eventually happy that he is still alive. The chemotherapy regimen prescribed by the oncologist successfully puts a teenager's Hodgkin's lymphoma into remission and she goes on to graduate from college and becomes a special education teacher. The orthopedist diagnoses a Ewing's tumor and performs the amputation that allows a young man to be alive at the birth of his son and to watch that child grow up. These are the rewarding, validating experiences that keep doctors coming to work each day and night and weekend and holiday, while other professionals are sleeping soundly or out playing golf.

But it is only the EP, the trauma surgeon, and the intensivist who are presented with patients on the brink of death or already dead and who bring them back to the land of the living on a daily and routine basis. We watch death defied before our very eyes, but most important, under our very hands. It is extremely difficult to replicate that rush in anything one can do in "the real world."

STRESSORS OF EMERGENCY PHYSICIANS

The stressors of EPs can be divided among their work, their patients, other doctors, and everything else. Yes, we take care of the most difficult patients. We serve as their last hope before they die. As emergency docs, we become accustomed to being around death, and it is no longer a stressor for us. Blood and smells that are unpleasant to most other people become a part of the background environment of the ED. And it is not the distressed patients. Like anyone who is distressed, they require patience and kindness as well as direct answers.

The areas of stress for an ER doc are (1) absorbing the emotional intensity of patients and loved ones, (2) working in a fishbowl, (3) enduring unrealistic expectations, (4) exposure to the worst qualities of human nature, and (5) every action has life-and-death consequences that include medical malpractice risks.

Absorbing the Emotional Intensity

As the person most responsible for saving a patient or a cherished family member or friend, the EP is the focus of a considerable amount of emotionally charged attention. We feel the pressure of the patient's or the family's wish to hear good news. Early in our careers, we may have a flight response, and the need to get away from the patient or the family quickly often results in the inappropriately short and blunt announcements of bad news that residents and junior attending physicians make. Later in our careers, we may find that we have hardened ourselves against the all-too-frequent pain of death notifications or the diagnosis of terminal disease, and may again be so blunt as to appear uncaring. Patients and their supporters often present with an almost desperate requirement that we physicians know it all and know it now. But our stressors are not limited to emergency patients.

EPs are on display to everyone—especially wearing scrubs. We are observed and judged by the public. On duty, we are expected to know everything about all medical emergencies, often without getting a substantial history and before doing a complete physical exam. This is true within the House of Medicine, where our colleagues can be potential critics, as well as with the public, whose sometimes unrealistic expectations are influenced by numerous popular television shows.

Enduring Unrealistic Expectations

All physicians feel the pressure to uphold a standard—following the Hippocratic oath to first do no harm. Yet often, emergency physicians are held to an unrealistic standard. Many patients and those who love them expect that the ED will provide assessment and treatment of the highest standard in the world, because that is what is deserved by the person they love. In the current health care environment, it is not uncommon for a patient to come to the ED because they cannot get a clinic or private office appointment after waiting for weeks or even months. So the EP who works up the complaint, even if the workup is not conclusive, becomes the best doctor in the world. Other doctors may be less impressed, viewing EPs as doing too little, interacting with patients too briefly, and releasing the patient to her or his own personal physician to do the definitive care. Moreover, when an on-call physician gets a call from an EP, it can mean only one of two things: either the physician needs to come to the ED to do an admission, and that means more work (often unpaid), or that physician's service has had a complication. Neither of these are good news.

Enduring the Worst of Humanity

While death is a normal part of a human life and injuries happen to everyone, no matter how cautious, on any given shift n an urban trauma hospital, we see deaths and injuries that are far from normal. They are the result of unbearable cruelty, hatred, carelessness, or just plain stupidity. These are the stories that are so funny that we have to laugh out loud, or so heartbreaking that we might reflect upon them throughout our careers. Although the ED offers opportunities to see the valiant and courageous acts that characterize human beings, we also see the worst that humanity has to offer: Stupidity, cruelty, and preventable death.

Our Patients

Emergency physicians like to say that we do not have private patients, yet many of the homeless, chronically ill, mentally ill, and addicted become what we refer to as "Frequent Flyers." The Frequent Fliers are the people who are scorned by society. They cannot find a private doc in the community who can tolerate them for more than one visit. Frequent Fliers are chronically noncompliant with medications and instructions, they abuse their bodies and their souls, and they fail to adhere to the basic demands of society.

Frequent Fliers come into the ED demanding food, a shower, a bed, and pain medication. They refuse to follow the rules. They will urinate and defecate in the corner of the Department, and then go into the bathroom to smoke cigarettes and shoot heroin. And they often know each other from the street, and will fight with each other during their time in the ED.

Emergency physicians often joke about whether we are doctors or kindergarten teachers when we are taking care of these patients. "Be nice," one of my colleagues often tells patients. "You can't steal food from other patients' trays or curse at them. You have to be nice." We bargain with them, telling them that they can have a bed for the night and breakfast in the morning if they stay in the bed and stop asking for Vicodan and using foul language.

You know you've met an Emergency Physician when someone calls out, "Yo, bitch," and she turns around and responds, "Do you need something?" There is little appreciation for what we do for these patients, and certainly, we are not practicing medicine during most of their care. Urban teaching hospitals don't have budgets for full-time social workers and most cities do not have sufficient resources to cope with patients such as these. In the best of circumstances, when a thoughtful nurse or medical student takes time to call around to find a homeless shelter with an available bed for one of them, the patient will often opt not to go. "Yeah, but they don't let me drink in there, doc. How can I go there if they don't let me drink?"

Even the patients who do not come with significant social problems, the ones we call "citizens" (the people with jobs and bills and homes and families and responsibilities) are not at their best when they come to us. Our patients do not shower, put on their Sunday best, and show up for their clinic appointment. They are pulled from burning buildings, dragged bleeding from the scene of a domestic dispute, brought from the job site where they suddenly developed crushing chest pain, or carried off of their favorite easy chair after experiencing facial numbness and slurred speech while watching soap operas in their nightgowns.

Our patients are most often unprepared, angry, and frightened by their appearance in the ED and that sets the scene for both the best and the worst behaviors that human beings are able to exhibit. Their lives are interrupted, their bodies have failed them, they have lost control, and, as human beings are wont to do, they vent their frustrations on the people whose very presence highlights their vulnerability: the ED staff. Just as our patients had no idea when they got up in the morning that they would find themselves in the Emergency Department that day, we had no idea that they would come in either. While the excitement and stimulation of not knowing what the shift will bring is part of what we love about EM, it is also one of the stressors. We need to know everything and we need to know it now. We cannot spend the day before reading up on the operation that we are going to do the next day. We cannot sit through a morning of teaching rounds, discussing a differential diagnosis with colleagues and looking symptoms up on the Internet. It is true that we often have time to review a procedure in a text before doing it or check something online, but we have to be prepared for the fact that all too often, we have to know a lot of things cold. In a true emergency, there is no time to look things up or seek another's opinion.

Our patients often feel stripped of their identities when they are asked to strip off their clothes and don a hospital gown. They take on the identity of a patient and a diagnosis, and what is said and done to them is hardly private in most crowded public teaching hospital emergency departments. Similarly, the doctors who say and do it have little privacy as well, and this is a stressor to emergency physicians. We practice in the proverbial fishbowl. There is no time to prepare before breaking the news that the chest x-ray we just ordered because a patient came in with a cough and chest pain is highly suggestive of malignancy. There is no way to rehearse our reaction when the patient with a small bowel obstruction hurls a liter of feculent vomitus at the doctor's chest. We put in our central lines and chest tubes in the presence of family members and colleagues, nurses and students, janitors, EMTs, and the police.

If our technique is not elegant, if we are not successful on the first effort, everyone knows it and it is the talk of corridors and the hospital cafeteria for the next several hours, if not days. No one mentions the fact that while other physicians most often perform their procedures in a controlled setting, EPs most often perform procedures on hypotensive, shocky patients who are either bleeding out from trauma, HIV positive, or septic and trying to die, which would be why they need an emergency procedure in the first place. ED docs are on display and are judged by patients, families, colleagues, the medical system, insurance, government programs, licensing boards.

Everything we do is potentially public. All of our patients, once stabilized, are handed off to other physicians. They are either admitted to the hospital or discharged for follow-up care by another doctor. So, whatever we have done for the patient during his time in the ED is under scrutiny. And usually, whatever we have done is not considered sufficient. Most of us find it endlessly amusing when residents on the in-patient units tell EM residents that they cannot come down to see the patient until all the laboratory results are back. When has an emergency physician ever had lab results prior to seeing a patient?[1] Because patients come to us when they have complications, they will often perceive that we are the all knowing physicians and that their own doctors are less competent. Because they come to us straight from their communities after motor vehicle collisions or gunshot wounds or strokes and we save their lives, they believe us capable of all things. Thus, patients' expectations of emergency physicians are high.

It is not infrequent that they come in saying that they have already to been to many doctors and clinics, none of whom could ascertain the source of their symptoms, so they have come to the ED anticipating that they will be diagnosed and cured. In their own lives, the problems they are experiencing are just as important as any gunshot wound or

---

[1] Not only do the inpatient physicians want a definitive diagnosis, which, incidentally, is not always necessary when one knows the patient needs to be admitted and to what service the patient needs to go, but they want the patient "packaged." This means that every possible lab has been ordered, every possible procedure

myocardial infarction. They cannot imagine that any physician would think otherwise. Thus, we are set up to disappoint these patients. We end up saying: "No, we cannot get an emergency MRI on a Saturday at three o'clock in the morning for the progressive hearing loss you have been having over the past year." Or we might say: "Well, I have found a hernia here and that is the likely cause of your intermittent abdominal pain and nausea, but no, we are not going to have the surgeon operate on you now, at Tuesday noon, when he has a full schedule of cases already." Or we might say, "Sure, I know the Internet says you need a duplex scan for your four months of testicular pain, but trust me, if you had a necrotic testicle in there for four months, you would be septic by now. So no, you will not get a duplex scan."

What compounds the fact that patients are often disappointed in their high expectations, and consultants are often disappointed that we have not completed their workup for them, is the sense that many physicians have that anyone with an MD degree can do the job of the emergency physician.[2]

House of Medicine Strains

What remains a source of stress, even to seasoned physicians, is the constant need to try to "sell" the admission to the inpatient service. A statement we hear commonly is that "I can't admit the patient yet. The UA (urinalysis) is not back yet." To the internist, we sometimes say, "So, if she has a UTI (urinary tract infection), are you going to refuse to admit her for pneumonia?" or we ask the psychiatrist, "And if he has THC (a marker for

---

done, and every possible drug given. Most of us teach our residents that, in this era of cost containment, they ought not to order a study that will not alter our management of the patient in the ED. Young residents often will say something like, "Well, I just know the orthopedist is going to want a sed rate," to which we reply, "Let them get it upstairs." In a crowded ED where patients are waiting for hours to see a doctor, it does not make sense to order tests whose results will not be back for hours, or sometimes days, and will not alter the management or disposition of the patient. This only serves to slow patient through-put time. Other services, however, often interpret this as our lack of knowledge, and EPs, especially young residents and junior faculty, find this a source of stress.

[2] In times gone by, doctors who could not successfully complete a residency or who were on probation of licensure, or who were foreign trained and unable to get into a US residency program, were permitted to work in Emergency Departments. While this has changed in academic settings since the advent of EM residency programs, many US hospitals still permit doctors who are not board certified in EM to practice EM in their EDs. Pathologists who cannot read EKGs, radiologists who cannot suture complicated lacerations, and surgeons who do not know how to do appropriate fever workups on infants are out there making fundamental errors in the care of ED patients across the nation and are making inappropriate requests of consultants to do the exams and procedures that they cannot do. Since these doctors brazenly call themselves "Emergency Room doctors," they are giving real, board-certified, and residency-trained EPs a bad reputation at the same time as they are demeaning our training, our skill set, and our knowledge base.

marijuana use) in his urine, does that mean he can't be admitted to Psych? Since when do psych patients not use drugs in this city?"

Patient Advocacy

We ER docs regard patient advocacy as part of our responsibility. Especially if we care for the underserved and disenfranchised, we regard it as our duty, and almost a badge of honor, to ensure that the patient, who all too frequently is unable to be his own advocate, gets the care that he both needs and deserves. Sometimes, "selling" the patient to a colleague who already has a full panel of patients and has done six or seven admissions that night sets the EP up as an adversary.

When the beeper goes off and the resident or hospitalist sees the extension of the ED, a typical first response is to curse and get that sinking feeling. The EP is rarely calling to say hello or "Meet me for a coffee is either of us gets a free minute tonight." No, the EP is calling to give the on call physician more work.

A call from the Emergency Department means that the on call doctor must haul himself out of the comfort of his bed or away from attending to his patients on the floor. Even worse, (a) it means that he or a member of his department has committed an error in patient management, (b) a patient was discharged prematurely from the Medicine service without getting his stress test and now he is back with chest pain, (c) the patient who underwent a laporotomy now has a wound infection and dehiscence, (d) the patient who was discharged after a dilatation and curettage has symptoms of a uterine rupture. Every doctor's worst nightmare complication is announced to him by an emergency physician. Is it any wonder that they are so ready to announce our complications?

My Work Is Up Close and Personal

Perhaps the worst stressor in emergency medicine is the daily exposure to the very worst deeds of which human beings are capable. The Emergency Department is a violent place in a violent society. Americans seem to glorify violence and aggression in sports and entertainment. We read explicit details of violent crimes in the paper and see pictures of corpses scattered in the streets of war torn cities on the evening news. When we want to be entertained, we go to movies where the "heroes" shoot and maim people while the audience claps. How could the ED be any worse?

The major differences between the violence to which the average American is exposed in the comfort of his living room or at the movies and the violence to which we are exposed in the ED is this: The violence we see in the ED is real.

I see and smell and feel the blood. It is splashed on my clothes and my shoes and my facemask. I feel the warmth and stickiness of it as my patient's blood pressure is dropping and his lips are becoming cyanotic. And he is a real person, with parents and a spouse and children who care about him and whose lives will forever be altered by the tragedy that is taking place. I will have to answer to them about the events that brought their loved one here, about what I did and how I did it, and what the effects of my actions were. Perhaps my patient will look into my eyes with panic and desperation on his face, clutching my arm and whispering, "Don't let me die, doctor. Promise me you will not let me die."

Or perhaps I will look at the battered and slashed body of someone who was tortured for hours in ways that are unimaginable by a perpetrator who has turned his back on all that had once made him human, and she will look into my eyes with panic and desperation on her face and whisper, "Please let me die, doctor. I just want to die."

These are real people and they are my responsibility. What my mind knows and what my hands can do are often all that stands between life and death for my patients. In those moments, there is nothing except me and my patient. I am no longer a person or a woman or a mother or a wife. I have no conscious awareness of anything but my patient. Every inch of his body, how it feels, how it looks, how it smells, how it sounds, how it moves, how its vital signs fluctuate are the entire universe to me. The colors are vivid and the sounds are loud and the sensations intense. That body and I are locked in a dance, and I must move it to my will.

This is my personal battle. My patient is my partner, and in those moments his survival is as vital to me as my own. There is an intimacy that cannot be understood by anyone who is not a physician who has experienced a critical resuscitation.

I fall in love with my patients in these moments. When they survive, I feel an incredible sense of joy. When they die, I feel a deep sense of loss. When I have told a family of the death of their loved one and they begin to cry, often I find that my eyes have begun to tear as well. These tears are real. During the resuscitation, their loved one was the focus of all of my energy and all my love and during the time I spend with them, I sense the magnitude of their loss.

STRESSORS OF EMERGENCY PHYSICIANS PERSONAL LIFE

Most ER docs learn that shift work is not good for relationships. It is also not good for sleep hygiene. In addition to the consequences of shift work, ER docs generally are challenged in three other ways in terms of their personal lives: Most of us are thrill-seeking, high energy, and easily bored.

We have trouble sitting still and really listening to our family members and friends. We also have an unusual sense of humor, which is essentially contextual. The humor of emergency docs and nurses is associated with remaining resilient on the job, but it frequently carries over to personal relationships. Spouses tire of the stories and sometimes do not appreciate the humor. And as we do at work, we tend to apply the quick fix to our personal relationships.

Much of what goes on in Emergency Medicine takes its toll on the personal lives of emergency physicians. One of these things is shift work. A great thing about EM is that we always know when we are off. Those of us who are parents can schedule work days around children's birthdays, school plays, and football games. But the downside of this is that at least half, and often more, of our shifts are worked on weekends, holidays, or overnight. Alterations between daytime and nighttime wakefulness causes havoc on the body's circadian rhythms. An overnight shift means the need to nap the day of the shift and the day after.

Often it takes several days to get back into the routine of sleeping nights, and then it is time for another night shift. Not being in bed when your spouse is in bed can cause a strain on the marriage, and those same kids who are delighted that your are off from work on their birthdays are not so delighted if they are asked to play quietly on the days you are sleeping or wait to open Christmas presents until the night of December 25th because you had to work all day.

The Toll on the Personal Lives

We are not psychologically injured by the suffering around us. But it makes us less responsive at home. We become and remain inured to it. It is hard to impress us with death, dying, destruction, and chaos, or nearly anything in or out of the ER. It is difficult to thrill us but we do enjoy it when it happens. Hardened by hardiness requires not having the luxury of being able to discuss your day with your spouse because the experiences may be emotionally disturbing.

Most emergency docs find it hard to sit still. It's just not in our natures. When family members want to have a long, deep conversation, we want to cook dinner while we are listening. We are well aware of our ability to multitask and to do a good job at several things at once, but a seventh grader who has a crush on a classmate who doesn't know he's alive doesn't see it that way. There's a lot of "You're not listening to me" and "I can listen to you and do this at the same time" that goes on, and often, a lot of hurt feelings.

The tendency toward rapid decision making and disposition that serves us so well at work is actually counterproductive in personal life. Even though we may have the answer when the child is on sentence number two, children need to feel that they are heard, that they are the center of attention, and that their thoughts about their lives and family matters are important. Our tendency to direct them to the essentials the way we cut through the patient's history to get to the essential elements can be counterproductive to communication.

Emergency doctors may also have trouble exposing their own vulnerability. At work, we are in charge. We have to be decisive and then committed to our decisions. We must also be, or at least look, competent and confident. Patients depend on the doctor's competence and confidence.

At home, we need to consider the needs of those with whom we share our lives, and we need to even the playing field by allowing ourselves to be vulnerable, admitting a lack of knowledge and ability. A spouse likes to feel needed, if not indispensable, and to feel that they do things for us that we cannot or would not do for ourselves. Often, we are moving too fast to let the people we love be good to us. Often, we are moving too fast to be good to the people we love. Favorite EP expressions are "I'm not impressed" and "I'm underwhelmed." My colleague's son once told me, "Dad is always saying stuff like, 'You call that a cut! You're hardly bleeding' or 'So what your leg hurts. Rub it. It's probably a charley horse.' I feel like I'd have to be carrying my decapitated head around under my arm for him to believe I had anything wrong with me." We really are just so underwhelmed by the real world. Barring some of the wonderful things our kids do, it is hard to impress an EP. How many people walk past screaming and crying individuals on gurneys without feeling compelled to go in and see what's going on? If an EP feels the pain of every patient, he will never get his job done. A certain amount of tolerance for the suffering of others makes it possible for us to treat them.[3]

Much of what we see and hear in the course of our work cannot be shared with friends and family. When I was a resident, I was discussing a patient with ischemic bowel at the dinner table and mentioned how the unusual current jelly stool that is described in the text books was produced by the patient. My daughter pounded her hand on the table and said, "Mom, please! Not everyone sitting here is a doctor. Some of us can't talk about poop and eat at the same time!" Sometimes what we cannot tell our families is just too horrible. I think that some of the things that doctors see, the things that speak to the basest nature of man, should not be generally known.

---

[3] If I don't break the loculations in a buttock abscess, it is certain to recur. If I do break the loculations, given the fact that anesthetics have poor absorption in the presence of pus and they don't eliminate sensations of pressure, the patient is going to feel pain and, most often, will scream and/or cry. We learn early to ignore the patient's response to pain that we inflict on them in order to heal. And similarly, that $500,000.00 research grant gets me far more excited than the bouquet of roses I get on Mother's Day. Sad, but true.

My soul has been changed by the things I know and the things I have seen, and I want to protect my husband and my children from the knowledge that the world is such a vicious and cruel and dangerous place. Relatively early in my career, I cared for a young woman who had been kidnapped and subjected to repeated and brutal sexual and psychological abuse for hours. I could not comprehend such cruelty, and I knew that beyond the physical scars that this woman would carry, her life was ruined. She would never know the sleep of peace. She would never walk down the streets of the city confidant and secure. She would never have sex with her lover and give herself over to the pleasure of it. She would probably never be able to bear a child.

For weeks after, I would sit at the foot of my sleeping daughter's bed and wonder if I had made a mistake in giving her life. What kind of a world had I brought her into? There would be no way that I could protect her from a capricious, spontaneous act of violence by a sociopath with a diseased mind and a damaged soul. Could all the joy that one could experience in this life be worth the price that my patient had paid? How could I go on living if my child were to suffer such pain and I had been responsible for bringing her into this world to experience it?

PROTECTIVE FACTOR OF FAITH IN HUMANITY

Yet through all of the fears, the abuses, the death, and the sadness, there are hope, heroes, and humor. So often, we are inspired by the strength and dignity displayed by individuals struggling with physical pain or the loss of their hopes and dreams in the short time that it takes to deliver a terminal diagnosis. We are sustained by the courage of our EMT and nursing colleagues, who hold the needs of the patients above their own. We are relieved when a patient's poor judgment or foolish act results in no significant harm and can be the funny story that we pass on at change of shift. We tend to laugh a great deal in emergency medicine.

Indeed, we see good things in the ED: The great grandmother who had had the perfect day attending church, eating her favorite meal, and spending time in the park with her family before having the perfect death, with them all around her caressing and kissing and speaking their love to her when it became clear that her 98-year-old heart did not have the ability to respond to our drugs, or the elderly music teacher who had never married, but whose former student, eternally grateful for the spark she lit in him that grew into his career with the NY Philharmonic Orchestra, had her power of attorney and hired loving, doting home health aides who cared for her around the clock, even while she was hospitalized and even though she could only speak the monosyllable "ba, ba, ba."

It is this evidence of love, of all that is good about mankind, that keeps us going, though it is rare in the world we inhabit. Although certainly not all of us tend toward the spiritual, many of us are aware that we participate in miracles daily. We are spurred on in our work, often in the saddest and most violent circumstances, because we know that while there is life, there is hope. We accept far more than we judge. I know that man is made in the image of God, and that as long as I can keep my patients alive and show them love and consideration and respect, there is that possibility that what is good in them, what is God in them, may triumph and bring nobility to their lives and the lives of those around them. I go to work each day for this.

REFERENCE

Newman, D. H. (2008). *Hippocrates' Shadow: Secrets from the House of Medicine [Hardcover]*. NY: Scribner.

/// 25 /// CONCLUSIONS

CHARLES R. FIGLEY, PETER HUGGARD, AND CHARLOTTE E. REES

First Do No Self-Harm, we hope, will become a clarion call for the improved health of physicians across their education continuum. We hope that improved health will be associated with more evidence-based programs in stress management and self-care, ultimately creating a caring environment for those who attend to the medical needs of others. In our introduction to the book, we announced five inter-related questions that the chapters across the four sections would address: What stressors do physicians experience across the education continuum? What are the consequences of stress for multiple stakeholders such as physicians, colleagues, and patients? How do physicians cope with stressful demands? What strategies can be used to promote resilience among physicians? How can we tackle the culture of stoicism and emotional silence in the House of Medicine that encourages physicians' self-harm? In this editorial postscript, we attempt to summarize some of the answers to these questions and then set our sights forward to imagine the future of physician stress-resilience research. We identify important questions that still remain within the different and complementary lenses (individual, relational, and systems-based) discussed in this book. We end our book on perhaps a counterintuitive note: drawing on positive psychology, we critique our problematizing of stress across the book and instead highlight its positive side.

WHAT STRESSORS DO PHYSICIANS EXPERIENCE ACROSS THE MEDICAL CONTINUUM?

Throughout this book, we have seen that physicians experience a multiplicity of stressors, some of which are generic across different stages of training and specialties, and others peculiar to particular stages and specialties, and to their individual experiences. Although the stressors outlined across Sections 1–4 can be clustered into four domains—personal, work-related, work-home balance, and educational—rather than being isolated and mutually exclusive, these domains interact and overlap. Stressors relating to personal factors include criteria such as age, gender, ethnicity, marital and parental status, personality, financial pressures, personal and professional identities, as well as life events such as illness and death in the family.

Work-related factors include high intensity of work, heavy professional responsibilities, reduced physical and social resources, limited control, autonomy, and power to alter work conditions, interpersonal conflict with colleagues, challenging interactions with patients such as dealing with patients' emotional and psychological distress, death and dying, mistakes, dealing with ethical and professionalism dilemmas, and medico-legal threats such as patient complaints.

Work-home balance includes conflicting work-home time demands, lack of flexibility in work schedules, and balancing demanding hours in both paid (e.g. physician) and unpaid work (e.g. childcare, household duties). Stressors peculiar to educational phases of physicianship include study overload, academic and clinical performance pressure, grade competition, sleep-deprivation, learning methods requiring tolerance of uncertainty (e.g. small group learning), experiences of professionalism dilemmas such as balancing personal learning needs with patient care, interpersonal conflict with seniors such as student abuse, educational transitions requiring learners to navigate their way through alien contexts, learners negotiating tensions between their developing personal and professional identities, and their identities as "student" or "junior doctor" resulting in their feeling like peripheral participants within transitory health care teams. What is clear from these chapters is that stressors emerge through a complex interplay between individual, relational, and systems-based factors.

WHAT ARE THE CONSEQUENCES OF STRESS FOR MULTIPLE STAKEHOLDERS?

Throughout the book, we have seen a multiplicity of negative consequences of stress, not only for those physicians directly affected but also for people indirectly affected such as family members, colleagues, and patients. We know that high levels of stress in physicians can contribute to a broad range of negative psychological outcomes such as increased anxiety, depression, burnout, compassion fatigue, and vicarious traumatization. Stress can also lead to negative health-related behaviors such as substance abuse, unhealthy eating, and lack of exercise.

High levels of stress, left unchecked, can influence physicians' job satisfaction and productivity, their career choices such as their decision to enter/avoid certain specialties, and can influence adversely their retention within medicine entirely. Ultimately, the stress experienced by physicians can impact negatively on their interpersonal relationships. With family members, unresolved stress and its consequences can lead to marital separation and divorce. With colleagues, stressed physicians can have poor communication, leading to poor patient care. Indeed, several chapters within this book discuss the negative impact of physician stress on the doctor-patient relationship itself. For example, physicians with unresolved stress can use the silencing response—silencing patients—as a means of coping, thereby affecting the doctor-patient relationship and the quality of patient care adversely.

So we know from these chapters that physician stress has consequences for the individual, for relationships, and for systems of care. Arguably, the most important message across this book relating to the consequences of stress is that physicians must *first do no self-harm* in order to avoid causing harm to patients and further harm to themselves.

HOW DO PHYSICIANS COPE WITH STRESSFUL DEMANDS?

The classic individualist definition of coping is the "constantly changing cognitive and behavioral efforts to manage specific external and/or internal demands that are appraised as taxing or exceeding the resources of the person" (Lazarus & Folkman 1984, p. 141).

Throughout this book, chapter authors talk about a multitude of cognitive and behavioral efforts that physicians make to cope with the demands of medical practice. Methods of coping that could be described as positive include physicians taking part in self-care such as taking regular breaks and engaging in healthy behaviors like exercising, engaging in self-reflection in order to facilitate insight into stress and resilience, discussing their stressful experiences with others such as colleagues and family members, drawing on professional supervision and mentorship, participating in educational and treatment programs specifically designed to enhance resilience, and finally, laughter and humor (McCann et al.).

Methods discussed throughout the book that could be described as negative or maladaptive include denial, avoidance, and emotional silence (McCann et al. in press). While coping is typically depicted through an individual lens throughout this book—in line with Lazarus & Folkman's (1984) classic definition—many of the coping methods discussed are essentially relational such as seeking social support; what Kuo (2012) terms "collective coping." Indeed, we know from other research that coping methods employed by health care professionals are not only influenced by individual factors but are also influenced by professional culture, which serves to either encourage or discourage particular methods of coping within the medical workplace (Hannigan et al. 2004; Courvoisier et al. 2011).

WHAT STRATEGIES CAN BE USED TO PROMOTE RESILIENCE AMONG PHYSICIANS?

A number of strategies to promote resilience among medics are discussed throughout these book chapters. In line with the findings of a recent review of resilience in health care professionals (McCann et al.), our chapters suggest a number of key factors relating to physician resilience: maintaining a work-life balance, professional identity, self-reflection and insight, beliefs and spirituality, and laughter/humor. One of the key cross-cutting themes relating to resilience in our book, which is worthy of further consideration here, is the importance of narrative in terms of helping physicians understand their stressful experiences and their developing professional identities. Narratives are essentially stories of experience through which we can make sense of stressful and emotional experiences.

Creating and sharing coherent and emotionally integrated narratives may help individuals gain control over stressful experiences, leading to enhanced well-being (Bohanek et al. 2005, Rees et al. in press). Therefore we would urge physicians to work through their stressful experiences by sharing their written or oral narratives of these experiences, and doing so *with* emotion, rather like our Section 4 authors have done in this book. Through the use of prompt questions (e.g. what is the essence of your stressful experience? When and where did it occur? Who was present? What happened? What did you do and why? How did you feel? What did you learn?), physicians can be helped to produce rich narratives of their stressful experiences. By doing so *with* emotion rather than suppressing emotion (as is culturally the norm in medicine) they can avoid intrusive negative thoughts, impaired memory for such stressful events, and loss of sensitivity (Rees et al. in press).

HOW CAN WE TACKLE THE CULTURE OF STOICISM?

In medical education, we talk a lot about the hidden curriculum: the titanic system of unwritten social and cultural rules, assumptions, expectations and values through which medical students become socialized into the culture of medicine (Wear & Skillicorn, 2009). We know from educational research that medical students learn numerous things as part of this hidden curriculum, which ultimately sheds light onto the culture of medicine. Examples include ethical erosion, getting ahead through competition, acceptance of hierarchy and therefore obedience to authority and reluctance to voice concerns, loss of idealism, and importantly within the context of this book, emotional silence (Lempp &

Seale 2004; Rees et al. in press). The chapters in this book talk about this culture of sto-icism: "a lifetime of joyless striving" (see the Introduction to Section 2) that serves to reinforce emotional silence as the norm.

Physicians-in-training learn very quickly that to survive in the House of Medicine they must work long hours, demonstrate unfailing dedication to the job, and avoid show-ing any form of weakness, whether this be emotional distress or mental health problems. Hiding emotional distress and mental health problems because of fear of stigma and its impact on career prospects is a very real concern for physicians, and this fear creates a culture of secrecy and taboo—a wall of silence if you will—which further reinforces the culture of stoicism (North East London Strategic Health Authority 2003; McCann et al. in press). How we break this culture of stoicism is the real challenge.

The inquiry into the extended suicide of Daksha Emson (a consultant psychiatrist in the UK with severe and enduring bipolar disorder) and her daughter Freya reported that the NHS needed to dramatically reduce the stigma of mental illness among its employees by issuing an antidiscriminatory code of practice and facilitating compulsory anti-stigma training to all senior clinical staff and managers.

The inquiry report also suggested that all managers needed to create a climate (through the code and staff training) in which physicians could seek support without the fear of the consequences of stigma. With initiatives such as this it may be possible to change the culture of stoicism to a culture of self-care in which the House of Medicine and its inhabitants are committed to self-help, self-health, and self-compassion (Bishop & Rees 2007; McCann et al. 2011).

THE FUTURE OF STRESS-RESILIENCE RESEARCH

While the majority of the literature on physician stress is typically underpinned by an individualist lens focusing on the measurement of the individual's stress, coping, and resilience, the chapters within this book present empirical research and practitioner-orientated insights about stress, coping, and resilience through one or more of three lenses: individual, relational, and cultural.

Furthermore, the research across these chapters has brought various theories to bear on physician stress and resilience such as emotional intelligence, narrative theory, com-plexity theory, socio-cultural learning theory, and identity theory alongside elements associated with positive psychology such as mindfulness, wisdom, and growth (see, for example, Chapter 15: Promoting Resilience and Posttraumatic Growth in Physicians). We know from these chapters (and other research) that stressors, the consequences of stress, coping, and resilience all operate through a complex interplay between the individual and his or her relationships with others, and within the wider cultural context of the medical workplace. Although we do not think that one lens should be privileged over another (they are all equally important), we would call for more research that considers those relational and cultural aspects of physician stress and resilience in order to address gaps in the research literature.

Indeed, a recent review of the literature on stress resilience in health care professionals highlights numerous research questions still unanswered by the research literature, all of which include relational (e.g. "What types of relationships enable support to be accessed and used effectively?") or cultural foci (e.g. "How does indoctrination into, and the culture of, a chosen health profession influence an individual's ability to deal with stress and adversity?" McCann et al. in press). We think student and physician stress and resilience is still a fertile field for research and a multiplicity of approaches are still needed.

RESEARCHING THE INDIVIDUAL

Looking to the future of individualist research, neuroimaging technology and protocols should help us determine the limits of human performance among medical professionals and improve the quality of training and education. It is well-known that noticing other people experiencing pain activates the central nervous system's pain matrix in the observer (Decety, Yang & Cheng, 2010). The ability to regulate emotional reactions to pain, be it direct or indirect, is critical to physicians who experience repeated exposure to the suffering of patients (Figley, 1995). In a recent study conducted by the renowned neurobiologist Jean Decety, researchers took brain-wave readings from participants (including physicians) as they watched another person prick himself with a pin, or dab himself with a cotton swab. The researchers determined the "pain empathy response" to witnessing the stressor (the pinprick and the swab) and found that there was no early or late stimulus response among the physicians due in large part to their many years of experience managing sickness and pain. Indeed, the pain-empathy response among physicians appears to disappear over their career because of their adaptation to stressful adversities. Further research is therefore required to develop more understanding around the processes of emotion-regulation development in physicians.

RESEARCHING RELATIONSHIPS

Although qualitative methodologies are being increasingly used in stress resilience research nowadays, most qualitative research employs interviews to elicit students and physicians' views and experiences of stress, coping, and resilience. While eliciting

narratives of experience can help reveal relational aspects of stress, resilience, and coping (e.g. collective coping), we think that observational methods are needed to further
illuminate relational features of stress such as in doctor-patient and doctor-colleague
relationships. Underpinned by symbolic interactionism, which looks at how meaning,
identities, social order, and so on are constructed through social interaction (Sandstrom
et al. 2006), and using innovations in visual methodologies such as video ethnography
and video reflexivity, stressful incidents within the medical workplace such as stressful
doctor-patient or doctor-colleague encounters could be observed, recorded, and played
back to individuals and/or clinical teams (Pink 2007; Iedema et al. 2006). Such video
reflexivity sessions should stimulate discussion about relational aspects of stress, coping,
and resilience, and indeed, help to inculcate change in these relational features (Iedema
et al. 2006).

RESEARCHING CULTURE

Although narratives of stressful experiences can help partly reveal the culture of the
medical workplace, we think more could be done to help illuminate the cultural aspects
of stress, coping, and resilience. In discussing how to reveal the hidden curriculum (i.e.
the structures and cultures of medical education), Hafferty (1998) suggests that four
areas should be examined to uncover implicit messages about what is and what is not
valued within the institution: institutional policies, evaluation/assessment activities,
resource-allocation decisions, and institutional slang.

Likewise, we think we can get to the heart of the medical culture and its interplay with
student and physician stress and resilience by (1) critically examining institutional policies on stress, coping, and resilience, (2) exploring whether students and trainees have
formal teaching about stress, coping, and resilience and if so what, (3) exploring whether
students and trainees have their stress, coping, and resilience "measured" as part of their
personal and professional development and if so, how, (4) examining if and how resources
are allocated to educational and treatment programs for stress, coping, and resilience, and
(5) exploring the institutional slang surrounding stress, coping, and resilience.

THE POSITIVE FACE OF STRESS

Although this book essentially problematizes stress within the context of medical education and practice, numerous authors across the book comment on the positive face of
stress. Indeed, much recent research has focused on the positive consequences of what
may be a stressful and traumatizing experience. When one responds by engaging with the

challenges experienced through traumatizing events, positive change, referred to as vicarious transformation, vicarious resilience, or posttraumatic growth can occur (Pearlman & Caringi, 2009; Hernandez et al. 2007; Kearney et al. 2009).

There is evidence from research with physicians and other clinicians that such growth can result in maximizing well-being (Kearney et al. 2009), creating positive shifts in a sense of meaning and feelings of enrichment (Harrison & Westwood, 2009), and creating moments of connection and making these moments matter (Perry, 2008). However, to engage fully with these traumatizing experiences, and to experience such personal growth, both the individual physician and the collective House of Medicine will need to actively invite into their lives participation in activities that potentially make them vulnerable as they seek to develop self-awareness. This book is one attempt to trigger such self-awareness in medical students and physicians.

As noted at the start of this book, we three co-editors dedicate this book to all members of the House of Medicine, including our physician friends and colleagues, who struggle every day to manage the demands of their job. These jobs have very little room for failure: Physicians make life and death decisions daily. We hope that this book will provide the clarion call to action: to face head-on the deficits of medical education, training, and practice, and to tackle the culture of medicine, so that the House of Medicine is a safe and healing place for both patients and their physicians. Cicero was right when he said, "In nothing do men more nearly approach the gods than in giving health to men." The time has come to recognize that as we do no harm to healers we enable healers to do their work.

REFERENCES

Bohanek, J.G., Fivush, R., & Walker, E. (2005). Memories of positive and negative emotional events. *Applied Cognitive Psychology, 19*, 51–66.

Bishop, J.P. & Rees, C.E. (2007). Hero or has-been: Is there a future for altruism in medical education? *Advances in Health Sciences Education, 12*(3), 391–399.

Courvoisier, D.S., Agoritsas, T., Perneger, T.V., Scmidtm R,E,, & Cullati S. (2011). Regrets associated with providing health care: Qualitative study of experiences of hospital-based physicians and nurses. *PLoS ONE, 6*(8). Accessed on September 14, 2012 from http://www.plosone.org/article/info%3Adoi%2F10.1371%2Fjournal.pone.0023138

Decety, J., Yang, C-Y & Cheng, Y. (2010). Physicians down-regulate their pain empathy response: An event-related brain potential study. *NeuroImage, 50*(4), 1676–1682.

Figley, C. R. (Ed.) (1995). *Compassion Fatigue: Theory, Research, and Treatment.* NY: Brunner/Mazel.

Graschew, G. & Roelofs, T.A. (Eds.). (2011). Advances in telemedicine: Applications in various medical disciplines and geographical regions. Accessed on September 12, 2012 from: http://www.intechopen.com/books/advances-in-telemedicine-applications-in-various-medical-disciplines-and-geographical-regions

Hannigan, B., Edwards, D., & Burnard P. (2004). Stress and stress management in clinical psychology: Findings from a systematic review. *Journal of Mental Health, 13*(3), 235–245.

Hafferty, F. (1998). Beyond curriculum reform: Confronting medicine's hidden curriculum. Academic Medicine, 73(4), 403–407.

Harrison, R.L. & Westwood, M.J. (2009). Preventing vicarious traumatization of mental health therapists: Identifying protective practices. Psychotherapy Theory, Research, Practice, Training, 46(2), 203–219.

Hernández, P., Gangsei, D., & Engstrom, D. (2007). Vicarious resilience: A new concept in work with those who survive trauma. Family Process, 46(2), 229–241.

Iedema, R., Long, D., Forsyth, R. & Bonsan, L.B. (2006). Visibilising clinical work: video ethnography in the contemporary hospital. Health Sociology Review, 15(2),156–168.

Kearney, M.K., Weininger, R.B., Vachon, M.L.S., Harrison, R.L. & Mount, B.M. (2009). Self-care for physicians caring for patients at the end of life. JAMA, 301(11), 1155–1164.

Kuo, B.C.H. (2012). Collectivism and coping: Current theories, evidence, and measurements of collective coping. International Journal of Psychology, DOI:10.1080/002027594.2011.640681.

Lazarus, R.S., Folkman S. (1984). Stress, Appraisal and Coping. New York: Springer.

Lempp, H., & Seale, C. (2004). The hidden curriculum in undergraduate medical education: Qualitative study of medical students' perceptions of teaching. BMJ, 329, 770–773.

McCann, C., Beddoe, L., McCormick, K., Huggard, P., Kedge, S., Adamson, C., & Huggard, J. (2012). Resilience in the health professions: A review of recent literature. International Journal of Wellbeing (Open Source Journal), 3: 1 (accessed March 22, 2013: http://www.internationaljournalofwellbeing.org/index. php/ijow/search/advancedResults.

North East London Strategic Health Authority. (2003). Report of an independent inquiry into the care and treatment of Daksha Emson MBBS, MCPsych, MSc and her daughter Freya. London: North East London Strategic Health Authority.

Pearlman, L.A., & Caringi, J. (2009). Living and working self-reflectively to address vicarious trauma. In C.A. Courtois & J.D. Ford (Eds.), Treating complex traumatic stress disorders: An evidence-based guide (pp. 202–224). New York: Guilford Press.

Perry B. (2008). Why exemplary oncology nurses seem to avoid compassion fatigue. Canadian Oncology Nursing Journal, 18(2), 87–99.

Pink S. (2007). Doing visual ethnography: Images, media and representation in research (2nd ed.) London: Sage.

Rees, C.E., Monrouxe, L.V., & McDonald, L.A. (2012). Narrative, emotion and action: Analyzing "most memorable" professionalism dilemmas. Medical Education (in press).

Sandstrom, K.L., Martin, D.D., & Fine GA. (2006). Symbols and Selves and Social Reality. A symbolic interactionist approach to social psychology and sociology (2nd ed.). Los Angeles: Roxbury.

Wear, D., & Skillicorn, J. (2009). Hidden in plain sight. Academic Medicine, 84(4), 451–458.

INDEX

Printed in the USA/Agawam, MA
September 13, 2018

683190.007